Research, Applications, and Interventions
for Children and Adolescents

D1799753

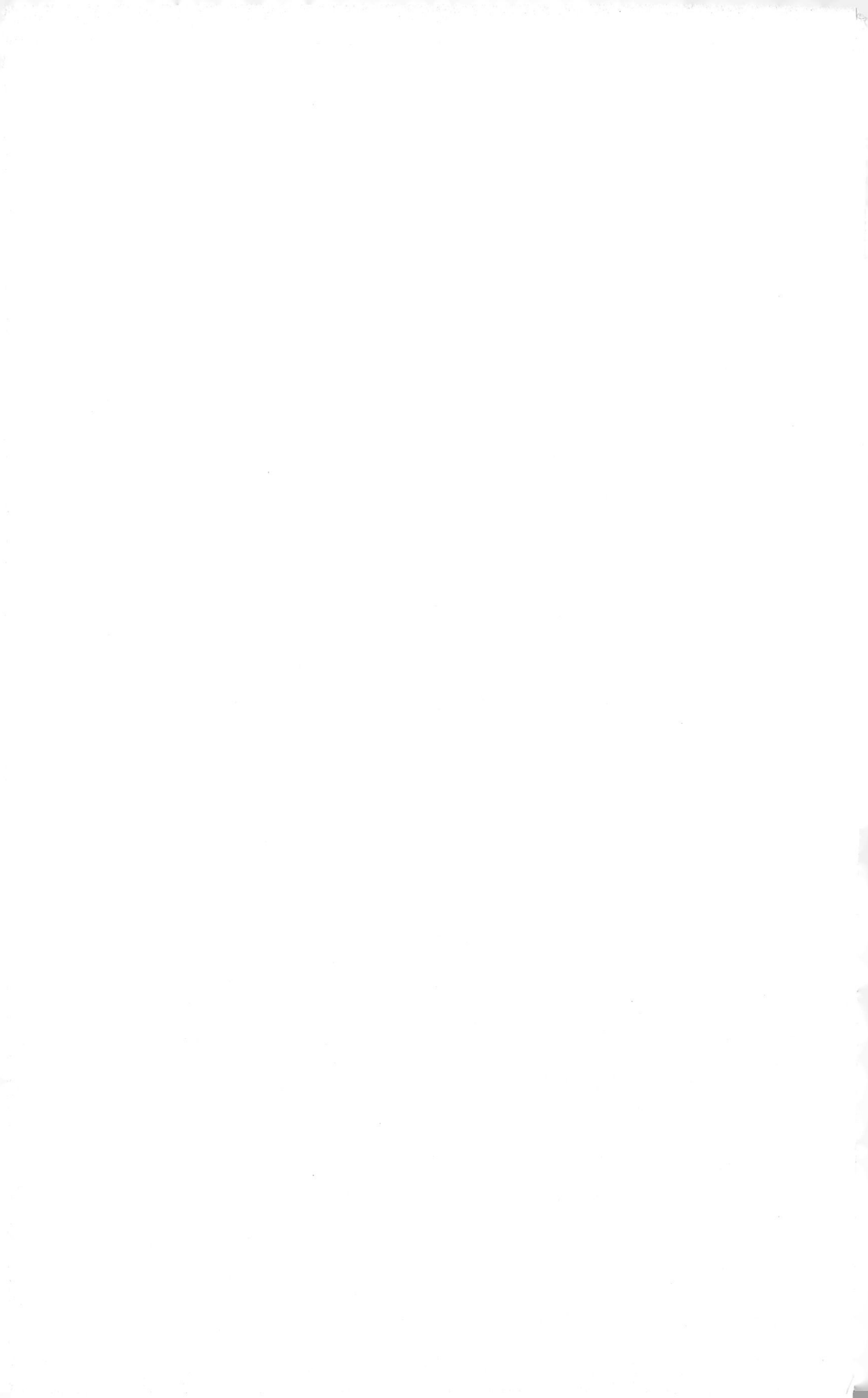

Carmel Proctor • P. Alex Linley
Editors

Research, Applications, and Interventions for Children and Adolescents

A Positive Psychology Perspective

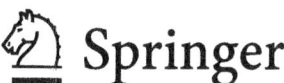 Springer

Editors

Carmel Proctor
Positive Psychology Research Centre
St. Peter Port, Guernsey

P. Alex Linley
Centre of Applied Positive Psychology
Coventry, UK

ISBN 978-94-017-8253-1   ISBN 978-94-007-6398-2 (eBook)
DOI 10.1007/978-94-007-6398-2
Springer Dordrecht Heidelberg New York London

© Springer Science+Business Media Dordrecht 2013
Softcover re-print of the Hardcover 1st edition 2013
This work is subject to copyright. All rights are reserved by the Publisher, whether the whole or part of the material is concerned, specifically the rights of translation, reprinting, reuse of illustrations, recitation, broadcasting, reproduction on microfilms or in any other physical way, and transmission or information storage and retrieval, electronic adaptation, computer software, or by similar or dissimilar methodology now known or hereafter developed. Exempted from this legal reservation are brief excerpts in connection with reviews or scholarly analysis or material supplied specifically for the purpose of being entered and executed on a computer system, for exclusive use by the purchaser of the work. Duplication of this publication or parts thereof is permitted only under the provisions of the Copyright Law of the Publisher's location, in its current version, and permission for use must always be obtained from Springer. Permissions for use may be obtained through RightsLink at the Copyright Clearance Center. Violations are liable to prosecution under the respective Copyright Law.
The use of general descriptive names, registered names, trademarks, service marks, etc. in this publication does not imply, even in the absence of a specific statement, that such names are exempt from the relevant protective laws and regulations and therefore free for general use.
While the advice and information in this book are believed to be true and accurate at the date of publication, neither the authors nor the editors nor the publisher can accept any legal responsibility for any errors or omissions that may be made. The publisher makes no warranty, express or implied, with respect to the material contained herein.

Printed on acid-free paper

Springer is part of Springer Science+Business Media (www.springer.com)

For all those who are striving to improve outcomes for children, giving every child, every chance, every day.

Foreword

What is the purpose of schools and indeed of education at large? Is it wholly, as governments would appear to think, to secure exam passes or is there a wider purpose?

For too long, I believe, schools and education have been overly concerned with academic attainment at the expense of character and well-being. This is not to say that a focus on academic attainment is wrong – far from it. But this extensive focus on academic attainment is, undoubtedly, to the detriment of other critical facets in the lives and development of children and young people – such as character and well-being – which leave the emerging generation short-changed in what they should expect from education and life development in general.

With the emergence of the discipline of positive psychology in the last 15 years, psychologists have decisively shifted their focus to attend to what is right with people, building on their strengths and celebrating their happiness and well-being, at the same time as being able to respond to their calls for help in times of distress and need. A similar paradigm shift is needed in education. We should recognize the damage that is being done to generations of children and young people by just "teaching to the test" and leaving to wither on the vine their crucial need for character development and life lessons in how to be happy and become productive and fulfilling members of the society.

This is why, at Wellington College, we have introduced a consistent focus on happiness into our curriculum, with extraordinary results, not only in the atmosphere of the school and the health of our young people, but also a very sharp rise in their academic performance. It is my hope that many more schools will embrace this shift in the emphasis of education and focus on developing the whole of the person in our children and young people. Schools will not find, as governments appear to believe, that academic results will fall. Rather, they will, I believe, see the results rise.

In this book, Carmel Proctor and Alex Linley bring a focus to how positive psychology can contribute to this debate, both in education and the classroom setting specifically, but also in our focus on the development and fulfillment of children and young people more broadly. The chapters cover topics including the strengths and well-being of children and adolescents, the role of family, peers and community in optimal development, the role and contribution of positive approaches to education, and positive youth development from the perspective of community activity and legal and policy positions. Taken together, they provide an excellent summary of the state of knowledge and practice in the research, applications and interventions of positive psychology as they apply to children and adolescents. Further research will inevitably be needed: this academic field, after all, is still young. But the authors make a compelling case, and they should be listened to with respect.

I thus encourage all those involved with the development of children and young people, and most especially educators and policy makers, to pay attention to the lessons of this volume in how we can create more optimal developmental contexts for our children and young people, building their character and well-being to equip them for the challenges and opportunities they will increasingly face in their journey through modern life.

Wellington College   Anthony Seldon

Contents

Part III   Family, Friends, and Community

Part IV   Positive Education

Part V   Positive Youth Development: Practice, Policy, and Law

Contributors

Afroze Anjum Psychological Services, South-West Education Office, Toronto District School Board, Toronto, ON, Canada

Michael T. Braun Department of Communication Arts, University of Wisconsin-Madison, Madison, WI, USA

B. Bradford Brown Department of Educational Psychology, 880A Educational Sciences, University of Wisconsin-Madison, Madison, WI, USA

R.J. Seán Cameron Business & Innovation Centre, The Pillars of Parenting, Wearfield, UK

Ann-Marie DiBiase Department of Graduate and Undergraduate Studies, Faculty of Education, Brock University, St. Catherines, ON, Canada

Lisa M. Edwards Department of Counselor Education and Counseling Psychology, Marquette University, Milwaukee, WI, USA

Sarah A. Fefer Department of Psychological and Social Foundations, University of South Florida, Tampa, FL, USA

John C. Gibbs Department of Psychology, The Ohio State University, Columbus, OH, USA

Lisa Suzanne Green Coaching Psychology Unit, University of Sydney, Sydney, NSW, Australia

Vanessa Gutierrez Department of Human and Community Development, University of Illinois at Urbana-Champaign, Urbana, IL, USA

Kimberly J. Hills Department of Psychology, University of South Carolina, Columbia, SC, USA

Andrew J. Howell Department of Psychology, Grant MacEwan University, Edmonton, AB, Canada

E. Scott Huebner Department of Psychology, University of South Carolina, Columbia, SC, USA

Xu Jiang Department of Psychology, University of South Carolina, Columbia, SC, USA

Hyeyoung Kang Department of Human Development, Binghamton University, State University of New York, Binghamton, NY, USA

Fahim Kazemi Health and Wellness Centre, University of Toronto Scarborough, Toronto, ON, Canada

Corey L.M. Keyes Department of Sociology, Emory University, Atlanta, GA, USA

Hans Henrik Knoop Department of Education, University of Aarhus, Aarhus N, Denmark

Nathaniel M. Lambert School of Family Life, Brigham Young University, Provo, UT, USA

Reed W. Larson Department of Human and Community Development, University of Illinois at Urbana-Champaign, Urbana, IL, USA

Roger J.R. Levesque Department of Criminal Justice, Indiana University, Bloomington, IN, USA

P. Alex Linley Centre of Applied Positive Psychology, The Venture Centre, Coventry, UK

Colin Maginn Business & Innovation Centre, The Pillars of Parenting, Wearfield, Sunderland, UK

Donna Mayerson VIA Institute on Character, Cincinnati, OH, USA

Jessica B. McClintock Department of Counselor Education and Counseling Psychology, Marquette University, Milwaukee, WI, USA

Ian Morris Wellington College, Crowthorne, Berkshire, UK

Ryan M. Niemiec VIA Institute on Character, Cincinnati, OH, USA

Jacolyn Maree Norrish MindSetGo, Melbourne, Australia

Holli-Anne Passmore Department of Psychology, Grant MacEwan University, Edmonton, AB, Canada

Stephen Cole Perry Department of Human and Community Development, University of Illinois at Urbana-Champaign, Urbana, IL, USA

Granville Bud Potter Columbus, OH, USA

Carmel Proctor Positive Psychology Research Centre, St. Peter Port, Guernsey, UK

Denise Quinlan Educational Assessment Research Unit, University of Otago, Dunedin, New Zealand

Marcela Raffaelli Department of Human and Community Development, University of Illinois at Urbana-Champaign, Urbana, IL, USA

Tayyab Rashid Health and Wellness Centre, University of Toronto Scarborough, Toronto, ON, Canada

Natalie Rusk Department of Human and Community Development, University of Illinois at Urbana-Champaign, Urbana, IL, USA

Shannon M. Suldo Department of Psychological and Social Foundations, University of South Florida, Tampa, FL, USA

Steve Tran Department of Human and Community Development, University of Illinois at Urbana-Champaign, Urbana, IL, USA

Amanda Veldorale-Brogan Department of Family and Child Services, College of Human Sciences, The Florida State University, Tallahassee, FL, USA

Kathrin Walker Extension Centre for Youth Development, University of Minnesota, Minneapolis, MN, USA

LaTesha Washington Department of Human and Community Development, University of Illinois at Urbana-Champaign, Urbana, IL, USA

Chapter 1
Surveying the Landscape of Positive Psychology for Children and Adolescents

P. Alex Linley and Carmel Proctor

1.1 Introduction

As we write, it has been almost 14 years since Martin Seligman inaugurated the emergence of positive psychology as a discipline, with his Presidential Address to the American Psychological Association. Despite the intervening decade and more, we are surprised at how little attention – in relative terms at least – has been dedicated to positive psychology theory, research, and applications as they pertain to children and adolescents. Looking back, this is perhaps reflective of positive psychology's *de facto* roots in social and clinical psychology, and its limited foundations in developmental and educational psychology, which are of course the disciplines where we might expect to find the most work in relation to children and adolescents.

While the first edition of the *Handbook of Positive Psychology* (Snyder and Lopez 2002), contained just three chapters on children and adolescents (Masten and Reed 2002; Roberts et al. 2002; Schulman 2002), it is notable that the second edition of this volume (Snyder and Lopez 2009), contained five chapters addressing the question of resilience in child development (Masten et al. 2009), the prevention of disorder and promotion of well-being through childhood development (Brown Kirschman et al. 2009), positive youth development (Lerner 2009; see also Chap. 15 by Rusk et al., this volume), family-centered positive psychology (Sheridan and Burt 2009), and positive schools (Huebner et al. 2009).

P.A. Linley (✉)
Centre of Applied Positive Psychology, The Venture Centre,
Sir William Lyons Road, Coventry CV4 7EZ, UK
e-mail: alex.linley@cappeu.com

C. Proctor
Positive Psychology Research Centre, P.O. Box 544,
St. Peter Port, Guernsey GY1 6HL, UK
e-mail: carmel@pprc.gg

C. Proctor and P.A. Linley (eds.), *Research, Applications, and Interventions for Children and Adolescents: A Positive Psychology Perspective*, DOI 10.1007/978-94-007-6398-2_1, © Springer Science+Business Media Dordrecht 2013

Clearly, then, there is an increasing shift towards greater attention being paid to positive psychology as it relates to children and adolescents. Broadly, this focus can be seen across three distinct but related areas: teaching, schools, and education; subjective experience (e.g., happiness, life satisfaction) and strengths; and intervention for positive development, whether at the individual, therapeutic, group, or policy level. In this introductory chapter, we will provide a brief synopsis of research and theory across each of these three domains, before moving on to show how the current volume builds on and extends this body of knowledge.

1.2   Positive Psychology in Teaching, Schools, and Education

The role of positive psychology in education started to become better recognized in the school literature, driven in part by the publication of positive psychology special issues of *School Psychology Quarterly* (2003) and *Psychology in the Schools* (2004). The role of positive psychology in education is primarily focused on encouraging and rewarding the multitude of talents and strengths a child has, by presenting opportunities for displays of these talents and strength each day, rather than for penalizing them for their deficits (Chafouleas and Bray 2004; Clonan et al. 2004; Huebner and Gilman 2003).

Theory and research in the positive psychology of education extends to all aspects of the educational experience and curriculum. For example, Clonan et al. (2004) outlined a vision of the positive psychology school, concentrating on areas of prevention (to reduce stress), consultation (across the curriculum and different service providers), and competency development (in academic skills and positive peer experience and interaction). However, the challenge for positive psychology is to establish what the key components of positive psychology "looks like" within a school, how the teaching and natural environment can be used to capitalize on positive psychological principles, and how a school can maintain and plan for sustained change (Clonan et al. 2004).

The focus of positive psychology applied to education has also been extended to consideration of the role of effective upward social comparisons in learning, growth, and development (Cohn 2004); teaching students to make wise judgments (Reznitskaya and Sternberg 2004), and the effective teaching of positive psychology as a subject in its own right (Baylis 2004; Fineburg 2004).

Furthermore, driven in part by the positive psychology movement, attention has also focused on what we might do to make schools happy places (Layard 2005; Martin 2005; Noddings 2003). This increasing focus on children and adolescents can be traced through the publication of the magnum opus of the field for work focused on positive psychology in schools, the *Handbook of Positive Psychology in Schools* (Gilman et al. 2009).

1.2.1   Applying Strengths in School and College

Within education, there have been specific attempts to apply and celebrate strengths in the classroom, with college students, with secondary students, and with younger children (Liesveld and Miller 2005). The Gallup Organization has developed and delivered the *StrengthsQuest* educational program (Clifton and Anderson 2002) across a variety of higher education colleges and universities. The program has been extended to secondary students (Anderson 2005), and preliminary reports from teachers using the program have been positive (e.g., Austin 2006; Henderson 2005).

Within the UK, a project has been run across a group of primary schools (ages 5 through 11 years), under the title of *Celebrating Strengths* (Fox Eades 2008). This project has linked strengths to specific festivals and events throughout the school calendar, and has included activities such as the strengths-based classroom (recognizing the strengths of all class members), victory logs (record books noting students' achievements), and celebrations of "what went well".

Again in the UK, in a quasi-experimental treatment-control study with a total of 319 adolescents aged 12–14 years, C. Proctor et al. (2011) showed that *Strengths Gym*, a series of character-strengths development interventions for adolescents, led to increased life satisfaction over a 6-month time period with corresponding increases not observed in a no-intervention comparison group (who were students at the same schools and in the same years, but not receiving the intervention).

Strengths Gym is a series of activities constructed around the 24 character strengths described by Peterson and Seligman (2004). The aim of the Strengths Gym program is to encourage students to build their strengths, learn new strengths, and to recognize strengths in others. The included activities for students are called Strengths Builders and Strengths Challenges. For each lesson, there is a definition of the character strength being focused on, two Strengths Builders exercises for students to choose from, and a Strengths Challenge as follow-up activity.

1.3 Subjective Experience and Strengths in Children and Adolescents

Just as positive psychology generally has helped increasing attention be paid to the questions of happiness and well-being, the same is also true for positive psychology research as it relates to children and adolescents. For example, C. L. Proctor et al. (2009) reviewed the literature on adolescent life satisfaction and concluded that, in general, research indicates that youths who report high levels of life satisfaction have better social and interpersonal relationships, engage in healthier behaviors, exhibit less antisocial and violent behavior, and develop fewer externalizing problems following stressful events than those with low life satisfaction. Building on this, C. Proctor et al. (2010) explored the benefits of very high levels of life satisfaction in youth and found that youths displaying very high levels of life satisfaction benefit form increased adaptive psychosocial functioning, intrapersonal, interpersonal, and social relationships, academic success, and decreased behavior problems (see also Gilman and Huebner 2006; Suldo and Huebner 2006). Further, life satisfaction has been found to be positively associated with multiple school related variables, including school satisfaction, teacher support, and perceived academic achievement, competence, and self-efficacy (see Suldo et al. 2006 for a review). Other notable work on positive subjective experiences in children and adolescents has been conducted by Froh et al. (2010) who have demonstrated that youths high in engaged living (social integration and absorption; i.e., having a passion to help others and be completely immersed in activity) are more grateful, hopeful, happier, prosocial, and report elevated life satisfaction, positive affect, self-esteem, school experience, and grade point average, as well as, tend to be less depressed, envious, antisocial, and delinquent.

Similarly, Nakamura and Csikszentmihalyi (2002) have long stressed the importance of encouraging adolescent participation in activities that facilitate "flow" – a mental state in which the challenge of an activity matches skill, such that neither anxiety or boredom occur. The flow state is an innately positive experience, one which is linked to academic success, diminished delinquency, physical health, and satisfaction with life (see Nakamura and Csikszentmihalyi 2002).

In relation to character strengths in young children, Park and Peterson (2006a) showed that it was possible to assess character strengths in children as young as 3 years of age through using parental descriptors which were then subject to content analysis. Park and Peterson (2006a) examined the associations between character strengths and happiness in some 680 children (aged 3–9 years), showing that the strengths of love, zest, and hope were significantly associated with happiness.

For the assessment of strengths in adolescents, Park and Peterson (2006b) developed the Values in Action Inventory of Strengths for Youth, and more recently, Brazeau et al. (2012) developed the Strengths Assessment Inventory – Youth, which assesses 11 content scales (e.g., Strengths at Home), and 12 empirical scales (e.g., Commitment to Family Values).

1.4 Intervention for Positive Development

Early work in the positive psychology canon in relation to positive development was focused on the role of resilience in childhood (Yates and Masten 2004) and positive youth development (Larson et al. 2004), both of which were themes that subsequently featured in the second edition of the *Oxford Handbook of Positive Psychology* (Snyder and Lopez 2009), as well as being the focus of a special issue of the *Journal of Positive Psychology* (Emmons 2011).

Earlier positive intervention work had been conducted by the Positive Parenting Program (Triple P) in Australia. The Positive Parenting Program is a family intervention program that is designed to prevent behavioral, emotional and developmental problems in children up to the age of 16. It aims to achieve this through promoting and developing the knowledge, skills and confidence of parents (Sanders 2003; Sanders et al. 2002).

Sanders et al. (2000) reported on the effectiveness of a 12-episode television series, *Families*, that was aimed at improving disruptive child behavior and family relationships. Each episode of *Families* lasted for approximately 20–30 min, and included a feature story about family issues, together with a segment of 5–7 min that presented parents with guidelines and instructions for using a range of parenting strategies to address common child behavioral problems, to prevent problems from occurring, and to help teach children to learn new skills and master difficult tasks. These segments also presented the viewer with a modeled demonstration of the suggested strategies. The initial report, based on 56 parents of children aged 2–8 years, showed that the prevalence of disruptive behavior dropped from 43 to 14%, with the effects being maintained at a 6-month follow up.

1.5 The Plan for This Volume

Our aim in preparing this volume was to bring together the latest evidence, thinking, and insights from positive psychology as they apply to children and adolescents. In establishing the content, we were mindful of the imbalance in the publication of research findings, applications, and interventions among children and adolescents in comparison to adults and aimed to fill the current need for a volume that would benefit a wide range of professionals working with children and adolescents.

Our contributors were invited to contribute chapters within their area of expertise as it relates to research, applications, and interventions for children and adolescents, drawing from their explicit experiences and research. Contributors were further encouraged to share their broader perspectives on their invited topics. The contributors represent a broad range of individuals, including clinical and academic psychologists, researchers, teachers, therapists, and program leaders, to name a few, and provide a unique and varied look at the current landscape. The result is a volume that brings together the latest knowledge on positive psychology as it pertains for children and adolescents.

This volume was not edited with preconceived or rigidly defined elements in mind, but with openness and freedom of content. The result is a body of work that not only contains exemplary reviews of the current literature and provides unique and varied demonstrations of applied positive psychological theory, but also contains personal experiences and events of immense importance to understanding positive psychology among this population as it occurs in the real world context.

Although this volume has been written from a positive psychology perspective, the content is by no means restricted to academics and professionals of psychology alone. The topics covered are broad and are of benefit to a wide range of professionals, including educators, clinicians, psychologist, social workers, students, and many others working with children and adolescents.

1.6 The Content of This Volume

In Part I (*Strengths and Well-Being*), Carmel Proctor (Chap. 2) presents a review of the literature on character strengths and a brief discussion and introduction to character strengths interventions in education. This chapter introduces the importance of good character as it pertains to positive youth development and well-being. Scott Huebner and colleagues (Chap. 3) address the assessment and promotion of perceived quality of life, or life satisfaction, among children and adolescents. A model for more comprehensive assessment of children's life satisfaction is presented along with research on key determinants of individual differences in life satisfaction among young people. These authors provide examples of interventions as they pertain to the empirically established determinants of life satisfaction and argue that more comprehensive assessments and targeted intervention programs are required across primary, secondary, and tertiary prevention contexts. Lisa Edwards and Jessica McClintock (Chap. 4) introduce us to hope and hope theory and its relationship to positive outcomes in youth. Theory, measurement, and research about hope among youth are reviewed and intervention programs developed for youth described along with direction for applications.

In Part II (*Interventions and Applications*) Andrew Howell and colleagues (Chap. 5) review research focused upon positive indicators of youth mental health. In this chapter, predictors of youth's scores on mental health dimensions of functioning and interventions aimed at boosting these scores are presented along with a discussion of the interplay between mental health and mental disorder dimensions of functioning in youth. Tayyab Rashid and colleagues (Chap. 6) address strengths-based assessment and the benefits of exploring character strengths by underscoring the shortcomings of a deficit model of assessment for children and adolescents. These authors present a model of assessing signature strengths and evaluate the impact on boosting life satisfaction, well-being, and social skills among young people. Nathaniel Lambert and Amanda Veldorale-Brogan (Chap. 7) conclude this section with their examination of gratitude and gratitude interventions focused research among children and adolescents.

In Part III (*Family, Friends, and Community*) Shannon Suldo and Sarah Fefer (Chap. 8) examine the links between parenting practices and youth well-being and well-being and parent–child relationships in the context of positive psychology. Aspects of the parent–child relationship and indicators of youth well-being are reviewed along with applications and interventions that promote positive outcomes for youth. Bradford Brown and Michael Braun (Chap. 9) review evidence of peers' contributions to healthy behavior and development and discuss implications for interventions and research. Colin Maginn and Seán Cameron (Chap. 10) present the Emotional Warmth Model of Professional Childcare. The Emotional Warmth Model seeks to address the problems experienced by looked-after children and draws on positive psychology to teach carers to find creative ways of helping children to utilize their strengths more effectively.

In Part IV (*Positive Education*) Ian Morris (Chap. 11) presents a case for well-being as the central aim of education and argues that schools must have an underpinning philosophy and practice of well-being to bring about the flourishing of both students and teachers. This topic is expanded further by Hans Henrik Knoop (Chap. 12) through his review of scientific evidence relating to positive education as an educational approach where individual strengths, well-being, and positive social relations are taught and used as the foundation for the pedagogy, with the aim of facilitating the flourishing of every student. Lisa Green and Jacolyn Norrish (Chap. 13) continue this theme by considering how positive psychology and coaching psychology can compliment each other in order to create comprehensive and sustainable applied positive education programs for schools in their effort to support the development of well-being among students.

In Part V (*Positive Youth Development: Practice, Policy, and Law*) John Gibbs and colleagues (Chap. 14) discuss the EQUIP program, a group-based cognitive-behavioral intervention designed to facilitate sociomoral development and positive youth development for behaviorally at-risk or antisocial youth. Natalie Rusk and colleagues (Chap. 15) review organized youth programs that provide opportunities for adolescents to develop life and career skills. Their focus is on adolescents' development of skills for managing emotions and how program leaders facilitate youth's active learning process through emotion coaching and effective organized programs facilitate positive youth development. Roger Levesque (Chap. 16) concludes the volume by reviewing how the legal system could benefit from optimal policies for ensuring positive youth development. Using the laws in the United States as examples of limitations and possibilities, the chapter provides the groundwork for understanding the foundations of which laws, policies, and practices relating to adolescents must rest, and the many ways that social institutions have the legal power to influence the development of youth.

This volume offers valuable information to a wide range of professionals in diverse fields and students in the social and behavioral sciences. It promises to be a valuable resource in the development of the field as it applies to youth.

References

Anderson, E. C. (2005). Strengths-based educating: A concrete way to bring out the best in students – and yourself. *Educational Horizons, 83*, 180–189.

Austin, D. B. (2006). Building on a foundation of strengths. *Educational Horizons, 84*, 176–182.

Baylis, N. (2004). Teaching positive psychology. In P. A. Linley & S. Joseph (Eds.), *Positive psychology in practice* (pp. 210–217). Hoboken: Wiley.

Brazeau, J. N., Teatero, M. L., Rawana, E. P., Brownlee, K., & Blanchette, L. R. (2012). The strengths assessment inventory: Reliability of a new measure of psychosocial strengths for youth. *Journal of Child and Family Studies, 21*, 384–390.

Brown Kirschman, K. J., Johnson, R. J., Bender, J. A., & Roberts, M. C. (2009). Positive psychology for children and adolescents: development, prevention and promotion. In C. R. Snyder & S. J. Lopez (Eds.), *Oxford handbook of positive psychology* (2nd ed., pp. 133–148). New York: Oxford University Press.

Chafouleas, S. M., & Bray, M. A. (2004). Introducing positive psychology: Finding a place within school psychology. *Psychology in the Schools, 41*, 1–5.

Clifton, D. O., & Anderson, E. C. (2002). *StrengthsQuest: Discover and develop your strengths in academic, career, and beyond*. Washington, DC: The Gallup Organization.

Clonan, S. M., Chafouleas, S. M., McDougal, J. L., & Riley-Tillman, T. C. (2004). Positive psychology goes to school: Are we there yet? *Psychology in the Schools, 41*, 101–110.

Cohn, M. A. (2004). Rescuing our heroes: positive perspectives on upward comparisons in relationships, education, and work. In P. A. Linley & S. Joseph (Eds.), *Positive psychology in practice* (pp. 218–237). Hoboken: Wiley.

Emmons, R. A. (Ed.). (2011). Positive youth psychology [Special issue]. *Journal of Positive Psychology, 6*(1).

Fineburg, A. C. (2004). Introducing positive psychology to the introductory psychology student. In P. A. Linley & S. Joseph (Eds.), *Positive psychology in practice* (pp. 197–209). Hoboken: Wiley.

Fox Eades, J. (2008). *Celebrating strengths: Building strengths-based schools*. Coventry: CAPP Press.

Froh, J. J., Kashdan, T. B., Yurkewicz, C., Fan, J., Allen, J., & Glowacki, J. (2010). The benefits of passion and absorption in activities: Engaged living in adolescents and its role in psychological well-being. *The Journal of Positive Psychology, 5*(4), 311–332.

Gilman, R., & Huebner, E. S. (2006). Characteristics of adolescents who report very high life satisfaction. *Journal of Youth and Adolescence, 35*, 311–319.

Gilman, R., Huebner, E. S., & Furlong, M. J. (Eds.). (2009). *Handbook of positive psychology in schools*. New York: Routledge.

Henderson, G. (2005). The power of teaching students using strengths. *Educational Horizons, 83*, 202–204.

Huebner, E. S., & Gilman, R. (2003). Toward a focus on positive psychology in school psychology. *School Psychology Quarterly, 18*, 99–102.

Huebner, E. S., Gilman, R., Reschly, A. L., & Hall, R. (2009). Positive schools. In C. R. Snyder & S. J. Lopez (Eds.), *Oxford handbook of positive psychology* (2nd ed., pp. 561–578). New York: Oxford University Press.

Larson, R., Jarret, R., Hansen, D., Pearce, N., Sullivan, P., Walker, K., et al. (2004). Organized youth activities as contexts for positive development. In P. A. Linley & S. Joseph (Eds.), *Positive psychology in practice* (pp. 540–559). Hoboken: Wiley.

Layard, R. (2005). *Happiness: Lessons from a new science*. London: Allen Lane.

Lerner, R. M. (2009). The positive youth development perspective: theoretical and empirical bases of a strengths-based approach to adolescent development. In C. R. Snyder & S. J. Lopez (Eds.), *Oxford handbook of positive psychology* (2nd ed., pp. 149–163). New York: Oxford University Press.

Liesveld, R., & Miller, J. A. (2005). *Teach with your strengths: How great teachers inspire their students*. New York: Gallup Press.

Martin, P. (2005). *Making happy people: The nature of happiness and its origins in childhood*. London: Fourth Estate.

Masten, A. S., & Reed, M.-G. J. (2002). Resilience in development. In C. R. Snyder & S. J. Lopez (Eds.), *Handbook of positive psychology* (pp. 74–88). New York: Oxford University Press.

Masten, A. S., Cutuli, J. J., Herbers, J. E., & Reid, M.-G. J. (2009). Resilience in development. In C. R. Snyder & S. J. Lopez (Eds.), *Oxford handbook of positive psychology* (2nd ed., pp. 117–131). New York: Oxford University Press.

Nakamura, J., & Csikszentmihalyi, M. (2002). The concept of flow. In C. R. Snyder & S. J. Lopez (Eds.), *Handbook of positive psychology* (pp. 89–105). New York: Oxford University Press.

Noddings, N. (2003). *Happiness and education*. New York: Cambridge University Press.

Park, N., & Peterson, C. (2006a). Character strengths and happiness among young children: Content analysis of parental descriptions. *Journal of Happiness Studies, 7*, 323–341.

Park, N., & Peterson, C. (2006b). Moral competence and character strengths among adolescents: The development and validation of the values in action inventory of strengths for youth. *Journal of Adolescence, 29*(6), 891–909.

Peterson, C., & Seligman, M. E. P. (2004). *Character strengths and virtues: A handbook and classification*. New York: Oxford University Press.

Proctor, C. L., Linley, P. A., & Maltby, J. (2009). Youth life satisfaction: A review of the literature. *Journal of Happiness Studies, 10*, 583–630.

Proctor, C., Linley, P. A., & Maltby, J. (2010). Very happy youths: Benefits of very high life satisfaction among youths. *Social Indicators Research, 98*, 519–532.

Proctor, C., Tsukayama, E., Wood, A. M., Maltby, J., Fox Eades, J., & Linley, P. A. (2011). Strengths gym: The impact of a character strengths-based intervention on the life satisfaction and well-being of adolescents. *The Journal of Positive Psychology, 6*, 377–388.

Reznitskaya, A., & Sternberg, R. J. (2004). Teaching students to make wise judgments: the "teaching for wisdom" program. In P. A. Linley & S. Joseph (Eds.), *Positive psychology in practice* (pp. 181–196). Hoboken: Wiley.

Roberts, M. C., Brown, K. J., Johnson, R. J., & Reinke, J. (2002). Positive psychology for children: development, prevention and promotion. In C. R. Snyder & S. J. Lopez (Eds.), *Handbook of positive psychology* (pp. 663–675). New York: Oxford University Press.

Sanders, M. R. (2003). Triple P – Positive Parenting Program: A population approach to promoting competent parenting. *Australian e-Journal for the Advancement of Mental Health, 2*(3).

Sanders, M. R., Montgomery, D. T., & Brechman-Toussaint, M. L. (2000). The mass media and the prevention of child behaviour problems: The evaluation of a television series to promote positive outcomes for parents and their children. *Journal of Child Psychology and Psychiatry, 41*, 939–948.

Sanders, M. R., Markie-Dadds, C., & Turner, K. M. T. (2002). The role of the media and primary care in the dissemination of evidence-based parenting and family support interventions. *The Behavior Therapist, 25*, 156–166.

Schulman, M. (2002). The passion to know: a developmental perspective. In C. R. Snyder & S. J. Lopez (Eds.), *Handbook of positive psychology* (pp. 313–326). New York: Oxford University Press.

Sheridan, S. M., & Burt, J. D. (2009). Family-centered positive psychology. In C. R. Snyder & S. J. Lopez (Eds.), *Oxford handbook of positive psychology* (2nd ed., pp. 551–559). New York: Oxford University Press.

Snyder, C. R., & Lopez, S. J. (Eds.). (2002). *Handbook of positive psychology*. New York: Oxford University Press.

Snyder, C. R., & Lopez, S. J. (Eds.). (2009). *Oxford handbook of positive psychology* (2nd ed.). New York: Oxford University Press.

Suldo, S. M., & Huebner, E. S. (2006). Is extremely high life satisfaction during adolescence advantageous? *Social Indicators Research, 78*, 179–203.

Suldo, S. M., Riley, K. N., & Shaffer, E. J. (2006). Academic correlates of children and adolescents' life satisfaction. *School Psychology International, 27*, 567–582.

Yates, T. M., & Masten, A. S. (2004). Fostering the future: resilience theory and the practice of positive psychology. In P. A. Linley & S. Joseph (Eds.), *Positive psychology in practice* (pp. 521–539). Hoboken: Wiley.

Chapter 3
Assessment and Promotion of Life Satisfaction in Youth

E. Scott Huebner, Kimberly J. Hills, and Xu Jiang

3.1 Assessment and Promotion of Life Satisfaction in Children

As the field of positive psychology advances, researchers have shown that positive mental health is more than the absence of psychopathology. Comprehensive models of mental health require considerations of well-being and ill-being constructs (Antaramian et al. 2010; Greenspoon and Saklofske 2001; Suldo and Shaffer 2008). Life satisfaction (LS) is one key well-being construct in positive psychology. Life satisfaction is defined as a cognitive judgment of one's perceived quality of life as a whole or with specific domains, such as family relations, work, and health (Diener 1984). Studies of the antecedents, correlates, and consequences of LS of adults have proliferated over the years. However, studies with children and adolescents have been limited. Fortunately, the number of studies of children's LS has grown significantly in the last decade (see C. L. Proctor et al. 2009a, b for a review).

Life satisfaction is an important factor in positive psychological development; it is not only a by-product of favorable life experiences, but is also a precursor of positive life outcomes. A meta-analysis of cross-sectional, longitudinal, and experimental studies of adults (Lyubomirsky et al. 2005) revealed that high subjective well-being (SWB; including LS) predicts subsequent positive marriages, friendships, work productivity, and mental and physical health. Longitudinal and experimental investigations of children's LS and positive emotions have been exceedingly scarce. However, short-term longitudinal studies have suggested that low LS in adolescents predicts decreases in emotional support from parents (Saha et al. 2010), decreases in student engagement in schooling (Lewis et al. 2011), and decreases in positive interactions with peers as well as increases in peer relational victimization

E.S. Huebner (✉) • K.J. Hills • X. Jiang
Department of Psychology, University of South Carolina, Columbia, SC 29208, USA
e-mail: huebner@mailbox.sc.edu; hillskj@mailbox.sc.edu; bnujiangxu@gmail.com

C. Proctor and P.A. Linley (eds.), *Research, Applications, and Interventions for Children and Adolescents: A Positive Psychology Perspective*, DOI 10.1007/978-94-007-6398-2_3,
© Springer Science+Business Media Dordrecht 2013

(Martin et al. 2008). As such, "high" LS is likely a protective factor in the development of healthy child and adolescent development (Suldo and Huebner 2004) as well as a desirable outcome in itself.

3.1.1 Measurement

Children's LS measures have been based on three distinct theoretical models: general, global, and domain-specific LS. First, there are instruments based on general models of LS that assume that overall or "general" LS is comprised of bottom-up judgments of specific life domains (e.g., family, peers, and school domains). Thus, a general or total LS score on such instruments reflects a simple (or weighted) sum of scores on items representing responses across a variety of specific domains. Second, there are instruments that attempt to assess satisfaction "as a whole" or overall LS based on a "global" model, which assumes that overall LS is best assessed by an exclusive emphasis on items that are domain-free (e.g., my life is going well) versus domain-specific (e.g., my *school* life is going well). In contrast to general LS scores, in which the number and nature of the domains are pre-determined by the researcher, global LS scales allow individual children to develop their overall judgments based on their own criteria (Pavot and Diener 1993). Third, multidimensional measures have been developed with the intent of eliciting children's judgments across various life domains that are considered to be important to most, if not all, individuals of the particular age group. In this fashion, such measures yield profiles of individuals' reports of LS, providing more differentiated, contextualized LS reports. Hence, a child who has average global LS, along with high *school* and low *family* satisfaction could be differentiated from a child who has average global LS, along with low *school* and high *family* satisfaction. In all cases, LS judgments generally comprise the full range of experiences from lower levels through a neutral level (neither satisfied nor dissatisfied) and through higher levels of LS. Such scales can provide finely nuanced differentiations (e.g., very high vs. moderately high LS) both above and below the neutral point. The resulting context-specific profiles thus provide more targeted information relevant to the design of more healthy environments for individual students or groups of students. Using the previous example, context-specific profiles allow the tailoring of interventions targeting the specific area of low satisfaction (e.g., low family satisfaction vs. low school satisfaction). Although such measures have existed for adult populations for many years, the development of psychometrically sound measures for children and adolescents has lagged considerably behind.

Based on the above considerations, and like others (e.g., Cummins 1997), we established a research agenda in the 1990s to develop several measures of global and domain-specific LS in our lab. These measures are discussed in detail in Huebner and Hills (in press). These instruments include, but are not limited to the Students' Life Satisfaction Scale (SLSS; Huebner 1991a) and the Multidimensional Students' Life Satisfaction Scale (MSLSS; Huebner 1994). The primary goals of the research were to develop LS scales for children ages 8–18 that: (a) tapped their global LS (i.e., SLSS); (b) provided an evidence-based profile of children's satisfaction with important, specific domains (e.g., school, family, friends) in their lives (i.e., MSLSS); (c) demonstrated acceptable reliability and validity; and (d) could be used effectively with children across a wide range of ability levels (e.g., children with mild developmental disabilities through gifted children). Space considerations do not allow us to elaborate upon the psychometric characteristics of the measures. However, more than two decades of research from our lab as well as others suggests that these self-report instruments demonstrate acceptable reliability and validity for a variety of purposes for children of approximately 8–18 years of age (Huebner and Hills in press; C. Proctor et al. 2009a, b).

These resulting measures have allowed us to study further the determinants and consequences of individual differences in children's global and domain-specific LS reports. The research has revealed a wide-ranging nomological network of related variables (Huebner 2004). In subsequent research and professional practice, we have used the SLSS and MSLSS in more comprehensive assessments to understand the nature, determinants, and consequences of LS. In professional practice, we have found that we can enhance the usefulness of the SLSS and MSLSS on occasion through conducting more detailed inquiries into the meaning of student responses. The standard measures do not allow examiners to determine the specific content and processes used by individual children to formulate their LS judgments. Open-ended, follow-up interview questions may thus facilitate greater understanding. Adapting procedures recommended by Harter (1985) for self-concept measures, we have used such questions as: "What made you agree/disagree that your life is good?" and "What made you agree/disagree that your family experiences are positive?" In addition to clarifying the meaning of a student's self-reports, such queries may clarify discrepancies between self-reports and reports from significant others, such as parents or teachers (Huebner et al. 2002).

We have also found that a modified version of Randolph et al. (2009) integrated model of objective and SWB can be useful to guide more complete assessments of students' LS. Their model includes four levels of indicators of well-being. The highest level refers to a student's overall quality of life. The second level includes the lower-order component of subjective global LS (along with measures of positive and negative emotions). The third level includes judgments of satisfaction regarding major, specific life domains, such as family, friends, school, self, and living environment (cf. Huebner 1994). The fourth level incorporates key, empirically-validated correlates under each domain. For example, several research-based variables could be assessed that contribute to satisfaction with school experiences, such as teacher behavior, school size, parental involvement, peer relationships, personality characteristics, and academic self-efficacy (see Baker and Maupin 2009 for a review). A similar set of variables could be generated for satisfaction with family, friends, and so forth. This last level includes, but is not limited to objective indicators. Although the hierarchical nature of the model may be debatable, the model reflects the possibilities for comprehensive assessments of the well-being of children for individual assessment purposes or group assessment purposes, such as school-wide or national assessments of children's well-being. Comprehensive well-being assessments can thus include subjective global and relevant subjective domain-based LS indicators.

Furthermore, these measures can then be complemented by considerations of key objective and/or subjective determinants guided by the extant research base. Depending upon the nature and levels of information desired, specific assessment plans can be constructed subsequently to meet specific goals for an individual child or groups of children. For example, the evaluation of the implementation of school-wide policies or programs to promote students' academic achievement levels might focus relatively more on school-related conditions and perceptions than community conditions and perceptions, depending upon the evidence base (e.g., strengths of the relationships or ability to alter more distal variables like community-school relationships) and the criterion variables of interest.

The use of this model is consistent with a positive psychology perspective in that it allows for a focus on positive conditions and experiences as well as negative conditions and experiences, accordingly LS indicators allow for differentiated responses above and below the neutral point. Based on the pattern of scores on the various measures, individualized interventions should be developed that target the identified likely determinants of low life LS as well exploit identified student or environmental assets relevant to a given individual or group. There are likely many different determinants of LS for specific individuals and groups of individuals. Thus, it seems imperative to conduct a thorough assessment in order to develop a meaningful understanding of the unique determinants and consequences. Because it is also unlikely that a particular intervention strategy will be effective for all children with low LS, it makes sense to develop a resulting individualized plan for a particular student or group of students who share a common set of antecedent conditions. Such an intervention may not only be helpful for children with existing low levels of LS, but also may also prevent the development of dissatisfaction and promote optimal levels in all students.

3.1.2 Research on Life Satisfaction of Children and Adolescents

Numerous predictors of individual differences in children's LS have been identified. However, some variables are more difficult, impossible, or impractical to alter, even in the most comprehensive LS promotion programs. Such variables range from demographic factors (e.g., ethnicity, socioeconomic status) to temperament/personality characteristics (e.g., extraversion, neuroticism). Thus, rather than offering an exhaustive review of the predictors of LS in children, the following review will focus on more readily alterable environmental variables (e.g., family, school setting) and self variables (e.g., cognitive, behavioral factors) within the context of the aforementioned model of Randolph et al. (2009). It should be noted, however, that some of the more non-malleable factors, such as personality characteristics, demographic variables, and cultural differences, might serve as moderators of the relationships between children's LS and "alterable" factors. Some examples will be discussed briefly in a later section.

the significance of LS in both low and high risk groups, interventions to address LS and other well-being variables are important at all points of the prevention-intervention continuum. Although psychological and physical health has historically been approached using a reactive, intervention focus (treating the ill), there has been a gradual and significant increase in attention to prevention. Many prevention frameworks have been developed and discussed in the literature and most reflect an overall notion of a multilevel system that increases in intensity based on risk and need. For example, the levels of a prevention framework typically reflect points of prevention beginning with primary prevention, secondary prevention, and tertiary prevention (also known as treatment). Primary prevention typically reflects pro-gramming efforts aimed toward an entire population of individuals (e.g., school-wide programming), whereas secondary prevention targets a select group of individuals with a specific set of risk factors (e.g., preschool for low-income families). Tertiary prevention targets a smaller group of individuals at imminent risk and/or current presentation of targeted difficulties. Response to Intervention is an initiative that has been widely adopted throughout school systems in the U.S. aimed toward early intervention and prevention. Response to Intervention is most often identified as a multi-tiered system with interventions that increase in intensity across the tiers, which parallels the aforementioned prevention framework (Fuchs and Fuchs 2009).

Possible secondary and tertiary interventions have been discussed extensively elsewhere (e.g., Suldo et al. 2011). For examples of secondary prevention, Huebner et al. (2007) and Huebner and Hills (in press) provide in-depth illustrative case stud-ies of how multidimensional assessments of children's LS yield profiles of individual and environmental deficits and assets that can be used to inform the development and evaluation of individualized intervention plans to promote improved well-being in youth. However, when low LS accompanies an existing psychiatric condition (e.g., mood disorders), more comprehensive assessments and intervention plans are obvi-ously needed. Sin et al. (2011) address some of the complexities associated with applying strategies that are effective for individuals or groups at the primary and secondary intervention levels relative to applying the same strategies at the tertiary level (e.g., individuals with clinical depression). Thus, the following section of this chapter will focus on primary prevention efforts, encompassing family, peers, school, and community environments. Furthermore, we will focus on primary pre-vention programs that can be delivered within the school context, which reflects a context in which children spend a considerable portion of their time, and one which provides access to almost all children and adolescents in developed countries. The examples are merely illustrative. The examples are not exhaustive, nor do they repre-sent the single "best" program. The components and effects of the programs may not be limited to a single environmental context; they may have cross-context effects. Individual program developers will have to choose programs to best fit their own circumstances. Again, a one-size-fits-all approach is not recommended.

A number of universal system-wide efforts have been developed to promote children's well-being and success in school and life. For the purposes of our discussion, they include interventions that address the following contexts: family, peer, school, community, and self. Extensive research on these programs has been conducted at school-wide levels across the U.S. and elsewhere.

3.1.5.1   Family-Related Variables

As noted in the previous section, strong family support and attachment processes are critically related to youth LS and positive youth outcomes. Given the strong link between family support for learning and family processes with positive youth outcomes, much effort has been aimed toward building relationships between families and schools. A multitude of programs exist to help facilitate the school-family connection. Families and Schools Together, or FAST, is one such effective universal prevention program that is suitable for a number of diverse populations. FAST is a multisession group for families of elementary school children to increase parenting skills and well-being. It includes a blend of developmentally appropriate intervention techniques to improve family functioning and reduce risk factors, such as school failure, violence, delinquency, substance abuse, and family stress (Substance Abuse and Mental Health Services Administration 2008). The FAST program works toward important goals outlined in the family-school partnership literature (e.g., Christenson and Sheridan 2001) that include a focus on: (a) shared school-family goals of improving student academic, social, behavioral, and emotional skills; (b) both education and positive socialization outcomes; (c) collaborative interactions between family members and schools; and (d) preventative solutions to promote student learning and overall development. Different FAST curricula have been developed to meet the needs of specific target populations. FAST has been replicated in 38 states in both urban and rural settings and in over 600 diverse school communities (Kratochwill et al. 2004) with evaluation of individual program sites yielding mixed results. However, an aggregated analysis (Crozier et al. 2010) and qualitative review (Terrion 2006) indicate that participation in FAST builds social capital by enhancing bonding among family members, enhancing bonding between the family and school, bridging FAST parents and social agencies, and increasing family empowerment and cohesion.

3.1.5.2   Peer-Related Variables

Children with adequate social skills are more likely to elicit positive attention from others and less likely to be victimized by peers, which also has positive effects on well-being. Without adequate social skills, children are more likely to have lower levels of well-being, including LS, and struggle with adjustment and mental health problems (Bukowski and Adams 2005). Many social skills interventions have been developed and tested at all levels of prevention and intervention. A number of quantitative reviews of Tier III/Targeted Intervention social skills studies that exclusively involve populations of children and adolescents with behavioral and emotional disorders suggest that this type is only minimally effective at this level (Bellini et al. 2007; Quinn et al. 1999) with many studies documenting iatrogenic effects. However, studies that have evaluated social skills programming at a broader, more universal level have yielded more positive results. January et al. (2011) reviewed 28 peer-reviewed journal articles published between 1981 and 2007 to assess the effectiveness of universal prevention programming (i.e., classroom-wide interventions) for the improvement of social skills. Their findings indicated small but positive effects on improving social skills among students, with early intervention most effective across studies. Results of this meta-analysis indicated that active (vs. passive) models of learning are most effective, with better outcomes when participants are engaged in the intervention and play an active and productive role in the learning process (January et al. 2011).

3.1.5.3 School-Related Variables

Positive Behavioral Interventions and Supports (PBIS; Sugai and Horner 2006; Gottfredson et al. 1993) is a universal, school-wide prevention strategy that is currently implemented in over 7,500 schools across the U.S. and several other countries around the world (Sprague and Walker 2010). The purpose of PBIS is to prevent and reduce disruptive behavior problems through the application of behavioral, social learning, and organizational behavioral principles. PBIS aims to alter school environments by creating improved systems and procedures that promote positive change in student behavior by targeting staff and student behaviors. This universal prevention model aims to systematically and consistently manage student behavior problems by creating a school-wide program that clearly articulates positive behavioral expectations, provides incentives to students meeting expectations, and encourages data-based decision-making.

Although specific PBIS models vary in terms of their theoretical orientation and specific focal activities, they share a common emphasis on altering the school context in order to influence children's behavior and academic performance. Most of the whole-school strategies aim to provide staff and student behavior with positively oriented, clearly articulated rules and consequences and well-established processes and procedures for problem solving (Sugai and Horner 2006). Bradshaw et al. (2009) conducted a 3-year randomized controlled effectiveness trial of PBIS in 37 elementary schools and found a significant, positive impact on school climate, which is a strong correlate with youth well-being and academic outcomes. Results from non-randomized (Taylor-Greene et al. 1997; Horner et al. 2005) and randomized (Bradshaw et al. 2011; Horner et al. 2009) studies indicate that implementation of school-wide PBIS is associated with reductions in office discipline referrals (Bradshaw et al. 2009; Taylor-Greene et al. 1997), school suspensions (Horner et al. 2005), and improvements in student academic performance (Horner et al. 2009; Sugai and Horner 2006).

3.1.5.4 Community-Related Variables

Bullying and other forms of peer victimization (e.g., sexual harassment) have become focal points of intervention in school and community settings. The evolution of the Internet and its online social community has expanded the risk for many youth. Interventions targeting the reduction of bullying behavior at an individual level have been found to be only somewhat effective; however, comprehensive bullying prevention programs implemented and evaluated in many countries have been shown to be quite effective at positively influencing knowledge, attitudes, and self-perceptions related to bullying. However, results are more variable in evaluating the effects of these programs on actual bullying behavior. A meta-analysis conducted by Merrell et al. (2008) suggests that these programs are only minimally effective in reducing bullying behavior; however, other studies have reported as much as a 50 % reduction (Olweus 1993) in bullying incidents. Olweus and Limber's (1999) bullying prevention program is one example of an effective, comprehensive program. Community-wide programs found to be effective, promote awareness, education, and adult involvement in order to create a community and school climate that discourages bullying. Further, effective bullying prevention also requires an ongoing commitment from adults in the community and school to reduce or eliminate bullying. Effective programs target all individuals involved: bully (perpetrator of bullying behavior), victim (recipient of bullying behavior), and bystanders (children and adults witnessing the bullying behavior), and commit to ongoing implementation and evaluation of the programming. Addressing the online community and the peer victimization risks presented in that context is also a critical component, especially for adolescents. Comprehensive programming that includes these components has been found to also positively impact prosocial behavior and increase students' satisfaction with their community and school (Olweus 1993).

3.1.5.5 Self-Related Variables

Social-Emotional Learning (SEL) programs aim to help youth acquire core competencies to recognize and regulate emotions, set and achieve positive goals, recognize and appreciate the perspectives of others, establish and maintain positive relationships, make responsible decisions, and handle interpersonal situations constructively. The immediate goals of SEL programs are to foster the development of five interrelated sets of cognitive, affective, and behavioral competencies: self-awareness, self-management, social awareness, relationship skills, and responsible decision making (Collaborative for Academic, Social, and Emotional Learning 2005). SEL programming incorporates systematic instruction in processing, integrating, and selectively applying social and emotional skills in developmentally, contextually, and culturally appropriate ways (Crick and Dodge 1994). These skills are taught, modeled, practiced, and applied to diverse situations so that students use them as part of their daily repertoire of behaviors (Collaborative for Academic, Social, and Emotional Learning 2005). A meta-analysis of school-based, universal SEL programs inside and outside the U.S. (Durlak et al. 2011) indicate that these programs yield significant positive effects on targeted social-emotional competencies and attitudes about self, others, and school, which are significantly related to overall well-being. This universal programming also enhanced students' behavioral adjustment in the form of increased prosocial behaviors, reduced conduct and internalizing problems, improved academic performance on achievement tests, and grades. SEL programming has also demonstrated similar results at other levels of prevention (e.g., Tier II; Catalano et al. 2004; Hahn et al. 2007; Wilson and Lipsey 2007).

3.1.6   Conclusion

Numerous scholars have argued for large-scale monitoring of children's well-being, including their LS reports (Diener and Seligman 2004; Huebner et al. 2009). Meaningful data regarding children's well-being should be a prerequisite for understanding and developing healthy environments for children. Although there are numerous contexts in which such large-scale, child well-being assessments could be implemented, the school context provides one manageable example. For example, school professionals in the U.S. currently provide services at all three previously mentioned levels of service delivery, all of which can be informed by LS and other well-being data. Services at Tier I, or primary prevention services, involve universal assessments and instructional/intervention activities for all children in a given context (e.g., grade level instruction in a school). An example of the use of LS data at his level can be found in studies of the Dual-Factor Model of Mental Health (Greenspoon and Saklofske 2001), in which researchers have identified the incremental utility of incorporating positive subjective indicators along with traditional negative ones (e.g., behavior problems, including internalizing and externalizing behavior) to identify meaningful groups of children that would not be identified using negative indicators alone. For example, Antaramian et al. (2010) identified a group of students who reported non-significant levels of behavior problems and low SWB (including low LS reports) that showed significantly lower school engagement levels and school grades compared to students who reported non-significant levels of behavior problems and high SWB. In a similar study, Suldo and Shaffer (2008) found a similar group of students who displayed lower academic, interpersonal, and physical functioning in school compared to students who reported non-significant levels of problem behaviors and high SWB. Services at Tier II, or secondary prevention services, involve more intensive, sometimes group level services, delivered in the context of regular education programs for students experiencing difficulties in the regular classroom. As noted above, Huebner et al. (2007) and Huebner and Hills (in press) provide case examples of the employment of LS measures to identify student assets and environmental resources, which were subsequently used in the design of an individualized, pre-referral intervention for a student. Services at Tier III, or tertiary intervention services, involve the identification and development of special education programs and program monitoring plans for students with disabilities. An example of the usefulness of SWB data at this level is provided by Brantley et al. (2002). In their study, secondary school students' reports of SWB were measured by multidimensional LS reports. Not only were differences revealed between students with and without mental disabilities, but complex differences were also revealed across domains within special education student groups as a function of amount of time they spent in separate special education classrooms. Such use of SWB data, in conjunction with objective data, is consistent with the arguments of researchers (e.g., Frisch 2006; Gilman and Huebner 2003) that LS data should be routinely collected to monitor the effects of academic, psychosocial, and medical interventions applied to individuals and groups of children. Their argument rests on the notion that assessments of the impact of interventions should include students' perceptions of their quality of life as well as targeted behaviors and academic outcomes. In this manner, an intervention that both improves functioning (e.g., reduces symptoms of an anxiety disorder or chronic health condition) and also improves subjective quality of life would be distinguishable and preferable to an intervention that improves functioning but is perceived to reduce SWB or quality of life of a student or students.

We advocate the collection of objective and subjective quality of life data within the context of a multi-trait, multi-method, multi-occasion assessment approach to evaluate the success of policies and procedures to promote children's overall quality of life. The multi-method aspect of the assessment plan would entail collection of objective well-being data as described above using objective sources (e.g., parent and teacher judgments) and indices (e.g., parenting behavior, peer relationships, teacher behavior) as well as SWB data. The multi-trait aspect would involve multidimensional indices, such as global and domain-based LS reports as well as perhaps other data (e.g., behavior problems) of interest in particular contexts. The multi-occasion component would involve the collection of systematic, longitudinal data across meaningful time periods to track changes in well-being. The collection of subjective data is critical to assess the goodness of fit between child-focused interventions and children's related well-being. Although efforts to improve the lives of children are likely to be based on "good" motivations and "good" expected outcomes, the results of such efforts should be carefully monitored to determine their actual (vs. intended) effects on the subjective and objective lives of children. Children's perceptions of the nature and impact of life conditions and interventions can differ from those of key adults (e.g., parents, teachers), underscoring the importance of taking children's perspectives into account when considering issues of importance to them (Ben-Arieh et al. 2009). The use of evidence-based, developmentally appropriate objective and subjective measures, assessed over multiple periods of time, would facilitate meaningful assessments of the status of children's well-being from their own perspective.

Appendix 3.1

Psychosocial correlates of lower levels of global life satisfaction

Correlates	
Family	Socioeconomic status
	Non-intact family structure
	Low parental involvement
	Low parental emotional support
	Low parental autonomy support
	Low parental monitoring/supervision
	Low parent attachment/trust
	Parent conflict
Peers	Low quality of peer relationships
	Low quantity of friends
	Bullying/overt victimization
	Bullying/relational victimization
	Loneliness
School	Low school grades
	Low academic self-concept
	Low school attachment/connectedness
	School dropout
	Low school engagement behavior
	Negative teacher-student relations
	Low parental involvement
Living environment/community	Residential moves
	Low extracurricular activity participation
	Non-residential neighborhood location/ characteristics
	Absence of non-parental adult role models
	Victim of violent behavior
Self	Externalizing/antisocial behavior
	Internalizing behaviors (suicidal ideation, depression)
	Risk behavior (e.g., drug use, risky sex behavior)
	Low self-esteem
	Low hope
	Low self-efficacy
	External locus of control
	Low religious behavior (attendance)
	Low volunteering behavior
	Low spirituality
	Few character strengths
	Maladaptive attributions

References

Ackerman, B. P., Kogos, J., Youngstrom, E., Schoff, K., & Izard, C. (1999). Family instability and the problem behaviors of children from economically disadvantaged families. *Developmental Psychology, 35*, 258–268.

Antaramian, S., Huebner, E. S., Hills, K. M., & Valois, R. F. (2010). A dual-factor model of mental health: Toward a more comprehensive understanding of youth functioning. *The American Journal of Orthopsychiatry, 80*, 462–472.

Baker, J. A. (1999). Teacher–student interaction in urban at-risk classrooms: Differential behavior, relationship quality, and student satisfaction with school. *The Elementary School Journal, 100*, 57–70.

Baker, J. A., & Maupin, A. N. (2009). School satisfaction and children's positive school adjustment. In R. Gilman, E. S. Huebner, & M. J. Furlong (Eds.), *Handbook of positive psychology in the schools* (pp. 189–196). New York: Routledge.

Baker, J. A., Dilly, L., Aupperless, J., & Patil, S. (2003). The developmental context of school satisfaction: Schools as psychologically healthy environments. *School Psychology Quarterly, 18*, 206–222.

Bellini, S., Peters, J. K., Benner, L., & Hopf, A. (2007). A meta-analysis of school-based social skills interventions for children with autism spectrum disorders. *Remedial and Special Education, 28*, 153–162.

Ben-Arieh, A., McDonnell, J., & Attar-Schwartz, S. (2009). Safety and home-school relations as indicators of children's well-being: Whose perspective counts? *Social Indicators Research, 90*, 339–349.

Bradley, R. H., & Corwyn, R. F. (2004). Life satisfaction among European American, African American, Chinese American, Mexican American, and Dominican American adolescents. *International Journal of Behavioral Development, 28*, 385–400.

Bradshaw, C. P., Koth, C. W., Thornton, L. A., & Leaf, P. J. (2009). Altering school climate through school-wide positive behavioral interventions and supports: Findings from a group-randomized effectiveness trial. *Prevention Science, 10*, 100–115.

Bradshaw, C. P., Mitchell, M. M., & Leaf, P. J. (2011). Examining the effects of school-wide Positive Behavioral Interventions and supports on student outcomes: Results from a randomized controlled effectiveness trial in elementary schools. *Journal of Positive Behavior Interventions, 12*(3), 133–148.

Brantley, A., Huebner, E. S., & Nagle, R. J. (2002). Multidimensional life satisfaction reports of adolescents with mild mental disabilities. *Mental Retardation, 40*, 321–329.

Brown, A. C., & Orthner, D. K. (1990). Relocation and personal well-being among early adolescents. *Journal of Early Adolescence, 10*, 366–381.

Bukowski, W. M., & Adams, R. (2005). Peer relationships and psychopathology: Markers, moderators, mediators, mechanisms, and meanings. *Journal of Clinical Child and Adolescent Psychology, 34*, 3–10.

Callahan, M. R., Tolman, R. M., & Saunders, D. G. (2003). Adolescent dating violence victimization and psychological well-being. *Journal of Adolescent Research, 18*, 664–681.

Casas, F., Cristina, F., Mònica, G., Sara, M., Carles, A., & Sandra, S. (2007). The well-being of 12- to 16-year-old adolescents and their parents: Results from 1999 to 2003 Spanish samples. *Social Indicators Research, 83*, 87–115.

Catalano, R. F., Berglund, M. L., Ryan, J. A., Lonczak, H. S., & Hawkins, J. D. (2004). Positive youth development in the United States: Research findings on evaluation of positive youth development programs. *Annals of the American Academy of Political and Social Sciences, 591*, 98–124.

Chen, S., Cheung, F. M., Bond, M. H., & Leung, J. (2006). Going beyond self-esteem to predict life satisfaction: The Chinese case. *Asian Journal of Social Psychology, 9*, 24–35.

Christenson, S. L., & Sheridan, S. M. (2001). *School and families: Creating essential connections for learning*. New York: Guilford Press.

Collaborative for Academic, Social, and Emotional Learning. (2005). *Safe and sound: An educational leader's guide to evidence-based social and emotional learning programs, Illinois edition*. Chicago: Collaborative for Academic, Social, and Emotional Learning.

Crick, N. R., & Dodge, K. A. (1994). A review and reformulation of social information-processing mechanisms in children's social adjustment. *Psychological Bulletin, 115*, 74–101.

Crozier, M., Rokutani, L., Russett, J. L., Godwin, E., & Banks, G. E. (2010). A multisite program evaluation of families and schools together (FAST): Continued evidence of a successful multi-family community-based prevention program. *The School Community Journal, 20*, 187–207.

Cummins, R. A. (1997). *Manual for the comprehensive quality of life scale-student (grades 7–12); COMQOL-S5* (5th ed.). Melbourne: School of Psychology, Deakin University.

DeSantis-King, A., Huebner, E. S., Suldo, S. M., & Valois, R. F. (2006). An ecological view of school satisfaction in adolescence: Linkages between social support and behavior problems. *Applied Research in Quality of Life, 1*, 279–295.

Diener, E. (1984). Subjective well-being. *Psychological Bulletin, 95*, 542–575.

Diener, E., & Seligman, M. E. P. (2004). Beyond money: Toward an economy of well-being. *Psychological Science in the Public Interest, 5*, 1–31.

Durlak, J. A., Weissberg, R. P., Dymnicki, A. B., Taylor, R. D., & Schellinger, K. B. (2011). The impact of enhancing students' social and emotional learning: A meta-analysis of school-based universal interventions. *Child Development, 82*, 405–432.

Extremera, N., Durán, A., & Rey, L. (2007). Perceived emotional intelligence and dispositional optimism–pessimism: Analyzing their role in predicting psychological adjustment among adolescents. *Personality and Individual Differences, 42*, 1069–1079.

Flanagan, C., & Stout, M. (2010). Developmental patterns of social trust between early and late adolescence: Age and school climate effects. *Journal of Research on Adolescence, 20*, 748–773.

Frisch, M. (2006). *Quality of life therapy: Applying a life satisfaction approach to positive psychology and cognitive therapy*. New York: Guilford.

Fuchs, D., & Fuchs, L. S. (2009). Responsiveness to intervention: Multilevel assessment and instruction as early intervention and disability identification. *The Reading Teacher, 63*(3), 250–252. doi:10.1598/RT.63.3.10.

Gilman, R. (2001). The relationship between life satisfaction, social interest, and frequency of extracurricular activities among adolescent students. *Journal of Youth and Adolescence, 30*, 749–767.

Gilman, R., & Huebner, E. S. (2003). Review of life satisfaction research with children and adolescents. *School Psychology Quarterly, 18*, 99–102.

Gilman, R., & Huebner, E. S. (2006). Characteristics of adolescents who report very high life satisfaction. *Journal of Youth and Adolescence, 35*, 311–319.

Gilman, R., Dooley, J., & Florell, D. (2006). Relative levels of hope and their relationship with academic and psychological indicators among adolescents. *Journal of Social and Clinical Psychology, 25*(2), 166–178.

Gottfredson, D. C., Gottfredson, G. D., & Hybl, L. G. (1993). Managing adolescent behavior: A multiyear, multischool study. *American Educational Research Journal, 30*, 179–215.

Greenspoon, P. J., & Saklofske, D. H. (2001). Toward an integration of subjective well-being and psychopathology. *Social Indicators Research, 54*, 81–108.

Grossman, M., & Rowat, K. M. (1995). Parental relationships, coping strategies, received support and well-being in adolescents of separated or divorced and married parents. *Research in Nursing and Health, 18*, 249–261.

Hahn, R., Fuqua-Whitley, D., Wethington, H., Lowy, J., Crosby, A., Fullilove, M., et al. (2007). Effectiveness of universal school-based programs to prevent violent and aggressive behavior: A systematic review. *American Journal of Preventive Medicine, 33*(2, Suppl. 1), S114–S129.

Harter, S. (1985). *Manual for the self-perception profile for children*. Denver: University of Denver.

Ho, M. Y., Cheung, F. M., & Cheung, S. F. (2010). The role of meaning in life and optimism in promoting well-being. *Personality and Individual Differences, 48*, 658–663.

Homel, R., & Burns, A. (1989). Environmental quality and the wellbeing of children. *Social Indicators Research, 21*, 133–158.

Horner, R. H., Sugai, G., Todd, A. W., & Lewis-Palmer, T. (2005). School-wide positive behavior support. In L. Bambara & L. Kern (Eds.), *Individualized supports for students with problem behaviors: Designing positive behavior plans* (pp. 359–390). New York: Guilford.

Horner, R. H., Sugai, G., Smolkowski, K., Eber, L., Nakasato, J., Todd, A. W., et al. (2009). A randomized, wait-list controlled effectiveness trial assessing school-wide positive behavior support in elementary schools. *Journal of Positive Behavior Interventions, 11*, 133–144.

Huebner, E. S. (1991a). Initial development of the Student's Life Satisfaction Scale. *School Psychology International, 12*, 231–240.

Huebner, E. S. (1991b). Correlates of life satisfaction in children. *School Psychology Quarterly, 6*, 103–111.

Huebner, E. S. (1994). Preliminary development and validation of a multidimensional life satisfaction scale for children. *Psychological Assessment, 6*, 149–158.

Huebner, E. S. (2004). Research on assessment of life satisfaction of children and adolescents. *Social Indicators Research, 66*, 3–33.

Huebner, E. S., & Alderman, G. L. (1993). Convergent and discriminant validation of a children's life satisfaction scale: Its relationship to self- and teacher-reported psychological problems and school functioning. *Social Indicators Research, 30*, 71–82.

Huebner, E. S., & Gilman, R. (2002). An introduction to the multidimensional Students' life satisfaction scale. *Social Indicators Research, 60*, 115–122.

Huebner, E. S., & Hills, K. J. (in press). Assessment of subjective well-being of children and adolescents. In D. Saklofske, & V. Schwean (Eds.), *Oxford handbook of psychological assessment of children and adolescents*. Oxford: Oxford University Press.

Huebner, E. S., Brantley, A., Nagle, R. J., & Valois, R. (2002). Correspondence between parent and adolescent ratings of life satisfaction for adolescents with and without mild mental disabilities. *Journal of Psychoeducational Assessment, 20*, 424–433.

Huebner, E. S., Gilman, R., & Suldo, S. M. (2007). Assessing perceived quality of life in children and youth. In S. R. Smith & L. Handler (Eds.), *Clinical assessment of children and adolescents: A practitioner's guide* (pp. 347–363). Mahwah: Lawrence Erlbaum Associates, Inc.

Huebner, E. S., Gilman, R., Reschly, A., & Hall, R. (2009). Positive schools. In S. J. Lopez & C. R. Snyder (Eds.), *Oxford handbook of positive psychology* (2nd ed., pp. 561–569). New York: Oxford University Press.

January, A. M., Casey, R. J., & Paulson, D. (2011). A meta-analysis of classroom-wide interventions to build social skills: Do they work? *School Psychology Review, 40*, 242–256.

Karatzias, A., Power, K. G., Flemming, J., Lennan, F., & Swanson, V. (2002). The role of demographics, personality variables and school stress on predicting school satisfaction/dissatisfaction: Review of the literature and research findings. *Educational Psychology, 22*, 33–50.

Kelley, S., & Miller, L. (2007). Life satisfaction and spirituality in adolescents. *Research in the Social Scientific Study of Religion, 18*, 232–261.

Kratochwill, T. R., McDonald, L., Levin, J. R., Bear-Tibbetts, H. Y., & Demaray, M. K. (2004). Families and schools together: An experimental analysis of a parent-mediated multifamily group program for American Indian Children. *Journal of School Psychology, 42*, 359–383.

Ladd, G. W., Buhs, E. S., & Seid, M. (2000). Children's Initial sentiments about kindergarten: Is school liking an antecedent of early classroom participation and achievement? *Merrill Palmer Quarterly, 46*, 255–279.

Lewis, A. D., Huebner, E. S., Malone, P. S., & Valois, R. F. (2011). Life satisfaction and student engagement in adolescents. *Journal of Youth and Adolescence, 40*, 249–262.

Lyubomirsky, S., King, L. A., & Diener, E. (2005). The benefits of frequent positive affect. *Psychological Bulletin, 131*, 803–855.

Ma, C. Q., & Huebner, E. S. (2008). Attachment relationships and adolescents' life satisfaction: Some relationships matter more to girls than boys. *Psychology in the Schools, 45*, 177–190.

Malin, A., & Linnakylae, P. (2001). Multilevel modeling in repeated measures of the quality of Finnish school life. *Scandinavian Journal of Educational Research, 45*, 145–166.

Martin, K., & Huebner, E. S. (2007). Peer victimization and prosocial experiences and emotional well-being of middle school students. *Psychology in the Schools, 44*, 199–208.

Martin, K., Huebner, E. S., & Valois, R. V. (2008). Does life satisfaction predict victimization experiences in adolescence? *Psychology in the Schools, 45*, 705–714.

Maton, K. I. (1990). Meaningful involvement in instrumental activity and well-being: Studies of older adolescents and at risk urban teen-agers. *American Journal of Community Psychology, 18*(2), 297–320.

Substance Abuse & Mental Health Services Administration; Department of Health and Human Services. (2008, December). *Families and schools together.* Retrieved December 10, 2009, from National Registry of Evidence-Based Programs and Practices, http://nrepp.samhsa.gov/programfulldetails.asp?PROGRAM_ID=169#description

Merrell, K. W., Gueldner, B. A., Ross, S. W., & Isava, D. M. (2008). How effective are school bullying intervention programs? A meta-analysis of intervention programs. *School Psychology Quarterly, 23*, 26–42.

Neto, F. (2001). Personality predictors of happiness. *Psychological Reports, 88*, 817–824.

Ng, W., & Diener, E. (2009). Feeling bad? The "power" of positive thinking may not apply to everyone. *Journal of Research in Personality, 43*, 455–463.

Nickerson, A. B., & Nagle, R. J. (2004). The influence of parent and peer attachments on life satisfaction in middle childhood and early adolescence. *Social Indicators Research, 66*, 35–60.

Oberle, E., Schonert-Reichl, K. S., & Zumbo, B. D. (2010). Life satisfaction in early adolescence: Personal, neighborhood, school, family, and peer influences. *Journal of Youth and Adolescence.* doi:10.1007/s10964-010-9599-1.

Olweus, D. (1993). *Bullying at school: What we know and what we can do.* Cambridge: Blackwell.

Olweus, D., & Limber, S. (1999). Bullying prevention program. In D. S. Elliot (Ed.), *Blueprints for violence prevention.* Denver: C&M Press.

Park, N., & Huebner, E. S. (2005). A cross-cultural study of the levels and correlates of life satisfaction among adolescents. *Journal of Cross-Cultural Psychology, 36*, 444–456.

Park, N., & Peterson, C. J. (2006). Moral competence and character strengths among adolescents: The development and validation of the Values in Action Inventory of Strengths for Youth. *Journal of Adolescence, 29*, 891–909.

Pavot, W., & Diener, E. (1993). The review of the Satisfaction with Life Scale. *Psychological Assessment, 5*, 164–172.

Paxton, R., Valois, R. F., Huebner, E. S., & Drane, J. W. (2006). Opportunity for adult bonding/meaningful neighborhood roles and life satisfaction among USA middle school students. *Social Indicators Research, 79*, 291–312.

Phinney, J., & Ong, A. (2002). Adolescent-parent disagreements and life satisfaction in families from Vietnamese and European American backgrounds. *International Journal of Behavioral Development, 26*, 556–561.

Pinquart, M., Silbereisen, R. K., & Juang, L. P. (2004). Moderating effects of adolescents' self-efficacy beliefs on psychological responses to social change. *Journal of Adolescent Research, 19*, 340–359.

Proctor, C. L., Linley, P. A., & Maltby, J. (2009a). Youth life satisfaction: A review of the literature. *Journal of Happiness Studies, 10*, 583–630.

Proctor, C., Linley, P. A., & Maltby, J. (2009b). Youth life satisfaction measures: A review. *The Journal of Positive Psychology, 4*, 128–144.

Quinn, M. M., Kavale, K. A., Mathur, S. R., Rutherford, R. B., & Forness, S. R. (1999). A meta-analysis of social skills interventions for students with emotional and behavioral disorders. *Journal of Emotional and Behavioral Disorders, 7*, 54–64.

Randolph, J. J., Kangas, M., & Ruokamo, H. (2009). The preliminary development of the Children's Overall Satisfaction with Schooling Scale (COSSS). *Child Indicators Research, 2*, 79–94.

Saha, R., Huebner, E. S., Suldo, S. M., & Valois, R. F. (2010). A longitudinal study of adolescent life satisfaction and parenting. *Child Indicators Research, 3*, 149–165.

Sam, D. L. (1998). Predicting life satisfaction among adolescents from immigrant families in Norway. *Ethnicity and Health, 3*(1/2), 5–18.

Sastre, M. T. M., & Ferriere, G. (2000). Family "decline" and the subjective well-being of adolescents. *Social Indicators Research, 49*, 69–82.

Sin, N. L., Porta, M. D., & Lyubomirsky, S. (2011). Tailoring positive psychology interventions to treat depressed individuals. In S. I. Donaldson, M. Csikszentmihalyi, & J. Nakamura (Eds.), *Applied positive psychology: Improving everyday life, health, schools, work, and society* (pp. 79–96). New York: Routledge.

Sprague, J. R., & Walker, H. M. (2010). Building safe and healthy schools to promote school success: Critical issues, current challenges, and promising approaches. In M. R. Shinn & H. M. Walker (Eds.), *Interventions for achievement and behavior problems in a three-tier modeling including RTI* (pp. 225–258). Bethesda: National Association of School Psychologists.

Stevenson, W., Maton, K. I., & Teti, D. M. (1999). Social support, relationship quality, and well-being among pregnant adolescents. *Journal of Adolescence, 22*, 109–121.

Sugai, G., & Horner, R. (2006). A promising approach for expanding and sustaining school-wide positive behavior support. *School Psychology Review, 35*, 245–259.

Suldo, S. M., & Huebner, E. S. (2004). The role of life satisfaction in the relationship between authoritative parenting dimensions and adolescent problem behavior. *Social Indicators Research, 66*, 165–195.

Suldo, S. M., & Shaffer, E. J. (2008). Looking beyond psychopathology: The dual-factor model of mental health in youth. *School Psychology Review, 37*, 52–68.

Suldo, S. M., Shaffer, E. J., & Riley, K. N. (2008). A social-cognitive-behavioral model of academic predictors of adolescents' life satisfaction. *School Psychology Quarterly, 23*, 56–69.

Suldo, S. M., Huebner, E. S., Savage, J., & Thalji, A. (2011). Promoting subjective well being. In M. A. Bray & T. J. Kehle (Eds.), *The oxford handbook of school psychology* (pp. 504–522). Oxford: Oxford University Press.

Taylor-Greene, S., Brown, D., Nelson, L., Longton, J., Gassman, T., Cohen, J., et al. (1997). School-wide behavioral support: Starting the year off right. *Journal of Behavioral Education, 7*, 99–112. doi:10.1023/A:1022849722465.

Terrion, J. L. (2006). Building social capital in vulnerable families: Success markers of a school-based intervention program. *Youth Society, 38*(2), 155–176.

Valle, M. F., Huebner, E. S., & Suldo, S. M. (2004). Further evaluation of the Children's hope scale. *Journal of Psychoeducational Assessment, 22*, 320–337.

Valois, R. F., Zullig, K. J., Huebner, E. S., & Drane, J. W. (2001). Relationship between life satisfaction and violent behaviors among adolescents. *American Journal of Health Behavior, 25*, 353–366.

Valois, R. F., Zullig, K. J., Huebner, E. S., & Drane, J. W. (2004). Physical activity behaviors and perceived life satisfaction among public high school adolescents. *Journal of School Health, 74*, 59–65.

Vecchio, G. M., Gerbino, M., Pastorelli, C., Bove, G. D., & Caprara, G. V. (2007). Multi-faceted self-efficacy beliefs as predictors of life satisfaction in late adolescence. *Personality and Individual Differences, 43*, 1807–1818.

Wilson, S. J., & Lipsey, M. W. (2007). School-based interventions for aggressive and disruptive behavior: Update of a meta-analysis. *American Journal of Preventive Medicine, 33*(Suppl. 2S), 130–143.

Wilson, S. M., Henry, C. S., & Peterson, G. W. (1997). Life satisfaction among low-income rural youth from Appalachia. *Journal of Adolescence, 20*, 443–459.

Wong, S. S., & Lim, T. (2009). Hope versus optimism in Singaporean adolescents: Contributions to depression and life satisfaction. *Personality and Individual Differences, 46*, 648–652.

Young, M. H., Miller, B. C., Norton, M. C., & Hill, E. J. (1995). The effect of parental supportive behaviors on life satisfaction of adolescent offspring. *Journal of Marriage and Family, 57*, 813–822.

Zhang, L., & Leung, J. (2002). Moderating effects of gender and age on the relationship between self-esteem and life satisfaction in mainland Chinese. *International Journal of Psychology, 37*, 83–91.

Chapter 4
Promoting Hope Among Youth: Theory, Research, and Practice

Lisa M. Edwards and Jessica B. McClintock

4.1 Introduction

Over the centuries, countless theologians, philosophers, and authors have described hope. While numerous descriptions and definitions of this concept exist, psychologists have recently attempted to conceptualize and measure hope in an effort to understand its potential influence individuals' lives. The most well known operationalization of hope was provided by C. R. Snyder (1994) and has been used as the basis for numerous studies. This theory of hope is primarily cognitive in nature, and describes a motivational state based on goals, pathways, and agency goal-directed thinking. Research about hope over the past 20 years suggests it is an important construct that is associated with positive outcomes in both youth and adults. Specifically, hope has been linked to academic and athletic achievement, as well as health and mental health outcomes such as life satisfaction and wellness regimen adherence.

In this chapter, a review of hope theory and research among children and adolescents will be provided. First, Snyder's (1994) definition of hope will be described, as well as ways that it can measured in children and adolescents. Correlates and positive outcomes of hope among youth will be discussed, and specific examples of how researchers are applying hope theory to interventions will be presented. Finally, directions for future research and practice in this area will be discussed.

L.M. Edwards (✉) • J.B. McClintock
Department of Counselor Education and Counseling Psychology,
Marquette University, 168G Schroeder Complex, Milwaukee, WI 53209, USA
e-mail: lisa.edwards@marquette.edu; jessica.mcclintock@marquette.edu

C. Proctor and P.A. Linley (eds.), *Research, Applications, and Interventions for Children*   43
and Adolescents: A Positive Psychology Perspective, DOI 10.1007/978-94-007-6398-2_4,
© Springer Science+Business Media Dordrecht 2013

44 L.M. Edwards and J.B. McClintock

4.2 An Overview of Snyder's Hope Theory

Snyder et al. (1991) described hope as a motivational state based on three major components: goals, pathways, and agency. Snyder proposed that goals are the targets of mental action sequences, and that in order to necessitate hope, goals need to be sufficiently important to a person (Snyder et al. 1991). Furthermore, individuals must be able to imagine that they might be able to reach their goals; therefore goals must fall within the middle of a probability of attainment continuum (Snyder 2002).

In addition to the ability to clearly conceptualize goals, hope involves pathways thinking. Pathways thinking relates to the perceived ability to generate routes toward desired goals, which Snyder also describes as *waypower* (Snyder et al. 1991). Pathways thinking allows for individuals to find routes around obstacles to goals, which naturally occur as people often encounter challenges in their goal pursuit. For example, if a child is working to master a certain math skill (e.g., ratios), it might be difficult to find time to practice the skill, or to identify adults who are available to work with the child. Pathways thoughts would be those that the child uses to encourage him/herself to utilize study hall and free time to continue practicing, and to ask for help from afterschool tutors, siblings, and other family.

Agency, or the motivation to initiate and sustain movement towards goals, is the third component of hope (Snyder et al. 1991). Also known as *willpower*, agency allows people to remain determined and utilize their mental energy to move around obstacles and stay focused on achieving their goals. For the child who is learning about ratios, therefore, agency thoughts would be those reminders he or she uses to keep working towards the goals. Generally these reminders come in the form of self-talk (e.g., "I can do this", "I'm making progress", or "I'm going to keep working until I understand it").

Snyder et al. (2000b) note that pathways and agency thinking are additive and reciprocal, as well as positively related. However, these aspects of hope are not synonymous, as some individuals demonstrate the ability to sustain agency, but are unable to identify specific pathways towards goals, or vice versa. Further, neither component alone defines hope or would be sufficient to sustain successful goal pursuit (Snyder 2002). Snyder et al. (2000b) also distinguish hope from other common motivation-related constructs. For example, they note that while optimism, as conceptualized by Scheier and Carver (1985) describes generalized expectancies that one will experience good outcomes in the future, hope theory is more focused on identifying specific pathways around obstacles to reach goals. Self-efficacy, which relates to an individual's perceived capacity to carry out actions related to goals (Bandura 1982), is similar to agency, however it also does not address the pathways component of hope. Research has indicated that hope provides unique variance beyond optimism and self-efficacy in the prediction of well-being, thus providing additional support for its distinctiveness from these constructs (Magaletta and Oliver 1999).

4.3 Measuring Hope

Over the past 20 years, Snyder and colleagues (1994, 2000a, b) have developed useful measurements of hope for both adults and youth. In this section we review the Children's Hope Scale (Snyder et al. 1997) and the Adult Dispositional Hope Scale (Snyder et al. 1991) because they are the most popular measures of hope, and also because both can be used to assess hope in adolescence depending on the age of the adolescent.

4.3.1 Children's Hope Scale

The Children's Hope Scale (CHS; Snyder et al. 1997) is a 6-item self-report measure of hope for use with children ages 7–16. In accordance with Snyder's model of hope, three of the six items tap into agency ("I believe I'm doing fairly well"), and three are designed to assess pathways ("I have the ability to come up with many ways to solve any problems I may experience") (Snyder et al. 1991). Participants taking the CHS are instructed to rate statements using a 6-point Likert scale ranging from 1 (none of the time) to 6 (all of the time). The agency and pathways subscale scores can range from 3 to 18, while total scores (sum of both agency and pathways scores) can range from 6 to 36. According to descriptive statistics performed by Snyder et al. (1997) in the development of this scale, the average level of hope on the CHS is approximately 25 in samples of hundreds of children.

In order to determine reliability, the CHS was administered to school age children in four U.S. states, some of who were diagnosed with ADHD (Attention-Deficit/Hyperactivity Disorder) or had a history of severe health-related issues, such as cancer. Cronbach alphas for the CHS ranged from .72 to .86 with this sample, with a median alpha of .77 (Snyder et al. 1997). The test-retest correlations over a 1-month period were found to be both positive and significant, ranging from .70 to .80 (Snyder et al. 1997). Concurrent construct validity was supported in a number of ways. For example, parents' judgment of their child's hope level was found to be correlated positively with their children's scores on the CHS. Youth's CHS scores were also found to be correlated positively with scores on various measures of children's self-perceptions and control related attributions. Self-perceptions were assessed in the areas of scholastics, social acceptance, athletics, physical appearance, and behavioral conduct (Snyder et al. 1997; Lopez et al. 2000). CHS scores were negatively correlated with scores on the Children's Depression Inventory (CDI; Kovacs 1985). Evidence for discriminant validity was provided by showing that higher scores on the CHS were not associated with intelligence.

4.3.2 Adult Dispositional Hope Scale

The Adult Dispositional Hope Scale (ADHS; Snyder et al. 1991) is a 12-item self-report measure of hope for use with adults aged 15 and older. During administration the *Hope* scale is referred to as the "Goals scale" as a way to mask the purpose of the assessment. Participants taking the ADHS are instructed to rate statements using a 4-point Likert scale ranging from 1 (definitely false) to 4 (definitely true). Recently an 8-point Likert scale has been used to encourage score diversity. Four items measure agency ("I've been pretty successful in life"), four measure pathways ("I think of many ways to get out of a jam"), and four items are distracters ("I feel tired most of the time") (Snyder et al. 1991). Total ADHS scores range from 8 to 32 using a 4-point scale, and from 8 to 64 using the 8-point scale.

During the process of norming the ADHS Goals scale, Snyder et al. (1991) found that the average score for college and non-college student samples was 24 using the 4-point scale, and 48 using the 8-point scale. Reliability coefficients were determined by assessing six samples of undergraduate college students. Cronbach alphas ranged from .74 to .84 and test-retest correlations of .80 or above were found for a period of over 10 weeks (Snyder et al. 1991). Concurrent construct validity was assessed by comparing Hope scale responses to responses on similar scales of psychological processes (Snyder et al. 1991). For example, Hope scale scores were found to be correlated in the range of .50–.60 with measures of optimism (Scheier and Carver 1985; Lopez et al. 2000). Experimental construct validation was demonstrated by testing hope's application to daily life. For example, it was found that high-hope people view their goals in a more positive manner (Snyder et al. 1991). Finally, discriminant validity was supported by comparing ADHS scores to unrelated measures, such as the Self-Conscious Scale (Fenigstein et al. 1975), and no significant correlations were found (Lopez et al. 2000).

The adult and child dispositional hope scales were among the first to be developed, and have been utilized for the majority of studies about hope in youth and adults. Other scales that have received attention include: the Adult State Hope Scale (ASHS; Snyder et al. 1996), and the adult Domain Specific Hope Scale (DSHS; Sympson 1999). The ASHS evaluates goal-directed thinking in a given instant, and individuals who are given the scale are encouraged to have a here and now mind set (Lopez et al. 2000), while the adult DSHS measures hope in reference to six specific life domains: social, academic, family, romance/relationships, work/occupation, and leisure activities (Lopez et al. 2000).

It should also be noted that the adult goals scale has been translated into several languages, including: Arabic, Dutch, French, Slovak, Chinese, Korean, and Japanese (Abdel-Khalek and Snyder 2007). Only one published study was identified of a translation of the CHS, which was Portuguese (Marques et al. 2009b). A translation, back translation and validation process was used for this study with 367 Portuguese students, and results suggested that its psychometric properties were similar to the English version of the scale.

4.4 Hope and Positive Outcomes Among Youth

Hope has been shown to be related to many important outcomes in adults, from academic and athletic achievement in college students, to positive mental and physical health indicators. Readers interested in a review of these findings with adults are encouraged to read Snyder (2000a, b, 2002) for summaries. Though not as large as a body of literature as the research on adults, studies of hope among youth also support the importance of this construct in the lives of children and adolescents.

4.4.1 Academic Outcomes

It has been shown that hope has a significant effect on academic success in children and adolescents. Although hope scores are not significantly correlated with intelligence, children and adults with higher hope scores have been shown to perform better on standardized achievement measures, such as semester grades, graduation rates, and the Iowa Test of Basic Skills (Snyder et al. 1991, 1997, 2000a). More recently, Gilman et al. (2006) investigated the relationship between hope and academic and psychological indicators of school adjustment among 341 middle and high school students. The results indicated that youth with high hope reported higher academic and psychological adjustment. Similarly, Ciarrochi et al. (2007) investigated the role of three positive thinking variables (self-esteem, trait hope, and positive attributional style) as predictors of future high school grades, teacher-rated adjustment, and students' reports of their affective states in 784 high school freshmen. The results indicated that hope had a positive effect on total school grades as well as individual subjects (English, religious studies, math, science, and design) than positive attributional style or self-esteem.

4.4.2 Health Outcomes

Hope has also been shown to have positive health and medical outcomes for youth. A study conducted by Berg et al. (2007), examined the relationship between hope and pediatric asthma treatment adherence. A total of 48 participants were monitored on their adherence to an inhaled steroid using a metered-dose inhaler that measures the time and date of each use, with results indicating that hope was a significant predictor of adherence to the asthma treatment. In another study, Barnum et al. (1998) examined the relationship between hope and social support in the psychological adjustment of adolescents who have survived burn injuries. The participant sample consisted of 15 burn survivors and 14 friends of the survivors who comprised the control group. Results demonstrated that adolescent burn survivors with higher hope related to caregivers more positively and also engaged in fewer activities that undermined recovery.

4.4.3 Psychological Adjustment

Support for the relationship between hope and psychological adjustment also is suggested from research with youth. In the original CHS development and validation study, Snyder et al. (1997) found that hope scores were positively correlated with children's perceptions of athletic ability, physical appearance, social acceptance, and scholastic competence, and negatively related to depression. Similarly, Gilman et al. (2006) found that high hope youth reported higher scores on personal adjustment and global life satisfaction, and less emotional distress and Ashby et al. (2011) found that as hope scores increased among middle school students, scores of depressive symptoms decreased.

Hope has also been proven to deter youth from engaging in risky behaviors such as substance use. Carvajal et al. (1998) examined the relationship between intrapersonal factors (optimism, hope, and self-esteem) and youth substance abuse in a large sample of 1,985 adolescents. The results revealed that hope, along with optimism and self-esteem, were determinants of avoiding substance use in these youth. Hagen et al. (2005) also found that children that were more hopeful had fewer behavioral problems. Therefore, hope seems to serve as a form of protection from engaging in risky-behaviors.

Furthermore, hope has been found to play a role in school connectedness among youth. You et al. (2008) investigated the role of school connectedness in the relationship between hope and life satisfaction for middle and high school youth (N=866) with varying levels of exposure to peer victimization. The results showed that those students with higher life satisfaction were able to visualize various pathways to desired goals, which is a trait found in higher hope individuals. In addition, those who were victimized exhibited less hope and experienced less school connectedness.

Importantly, hope has been shown to be a protective factor in the lives of youth facing stressful life events (Valle et al. 2006). In one of the few longitudinal studies conducted about hope among youth, 699 middle and high school students were administered the CHS as well as measures of global life satisfaction, stressful life events, and problem behavior at the beginning and end of 1 year. Findings showed that participants with higher hope were more likely to report higher levels of life satisfaction a year later. Additionally, hope was shown to be a moderator of the relationship between stressful life events and global life satisfaction, highlighting its utility in the lives of youth.

4.5 Applying Hope to the Lives of Youth: Programs and Interventions

Research support for the utility of hope in the lives of youth has been accumulating over the past years. Additionally, professionals have begun to develop methods to accentuate and nurture hope among children and adolescents, though this area is just beginning to receive attention. In the following section, we review existing prevention and intervention efforts in this area that have focused on children and adolescents in particular.

4.5.1 Hope Therapy

Incorporating hope therapy into the therapeutic process is beneficial in helping clients build upon their innate strengths. Lopez et al. (2004) identified a number of strategies for integrating hope into the change process and heightening the hope that individuals already possess. The authors believe that hope is an important agent of change that can be very powerful in motivating clients. Therefore, in order to foster to the change process, *hope finding*, *bonding*, *enhancing*, and *reminding* are essential strategies for accentuating hope (Lopez et al. 2004).

Lopez et al. (2004) suggest that *hope finding* utilizes formal and informal strategies to reinforce client expectations that the therapist has the ability and motivation to foster change, thereby instilling hope in the client. For example, measures such as the ASHS and CHS can be used in the early phases of therapy to identify individuals' levels of hope. Informal strategies might include narrative approaches that illuminate the construct of hope to individuals of all ages in individual and psycho-educational programs.

The goal of *hope bonding* is to further build a strong hopeful therapeutic alliance. Formal strategies for hope bonding include building a working alliance between the therapist and client based on mutually agreed upon goals. The development of a variety of pathways to goal attainment is also essential in building a hope bond. Suggested informal strategies for hope bonding includes therapists encouraging the development of hopeful relationships that increase hope with an individual's life.

Hope-enhancing is the process of building upon the hope the client already possesses. Formal strategies for hope enhancing include psychoeducational programs that are aimed at assisting individuals in making positive decisions and increasing hope. For example, hope programs conducted in schools over short-term weekly sessions have been shown to enhance hope (Edwards and Lopez 2000; Pedrotti et al. 2000). Informal strategies include encouraging clients to develop attainable goals in a clear fashion, and constructing a variety of pathways or routes to the desired goals. Reframing obstacles and building motivation to maintain desired goals are additional strategies for enhancing hope.

Finally, *hope reminding*, or the encouragement of the daily use of hope, involves repetition and daily practice of hopeful cognitions. Finding the hope that individuals innately possess is important for constructing tools that will aid in change, and hope-reminding encourages clients to become their own hope-enhancing change agents. Formal strategies for helping clients in the hope-reminding process include a number of self-monitoring techniques or mini-interventions that can be used in and outside of sessions, including reviewing favorable hope narratives, constructing and completing a brief automatic thought record, reviewing personal hope statements, and bonding with hopeful individuals. Informal strategies include modeling interventions in sessions, and increasing client awareness of goal and obstacle thoughts. All of these strategies offered by the authors can be incorporated into a variety of therapy settings and used with many therapeutic orientations.

4.5.2   Hope Interventions and Programs

In addition to suggestions for incorporating hope into the therapeutic setting, a number of researchers have developed programs to incorporate hope into other settings outside of traditional therapy (Lopez et al. 2004). For example, at the University of Kansas a series of school-based programs were created to enhance hope in culturally diverse elementary and middle school students. These 5-week *Making Hope Happen* programs (Edwards and Lopez 2000; Pedrotti et al. 2000) included age-appropriate activities and lessons related to identifying hope in story/novel characters and students, as well as working towards individual goals. Evaluation of the elementary program suggested that hope was increased in these youth, however a control group was not utilized. Results from the middle school program indicated that hope was increased and maintained over 6 months, and that students who participated in the intervention scored significantly higher than a control group of students who had not received the programming.

In an effort to more rigorously evaluate this type of program for youth, Marques et al. (2009a) implemented a 5-week hope based intervention at the University of Kansas designed to enhance hope, life satisfaction, and self-worth, mental health, and academic achievement in middle school students. The intervention consisted of 62 participants (31 in the intervention group and 31 in a matched comparison group all from a community school). All the participants were Caucasian, with the majority being female (71 %), and with a mean age of 11 years. The intervention was conducted in groups of 8–12 students led by doctoral students in psychology. Participants learned hope vocabulary, concepts of hope, hope goal setting, how to create hopeful talk, and how to apply hope to the future.

Pretests and posttests, as well as 6 and 18-month follow-up assessments of various instruments: CHS; the Students' Life Satisfaction scale (Huebner 1991); the Global Self-Worth Sub-scale (Harter 1985); and the Mental Health Inventory (Ware et al. 1993), were administered to evaluate intervention outcomes. At 6-month follow up, the intervention group consisted of 28 students (9.68 % attrition rate) and the comparison group included 26 students (16.13 % attrition rate). The 18-month follow up included 27 students in the intervention group (12.91 % attrition rate) and the comparison group included 24 students (22.59 % attrition rate). Findings of this study (Marques et al. 2009a) revealed that at posttest those in the intervention group experienced improvements in hope, life satisfaction, and self-worth at the 18-month follow up. The results indicate that a brief hope intervention can increase psychological strengths, including hope and others, for up to 18 months and potentially beyond.

In another effort to increase hope in youth, Robitschek (1996) developed a ropes course designed to increase hope in at-risk youth who attended a summer jobs program. The program participants consisted of 50 boys and 48 girls, ages 14–18 (mean age = 14.86), who were participants in a city-funded summer jobs program for at-risk youth. Of the 98 participants there were 36 African Americans, 17 Caucasians, 41 Hispanics, 1 Native American, and 3 biracial adolescents. The intervention was comprised of a 1-day adventure program with a ropes course. The ropes course challenge consisted of individual and team-building activities, all of which were expected to enhance hope in some way.

In order to evaluate the program participants were given the ADHS (Snyder et al. 1991) at the beginning and end of the activity. Participants also completed a demographic questionnaire and thought-listing exercise. For the thought exercise participants were prompted to write down any thoughts they had about their experience on the ropes course. The results of the thought exercise reveal that the ropes course appeared to be a positive experience for the participants as a whole. In addition, hope scale scores increased (Agency mean score pretest mean 19.85, Agency posttest mean score 20.74; Pathways means score pretest 18.07, Pathways posttest mean score 19.85).

Another study that looked to increase hope in at-risk youth in a group setting was conducted by Brown Kirschman et al. (2010). The researchers incorporated hope into a 6-week summer camp aimed at developing dance and psychosocial competence skills. The authors hypothesized that participants would report higher levels of hope at the completion of the camp as compared to baseline hope scores. There were a total of 406 participants middle-school aged campers (312 female, 94 male). The age range of the participants was 11–14 years with a mean age of 12.13 years. Participants were selected based on their level of at-risk characteristics (low socioeconomic status, lack of identified role models, siblings/parent incarceration, siblings who were teenage parents). Participants self-identified as African American (76.2 %), Biracial (11.4 %), Caucasian (6.6 %), Hispanic (4 %), Asian (<1 %), and Native American (<1 %).

The study was conducted at a camp that was already in existence. The camp was designed through the collaboration of a dance company, social workers, art, music, and writing teachers, a clinical evaluation team, and professional dancers. A number of measures were given to participants the first day of camp, the last day of camp, and at a 4-month follow-up, including the CHS, the Survey of Exposure to Community Violence (Richters and Saltzman 1990), a skills rating form for abilities in ballet, tap, jazz, modern dance, percussion, and creative writing, a friendship follow-up measure to evaluate the frequency with which participants continued contact with fellow campers and staff, and the Youth Risk Behavior Surveillance System (Eaton et al. 2008). The results of the evaluations indicated increases in hopeful thinking and overall hope (pre-camp mean hope score 26.96, post-camp mean hope score 27.58). No further changes were observed at the 4-month follow-up. Once again the results provide support that hope is relevant with at-risk youth in a variety of settings.

Finally, McNeal et al. (2006) evaluated changes over a 6-month period in hope among youth in a residential care center for emotional and behavioral disorders.

The researchers hypothesized that hope scores would improve for youth in the program. The analysis consisted of 185 participants: 121 male (65 %) and 64 female (35 %), ranging in age from 10 to 17 years (mean 14.5 years). The participants identified ethnically as: Caucasian (64 %), African American (18 %), Hispanic (18 %), Biracial (3 %), Native American (3 %), and Asian (2 %). At admission into the residential facility 50 % met the criteria for disruptive behavior, 37 % had anxiety disorder, 27 % had a substance use disorder, 19 % suffered from depression/depressive mood, and 4 % had an eating disorder. To assess hope the CHS was given to participants. The Child Behavior Checklist (Achenbach 1991) assessed the occurrence of behavior and emotional problems in children from the point of view of their parents. The Diagnostic Interview Schedule for Children Version 2.3 (DISC-2.3; Schwab-Stone et al. 1996) measured prevalence of psychiatric disorders. The participants were given the CHS and DISC-2.3 at admission, 2 weeks into treatment, and at the 6-month follow-up. The results indicate that there was a significant improvement in hope scores over the 6 months of treatment. In particular, agency (willpower) hope scores were significantly improved for those with higher levels of psychopathology at admission.

As can be seen, these beginning efforts at enhancing hope among youth are diverse in scope and population. Nonetheless, they show promising findings and suggest that hope is a construct that can be enhanced through psychoeducational efforts, and that nurturing hope will have academic and psychosocial benefits for children and adolescents.

4.6   The Future of Hope: Recommendations and Possibilities

Research over the past 20 years has helped to demonstrate the importance of hope in the lives of youth and adults. With its association to many positive outcomes, hope has the potential to increase well-being and buffer the negative effects of stress. Among youth, professionals are beginning to harness the power of this construct through their work with programs that help children and adolescents apply hope theory to their everyday lives and contexts. While strides have been made in this area, there are still several ways in which the field can continue to grow.

One recommendation for future research lies with the refinement of hope measurement. Since nurturing hope from a young age might be particularly important, developing measures that can assess hope levels in young children are needed. The Young Children's Hope Scale (McDermott et al. 1997), which was designed to measure dispositional hope in preschool to fourth grade level children, was an effort in this direction; however, this scale was never published. Similarly, prevention and intervention efforts that target young children could be helpful in possibly decreasing later risky behaviors (e.g., substance abuse) and maximizing positive outcomes, such as life satisfaction, school achievement and connectedness, and positive emotions. Developing programs that teach young children about hope may bolster their levels of hope, and in turn inoculate them against the negative effects of life events (Valle et al. 2006).

Another recommendation for future research relates to gaining a better understanding of hope and how it operates in the lives of culturally diverse youth. The majority of research about hope among adults has been conducted with white, college aged populations, but there have been increasing efforts to study ethnically diverse samples within the United States (Chang and Hudson Banks 2007; Danoff-Burg et al. 2004). Research about hope among youth has generally included culturally diverse samples, but few efforts have been made to explore the cultural context of hope specifically. Indeed, researchers need to begin to understand whether hope levels vary across different ethnic groups, and whether or not hope functions differently in these groups. In other words, might some youth have higher or lower levels of hope than others? And how does hope relate to certain outcomes among youth of color? These questions provide many avenues for future research.

Finally, recent research findings have shown that incorporating hope into the lives of youth can have a positive impact on academics and overall psychological well-being (Gilman et al. 2006). Therefore, it seems warranted to continue to find avenues to integrate hope into prevention/intervention activities for youth as a whole, whether they are at-risk or not. Bringing hope into the everyday school setting, psychological treatment program, or even recreational activities for youth will likely empower them to overcome obstacles and reach their desired goals. With a generation of youth armed with hope, the world has a bright future.

References

Abdel-Khalek, A. M., & Snyder, C. R. (2007). Correlates and predictors of an Arabic translation of the Snyder Hope Scale. *The Journal of Positive Psychology, 2*, 228–235.

Achenbach, T. M. (1991). *Manual for the youth self-report and 1991 profile*. Burlington: University of Vermont Department of Psychiatry.

Ashby, J. S., Dickinson, W. L., Gnilka, P. B., & Noble, C. L. (2011). Hope as a mediator and moderator of multidimensional perfectionism and depression in middle school students. *Journal of Counseling and Development, 89*, 131–139.

Bandura, A. (1982). Self-efficacy mechanism in human agency. *American Psychologist, 37*, 122–147.

Barnum, D., Snyder, C. R., Rapoff, M., Mani, M., & Thompson, R. (1998). Hope and social support in the psychological adjustment of children who have survived burn injuries and their matched controls. *Children's Health Care, 27*(1), 15–30.

Berg, C. J., Rapoff, M. A., Snyder, C. R., & Belmont, J. M. (2007). The relationship of children's hope to pediatric asthma treatment adherence. *The Journal of Positive Psychology, 2*(3), 176–184. doi:10.1080/17439760701409629.

Brown Kirschman, K. J., Roberts, M. C., Shadlow, J. O., & Pelley, T. J. (2010). An evaluation of hope following a summer camp for inner-city youth. *Child and Youth Care Forum, 39*(6), 385–396. doi:10.1007/s10566-010-9119-1.

Carvajal, S. C., Clair, S. D., Nash, S. G., & Evans, R. I. (1998). Relating optimism, hope, and self-esteem to social influences in deterring substance use in adolescents. *Journal of Social and Clinical Psychology, 17*(4), 443–465.

Chang, E. C., & Hudson Banks, K. (2007). The color and texture of hope: Some preliminary findings and implications for Hope Theory and counseling among diverse racial/ethnic groups. *Cultural Diversity and Ethnic Minority Psychology, 13*, 94–103. doi:10.1037/1099-9809.13.2.94.

Ciarrochi, J., Heaven, P. C. L., & Davies, F. (2007). The impact of hope, self-esteem, and attributional style on adolescents' school grades and emotional well-being: A longitudinal study. *Journal of Research in Personality, 41*(6), 1161–1178.

Danoff-Burg, S., Prelow, H. M., & Swenson, R. R. (2004). Hope and life satisfaction in Black college students coping with race-related stress. *Journal of Black Psychology, 30*, 208–228. doi:10.1177/0095798403260725.

Eaton, D. K., Kann, L., Kinchen, S., Shanklin, S., Ross, J., Hawkins, J., Harris, W. A., Lowry, R., McManus, T., Chyen, D., Lim, C., Brener, N. D., Wechsler, H., & Centers for Disease Control and Prevention (CDC). (2008). Youth risk behavior surveillance—United States, 2007. *Morbidity and Mortality Weekly Report: Surveillance Summaries, 57*(4), 1–131.

Edwards, L. M., & Lopez, S. J. (2000). *Making hope happen for kids.* Unpublished protocol, University of Kansas, Lawrence.

Fenigstein, A., Scheier, M. F., & Buss, A. H. (1975). Public and private self-consciousness: Assessment and theory. *Journal of Consulting and Clinical Psychology, 43*(4), 522–527.

Gilman, R., Dooley, J., & Florell, D. (2006). Relative levels of hope and their relationship with academic and psychological indicators among adolescents. *Journal of Social and Clinical Psychology, 25*(2), 166–178.

Hagen, K. A., Myers, B. J., & Mackintosh, V. H. (2005). Hope, social support, and behavioral problems in at-risk children. *American Journal of Orthopsychiatry, 75*(2), 211–219.

Harter, S. (1985). Self-perception profile for children. In *Manual for the self-perception profile for children.* Denver: University of Denver.

Huebner, E. S. (1991). Initial development of the Students' Life Satisfaction Scale. *School Psychology International, 12*(3), 231–240.

Kovacs, M. (1985). The Children's Depression, Inventory (CDI). *Psychopharmacology Bulletin, 21*(4), 995–998.

Lopez, S. J., Ciarlelli, R., Coffman, L., Stone, M., & Wyatt, L. (2000). Diagnosing for strengths: on measuring hope building blocks. In C. R. Snyder (Ed.), *Handbook of hope* (pp. 57–84). San Diego: Academic.

Lopez, S. J., Snyder, C. R., Magyar-Moe, J. L., Edwards, L. M., Pedrotti, J. T., Janowski, K., Turner, J. L., & Pressgrove, C. (2004). Strategies for accentuating hope. In P. A. Linley & S. Joseph (Eds.), *Positive psychology in practice* (pp. 388–404). Hoboken: Wiley.

Magaletta, P. R., & Oliver, J. M. (1999). The hope construct, will, and ways: Their relations with self-efficacy, optimism, and general well-being. *Journal of Clinical Psychology, 55*, 539–551.

Marques, S. C., Lopez, S. J., & Pais-Ribeiro, J. L. (2009a). "Building hope for the future": A program to foster strengths in middle-school students. *Journal of Happiness Studies, 12*, 139–152.

Marques, S. C., Pais-Ribeiro, J. L., & Lopez, S. J. (2009b). Validation of a Portuguese version of the Children's Hope Scale. *School Psychology International, 30*(5), 538–551.

McDermott, D., Hastings, S. L., Gariglietti, K. P., & Callahan, B. (1997). *The development of the young children's hope scale.* Unpublished manuscript, University of Kansas, Lawrence.

McNeal, R., Handwerk, M. L., Field, C. E., Roberts, M. C., Soper, S., Huefner, J. C., & Ringle, J. L. (2006). Hope as an outcome variable among youths in a residential care setting. *The American Journal of Orthopsychiatry, 76*(3), 304–311.

Pedrotti, J. T., Lopez, S. J., & Krieshok, T. (2000). *Making hope happen: A program for fostering strengths in adolescents.* Unpublished protocol, University of Kansas, Lawrence.

Richters, J. E., & Saltzman, W. (1990). *Survey of exposure to community violence: Self-report version.* Rockville: J. E. Richters.

Robitschek, C. (1996). At-risk youth and hope: Incorporating a ropes course into a summer jobs program. *Career Development Quarterly, 45*(2), 163–169.

Scheier, C. S., & Carver, M. F. (1985). Optimism, coping, and health: Assessment and implications of generalized outcome expectancies. *Health Psychology, 4*, 219–247.

Schwab-Stone, M. E., Shaffer, D., Dulcan, M. K., Jensen, P. S., Fisher, P., Bird, H. R., et al. (1996). Criterion validity of the NIMH Diagnostic Interview Schedule for Children Version 2.3 (DISC-2.3). *Journal of the American Academy of Child and Adolescent Psychiatry, 35*(7), 878–888.

Snyder, C. R. (1994). *The psychology of hope: You can get there from here.* New York: Free Press.

Snyder, C. R. (Ed.). (2000a). *Handbook of hope: Theory, measures, and applications.* San Diego: Academic.

Snyder, C. R. (2000b). The past and possible futures of hope. *Journal of Social and Clinical Psychology, 19*, 11–28.

Snyder, C. R. (2002). Hope theory: Rainbows in the mind. *Psychological Inquiry, 13*, 249–275.

Snyder, C. R., Harris, C., Anderson, J. R., Holleran, S. A., Irving, L. M., Sigmon, S. T., et al. (1991). The will and the ways: Development and validation of an individual-differences measure of hope. *Journal of Personality and Social Psychology, 60*(4), 570–585.

Snyder, C. R., Sympson, S. C., Ybasco, F. C., Borders, T. F., Babyak, M. A., & Higgins, R. L. (1996). Development and validation of the State Hope Scale. *Journal of Personality and Social Psychology, 70*(2), 321–335.

Snyder, C. R., Hoza, B., Pelham, W. E., Rapoff, M., Ware, L., Danovsky, M., et al. (1997). The development and validation of the Children's Hope Scale. *Journal of Pediatric Psychology, 22*(3), 399–421.

Snyder, C. R., Ilardi, S. S., Michael, S. T., & Cheavens, J. (2000a). Hope theory: updating a common process for psychological change. In C. R. Snyder & R. E. Ingram (Eds.), *Handbook of psychotherapy: The process and practices of psychological change* (pp. 128–153). New York: Wiley.

Snyder, C. R., Sympson, S. C., Michael, S. T., & Cheavens, J. (2000b). The optimism and hope constructs: Variants on a positive expectancy theme. In E. C. Chang (Ed.), *Optimism and pessimism.* Washington, DC: American Psychological Association.

Sympson, S. C. (1999). *Validation of the domain specific hope scale: Exploring hope in life domains.* Unpublished doctoral dissertation, University of Kansas, Lawrence.

Valle, M. F., Huebner, E. S., & Suldo, S. M. (2006). An analysis of hope as a psychological strength. *Journal of School Psychology, 44*, 393–406.

Ware, J. E., Jr., Snow, K., Kosinski, M., & Gandek, B. (1993). *SF-36 health survey: Manual and interpretation guide.* Boston: Health Institute.

You, S., Furlong, M. J., Felix, E., Sharkey, J. D., Tanigawa, D., & Green, J. G. (2008). Relations among school connectedness, hope, life satisfaction, and bully victimization. *Psychology in the Schools, 45*(5), 446–460.

Part II
Interventions and Applications

Chapter 5
Flourishing Among Children and Adolescents: Structure and Correlates of Positive Mental Health, and Interventions for Its Enhancement

Andrew J. Howell, Corey L.M. Keyes, and Holli-Anne Passmore

5.1 Introduction

One of our colleagues posted an office whiteboard question, "What do you want your child to be?", and noted the complete absence of answers such as "not depressed or anxious"; not a single parent wrote "not a drug addict". We hope for *positive* futures for our children, not futures *absent of negatives*. No one will argue that avoidance of problems, such as substance abuse, suicide, or juvenile delinquency, is undesirable or unimportant. While we can say that "the kids are alright" because "at least 80 % of youth in a typical year remain free of mental disorder" (Keyes 2009, p. 9), this begs a number of questions: Is *alright* an adequate goal for our children's well-being? Does *alright* really equate to being mentally healthy?

The benchmarks for mental health that we outline in this chapter are positive, going beyond the absence of problems. In the past, research has focused on the measurement and reporting of negative indicators, such as the avoidance of substance abuse and delinquency (Gillham et al. 2002; Moore and Keyes 2003). This *pathology* or *deficit* model has been the traditional and predominant approach to studying how children develop (Halle 2003; Roberts et al. 2002), and a similar deficit framework has been dominant in the fields of early-childhood and youth development (Lerner 2009; VanderVen 2008). However, with the new millennium came an increased focus upon positive indicators of youth well-being, as the following two examples attest.

A.J. Howell (✉) • H.-A. Passmore
Department of Psychology, Grant MacEwan University, Edmonton, AB T5J 4S2, Canada
e-mail: howella@macewan.ca; hap@shaw.ca

C.L.M. Keyes
Department of Sociology, Emory University, Atlanta, GA 30322, USA
e-mail: ckeyes@emory.edu

C. Proctor and P.A. Linley (eds.), *Research, Applications, and Interventions for Children and Adolescents: A Positive Psychology Perspective*, DOI 10.1007/978-94-007-6398-2_5, © Springer Science+Business Media Dordrecht 2013

Land et al. (2011; see also Land et al. 2001) analyzed scores on the Child and Youth Well-Being Index, an index based on national surveys conducted in the United States over the period 1975–2007. The index consists of 28 indicators of well-being in seven domains (i.e., material well-being, health, safety/behavioral concerns, educational attainment, community connectedness, social relationships, and emotional/spiritual well-being). Results showed that overall well-being fluctuated during the 1970s, decreased through the 1980s, increased between 1994 and 2002, and then plateaued. Considering specific domains, improvements occurred since 1994 in safety/behavioral concerns and community connectedness, but decreases occurred in health and social relationships. The researchers concluded that there is room for significant improvement in the well-being of American children.

Land et al. (2011) employed both positive and negative markers of well-being (e.g., rate of weekly religious attendance and suicide rate were two of the markers of emotional/spiritual well-being). Scores across such markers were summed, suggesting that they signify a single underlying dimension ranging from ill-being (mental illness) to well-being (mental health). Greenspoon and Saklofske (2001), in contrast, examined whether mental disorder and mental health are *separable* dimensions of functioning as opposed to opposite poles of a single dimension. The mental disorder dimension identifies variation in the degree to which youth experience psychopathology, whereas the mental health dimension identifies variation in the degree to which youth experience the presence of well-being. Based on data of 407 children in grades 3–6, the *dual-factor* conceptualization was supported; that is, there were children who experienced both low psychopathology and low well-being, others who exhibited both high psychopathology and high well-being, and others who had scores on the two dimensions that opposed each other. Moreover, evidence emerged that the combination of low well-being with high psychopathology was most deleterious.

These studies serve as exemplars of a shift in focus of well-being research in children and youth over the past decade toward a greater consideration of positive markers of well-being. We now turn to examine further work emphasizing the importance of independently assessing positive and negative indicators of well-being.

5.2   Complete State Model of Mental Health in Youth

Furthering the conceptualization of mental health as distinct from mental illness, Keyes (2002, 2005a, b, 2007) described a *complete state model of mental health*, in which mental health and mental disorder are viewed as separate but (inversely) related dimensions of functioning. Mental health requires positive evidence of healthy functioning, and complete mental health involves the presence of mental health and the absence of psychopathology. Keyes (2002, 2005a, b, 2007) operationalized positive mental health as a combination of emotional well-being, psychological well-being, and social well-being. To that end, the Short Form of the Mental Health

Table 5.1 Type of well-being, DSM-type categorical diagnosis, and questions in the mental health continuum short form (MHC-SF)

Emotional well-being: flourishing requires "almost every day" or "every day" and languishing requires "never" or "maybe once or twice" during the past month on one or more of the three symptoms of emotional well-being

"How often during the past month did you feel ..."

1. Happy
2. Interested in life
3. Satisfied

Positive functioning: flourishing requires "almost every day" or "every day" and languishing requires "never" or "maybe once or twice" during the past month on six or more of the 11 symptoms of positive functioning

"How often during the past month did you feel ..."

4. That you had something important to contribute to society. (Social contribution)
5. That you belonged to a community (like a social group, your school, or your neighborhood). (Social integration)
6. That our society is a good place, or is becoming a better place, for all people (social growth)
7. That people are basically good. (Social acceptance)
8. That the way our society works made sense to you. (Social coherence)
9. That you liked most parts of your personality. (Self acceptance)
10. Good at managing the responsibilities of your daily life. (Environmental mastery)
11. That you had warm and trusting relationships with others. (Positive relationships with others)
12. That you had experiences that challenged you to grow and become a better person. (Personal growth)
13. Confident to think or express your own ideas and opinions. (Autonomy)
14. That your life has a sense of direction or meaning to it. (Purpose in life)

Continuum (MHC-SF) consists of items in Table 5.1 that represent emotional well-being (items 1–3; Bradburn 1969), psychological well-being (items 9–14; Ryff 1989; Ryff and Keyes 1995), and social well-being (items 4–8; Keyes 1998). The MHC-SF was created to address the problem of the diagnostic threshold and number of items in the MHC Long Form (MHC-LF). While the MHC-LF consisted of 40 items, the MHC-SF consists of 14 items, each representing a facet of emotional, psychological, and social well-being. The response option for the short form was changed to measure the frequency (from "never" to "every day") with which respondents experienced each sign of well-being during the past month. In the same way that depression requires symptoms of *an*–hedonia, mental health consists of symptoms of hedonia, or emotional well-being. But, feeling good is not sufficient for the identification of a clinical state, in the same way that feeling sad or losing interest in life is not sufficient for diagnosing depression. Rather, similar to the requirement that major depression consists of symptoms of *mal*–functioning, mental health must also consist of symptoms of positive functioning. Individuals with flourishing mental health must report at least 7 of the 14 signs of mental health "almost every day" or "every day," with at least one sign of mental health coming from the emotional well-being domain.

The MHC-SF has shown excellent internal consistency (>.80) and discriminant validity in adolescents (ages 12–18) and adults in the United States, the Netherlands, and South Africa (Keyes 2005b, 2006; Keyes et al. 2008; Lamers et al. 2010; Westerhof and Keyes 2010). The test-retest reliability of the MHC-SF over three successive 3-month periods averaged .68 and the 9-month test-retest was .65 (Lamers et al. 2010). The three factor structure of the long and short forms of the MHC – emotional, psychological, and social well-being – has been confirmed in nationally representative samples of American adults (Gallagher et al. 2009), college students (Robitschek and Keyes 2009), and in a nationally representative sample of adolescents between the ages of 12 and 18 (Keyes 2005b, 2009), as well as in South Africa (Keyes et al. 2008) and the Netherlands (Lamers et al. 2010).

Most recently, Lamers et al. (2012) evaluated the measurement invariance of the MHC-SF using data from a representative sample of 1,932 Dutch adults who completed the MHC-SF at four time points over 9 months. This study employed item response theory and analytic techniques to examine differential item functioning (DIF) across demographics, health indicators, and time points. The results indicated differences in the performance of one item (social well-being) for educational level, one item (social well-being) for sex, and two items (psychological well-being) for age. However, none of the items with differential performance were large enough to affect any mean comparisons. The MHC-SF is highly reliable over time, as there was no DIF on ten of the items across demographics, health indicators, and four time points. The four items with DIF were low and did not affect mean comparisons after appropriate adjustments, and the means and reliabilities of the subscales were consistent over time. Overall, the MHC-SF is a highly reliable and valid instrument to measure positive aspects of mental health.

We turn now to evidence in support of the complete state model of mental health. Keyes (2005a) demonstrated, on a national probability sample of 3,032 American adults using the MHC-LF, that the best-fitting structure underlying correlations among emotional, psychological, and social well-being and symptoms of depression, generalized anxiety, panic disorder, and alcohol dependence was that of two separate, but negatively correlated, factors corresponding to mental health and mental disorder. Importantly, additional analyses showed that the absence of mental health was oftentimes worse than the presence of mental disorder (e.g., on outcomes such as feeling cared for by others), and that mental disorder combined with the absence of mental health was associated with poorer levels of functioning than mental disorder alone (e.g., on outcomes such as lost work days).

Subsequent studies have examined the extent to which the separable dimensions of mental health and mental illness can be extended downward to younger age groups. Peter et al. (2011) administered a variant of Keyes' measure alongside measures of depression, anxiety, health, forgiveness, childhood trauma, and religious faith to 1,245 undergraduates (mean age=20). Measures of mental health and illness were moderately and inversely correlated, supporting the underlying structure of the two continua model. Eklund et al. (2011) assessed, among 240 college students aged 18–25, well-being and mental disorder symptoms. Students were classified as belonging to one of four groups representing high and low well-being crossed with high and low psychopathology. Dependent measures included measures of hope, grit, and gratitude, as well as measures of locus of control, attention problems, hyperactivity, and alcohol abuse. On positive outcome measures, the complete mental health group had higher scores on gratitude and hope than all other groups. On negative outcome measures, students with complete mental health and those with low levels of both life satisfaction and psychopathology had lower attention problems and lower external locus of control scores relative to the remaining groups.

In a national sample of 1,234 youths aged 12–18, Keyes (2006) measured mental health with the MHC-SF; psychopathology was assessed with measures of depression and conduct problems; and psychosocial functioning was assessed with measures of self-concept, self-determination, and closeness to others. Youths were classified categorically as flourishing (38 %), moderately mentally healthy (56 %), or languishing (6 %). Flourishing youth had the lowest rates of psychopathology and the highest levels of psychosocial functioning. A lower proportion of 15- to 18-year-olds compared to 12- to 14-year-olds fell into the flourishing category. Moreover, the sample was characterized with more emotional well-being than psychological well-being, and more psychological well-being than social well-being.

Suldo and Shaffer (2008) assessed mental health and mental disorder among 349 adolescents aged 10–16. The researchers included measures of life satisfaction, affect, and psychopathology, as well as measures of attitudes toward school, grade point average, math and reading achievement, and attendance history. Fifty-seven percent of children were classified as having complete mental health (i.e., high mental health and low mental disorder), 13 % were classified as being vulnerable (i.e., low mental health and low mental disorder), 13 % were classified as content but symptomatic (i.e., high mental health and high mental disorder), and 17 % were classified as troubled (i.e., low mental health and high mental disorder). In comparing those with complete mental health with those classified as vulnerable, the presence of mental health predicted more adaptive academic (e.g., attendance), social (e.g., fewer social problems), and physical functioning (e.g., lower role limitations).

In a follow-up study with the same sample, Suldo et al. (2011) examined the long-term prediction of outcomes (including attendance, disciplinary actions at school, grade point average, and standardized test scores on reading and math) as a function of both mental health and mental disorder. Students with complete mental health, and those classified as vulnerable or content but symptomatic, declined less in school grades relative to those classified as troubled. The best outcomes (e.g., high grades) were experienced by those with high mental health and low psychopathology. Those classified as content but symptomatic had the poorest attendance, perhaps reflecting a tendency for those with high well-being and high psychopathology to be characterized as prone to externalizing disorders (Suldo et al. 2011).

Finally, Shaffer-Hudkins et al. (2010) examined the relationship of both mental health and mental illness to *physical* health among 410 adolescents aged 10–16. Participants completed measures of life satisfaction, positive and negative affect, internalizing and externalizing psychopathology, and physical health. All indicators of mental health (i.e., life satisfaction, high positive affect, and low negative affect) were significant predictors of physical well-being. Both indicators of mental illness (i.e., internalizing and externalizing symptoms) also predicted physical well-being. In regression analyses in which indicators of both positive mental health and mental illness were used to predict physical well-being, all three mental health indicators and internalizing symptoms (but not externalizing symptoms) emerged as predictors of physical well-being.

This area of research indicates that positive markers of mental health are indeed distinct from negative markers of mental illness, that mental health and mental illness are inversely correlated at a modest level, and that incremental validity is obtained when both kinds of indicators are employed in research predicting outcomes associated with mental health and mental illness. This body of work therefore strongly supports the validity of the positive mental health dimension of functioning in youth.

5.3 Predictors of Well-Being in Youth

What variables predict scores on the mental health dimension of functioning identified in the dual-factor and complete state models? C. L. Proctor et al. (2009) conducted a comprehensive review of 141 studies concerning predictors of one aspect of well-being – life satisfaction – among youth. Concerning personality traits, significant positive associations emerged between life satisfaction and both extraversion and self-esteem, whereas negative associations emerged between life satisfaction and neuroticism. Exercise emerged as a positive predictor of life satisfaction, whereas poor physical health was a negative predictor, as were tobacco use, alcohol use, and illicit drug use. Leaving school prior to graduation and lower employability were associated with lower life satisfaction. Goal attainment, high personal standards, and the pursuit of intrinsic goals positively predicted life satisfaction. Hope and self-efficacy positively predicted life satisfaction. Life satisfaction was inversely associated with poor parental relationships and positively associated with healthy family functioning. Attachments to both parents and peers were predictive of higher life satisfaction, as was perceived parental social support. Youths residing in dense urban settings experienced lower satisfaction, as did youths subjected to numerous changes in residence. Other stressful life events also predicted lower satisfaction. Higher levels of life satisfaction were associated with lower occurrence of fighting and violence, lower bullying, and lower dating-related violence. Finally, numerous forms of psychopathology predicted lower life satisfaction among youth, including eating disorder, depression, suicidality, and insomnia. Similar to the finding of Keyes (2006) reported above, C. L. Proctor et al. (2009) noted that life satisfaction tends to decrease with the onset of adolescence.

This same research team examined *very high* life satisfaction among youth and its correlates (C. Proctor et al. 2010). C. Proctor et al. (2010) studied 410 adolescents aged 16–18 with measures of life satisfaction as well as measures of health-promotion behaviors, extracurricular activities, environmental views, and ratings concerning school satisfaction, life meaning, achievement, and gratitude.

Participants were classified into very satisfied, very unsatisfied, and average groups. The three groups significantly differed from each other on most variables. For example, the very satisfied students scored higher than the average students on measures of school satisfaction, parental relations, life meaning, gratitude, self-esteem, social acceptance, and academic achievement. This and similar research (e.g., Gilman and Huebner 2006; Suldo and Huebner 2006) provides evidence consistent with the complete state model of mental health in that gradations in positive mental health are associated in a dose–response manner with changes in important criterion variables. Next we consider examples of additional research exploring further correlates of well-being among children and youth.

5.3.1 *Psychological Need Satisfaction*

Predictors of well-being in youth have recently been examined through the lens of *self-determination theory* (e.g., Ryan and Deci 2000), which holds that the satisfaction of three fundamental psychological needs – for autonomy, competence, and relatedness – significantly contributes to well-being. Soenens and Vansteenkiste (2005) showed that, among two samples (N > 600 combined) of youth aged 15–22, perceptions of autonomy-support provided by parents and by teachers were predictive of need satisfaction in three important life domains (i.e., social competence, school, and job seeking), which was in turn predictive of positive adjustment (e.g., scholastic competence, vocational identity). Veronneau et al. (2005) measured need satisfaction in three different contexts (i.e., at home, at school, and with friends) as well as levels of depression, positive affect, and negative affect among 331 Canadian 3rd and 7th graders. The depression and affect measures were repeated after an interval of 6 weeks. Results showed that need satisfaction was related to concurrent and future well-being. For example, satisfaction of each of the three needs was related to concurrent positive affect, and satisfaction of the *relatedness need* predicted future positive affect. There was also evidence that need satisfaction in the context of home and school was more important than need satisfaction in the context of relationships with peers. In follow-up research, Milyavskaya et al. (2009) examined whether the experience of *balance* across the satisfaction of the needs for autonomy, competence, and relatedness was predictive of high levels of well-being and adjustment (i.e., the extent to which the needs were equally met across three diverse contexts of school, home, work, and peer relationships). They conducted three studies with several hundred adolescents in Canada, the United States, and China in which they assessed numerous variables including positive affect, negative affect, self-concept, need satisfaction, school adjustment, and teacher-rated adjustment. The experience of balanced need satisfaction across diverse contexts was predictive of high levels of well-being and other indicators of adjustment. Finally, among 255 adolescents aged 14–16, Eryilmaz (2012) measured need satisfaction as well as subjective well-being (i.e., positive affect, negative affect, life satisfaction), and strategies for enhancing well-being (e.g., reacting positively to an environment). Results showed positive associations between need satisfaction and subjective well-being; moreover, mediation analysis suggested that the use of strategies to enhance well-being predicted enhanced need satisfaction, and that enhanced need satisfaction in turn predicted high subjective well-being.

5.3.2 Character Strengths

Strengths of character have also been examined as predictors of well-being in children and youth. Park and Peterson (2006a) obtained open-ended character descriptions from parents of 680 children between 3 and 9 years of age. The descriptions were content-analyzed to reflect the presence or absence of the 24 strengths of character categorized by Peterson and Seligman (2004). Each description was also evaluated to yield a 7-point rating of the child's happiness. Results showed that hope, zest, and love were the three strengths of character significantly associated with happiness. Subsequently, Park and Peterson (2006b) devised a 198-item self-report inventory (called the Values in Action – Inventory of Strengths for Youth) to assess the 24 strengths of character based upon several hundred respondents aged 10–17. Factor analysis of the measure suggested four factors: temperance strengths (e.g., self-regulation, prudence); intellectual strengths (e.g., creativity, curiosity); theological strengths (e.g., hope, religiousness); and other-directed strengths (e.g., modesty, kindness). Four strengths of character were significantly associated with life satisfaction: hope, zest, love, and gratitude. Froh et al. (2011) showed, among 1,035 high school students, that the characteristic of gratitude significantly predicted life satisfaction and other outcomes such as grade point average. Gillham et al. (2011) showed that, among 149 high school students, other-directed strengths (such as kindness) predicted less depression, whereas transcendence strengths (e.g., religiousness) predicted greater life satisfaction.

5.3.3 Engagement

Froh et al. (2010) devised a 15-item measure, the Engaged Living in Youth Scale, to assess the extent to which engaged living is associated with well-being. Engaged living was defined as "having a passion to help others and be completely immersed in activities" (p. 311) and thus was conceptualized as involving both social integration and absorption. Results of five studies with youth ranging in age from 10 to 19 showed that both subscales were positively associated with measures of well-being (i.e., self-esteem, positive affect, life satisfaction, and happiness) as well as with gratitude, hope, meaning in life, and grade point average. Inverse correlations emerged between both subscales and measures of materialistic values, envy, antisocial behavior, negative affect, and depression.

5.3.4   Benefit Finding

Benefit finding refers to perceiving meaning or possibility in the face of adversity. Among a sample of 1,999 children with cancer, Phipps et al. (2007) demonstrated that scores on the Benefit Finding Scale for Children predicted aspects of well-being, including optimism and self-esteem; benefit finding was inversely associated with anxiety symptoms. Similarly, Michel et al. (2010) used the Benefit Finding Scale for Children with 48 youth aged 12–15 who had survived cancer and again demonstrated a positive association with optimism. In related research, Levine et al. (2008) demonstrated that growth following adversity, as assessed with the Post-Traumatic Growth Inventory, was most closely associated with responses to moderate posttraumatic stress levels (as opposed to low or high levels of posttraumatic stress). Unexpectedly, post-traumatic growth was inversely related to resilience among 2,908 Israeli adolescents who had experienced exposure to terror (Levine et al. 2009).

5.3.5   Spirituality and Religiousness

Spirituality (referring to non-institutionally based inner belief systems regarding life views and self-transcendence) and religiousness (referring to institutionally-based beliefs regarding supernatural powers, affiliation, and participation) have infrequently been studied as predictors of well-being in children, youth, and adolescents. Nonetheless, existing research has been supportive. For example, Dowling et al. (2004) demonstrated, in a study of 1,000 youth aged 9–15 years, that spirituality comprised an important component of "exemplary positive development" (p. 11). Kelley and Miller (2007) reported, in a sample of 615 adolescents aged 11–23, that life satisfaction was significantly and positively associated with frequency of daily spiritual experiences, and with measures of both religiousness and spirituality. Similar findings regarding spirituality and positive mental health were reported by Holder et al. (2010) in their study of 320 children aged 8–12 years. Holder et al. (2010) reported that "[i]n general, children who indicated that they were spiritual were happier based on self-reports and reports by their parents" (p. 144). However, Holder et al. (2010) found only a weak association between children's religious practices and their happiness.

5.3.6   Nature Involvement

Daily interactions with nature have been suggested to not only contribute to positive mental development and well-being in children and youth, but "to constitute an irreplaceable core for healthy childhood growth and development" (Kellert 2005, p. 81).

A growing body of evidence is accumulating regarding the positive association between contact with the natural environment and children and youth's well-being. For example, in a quasi-experimental study, Han (2009) demonstrated that the simple addition of six plants at the back of an 8th grade classroom of 35 students was associated with increased feelings of comfort and friendliness, compared to students in the control classroom with no plants. Additionally, at the end of 2.5 months, fewer sick hours and punishment incidents were recorded for students in the classroom with plants. Taylor et al. (2002) reported in their study of 169 children ranging in age from 7 to 12 years, that the "greener" the view from a girl's home, the higher the girl's score on an index measuring three types of self-discipline. The effect of near-home nature for boys, however, was not significant. Wells and Evans (2003) demonstrated, in their study of 337 rural children in grades 3–5, that higher levels of nearby nature corresponded to higher global self-worth.

This area of research has documented that youth scoring highly on the positive mental health dimension differ systematically from those experiencing lower mental health on personality traits (e.g., extraversion, neuroticism), cognitive content (e.g., hope, optimism, benefit finding), social support (e.g., relationships with parents), activities (e.g., nature involvement, exercise), and transcendent experiences (e.g., spirituality, purpose in life). While the correlational nature of this research precludes the drawing of causal conclusions, these factors are at least suggestive of targets of interventions aimed at boosting well-being, to which we now turn.

5.4 Well-Being Therapies for Children and Adolescents

Enhanced understanding of the structure and predictors of childhood positive mental health has ultimately helped to foster the development of interventions to boost well-being among this segment of the population. Here we provide a sample of well-being therapies for youth.

5.4.1 Positive Action

Flay (e.g., Flay and Allred 2003) devised a *Positive Action* program for elementary school students with six central components: self-concept, positive action, responsible self-management, getting along with others, being honest, and continuous improvement. In an evaluation of the program comparing schools that adopted the Positive Action program and matched schools that did not, benefits of the program were revealed on measures of reading and aptitude test scores, and on behavioral measures of violence, suspensions, and truancy (Flay and Allred 2003). Moreover, performance by students in subsequent grades (e.g., high school) was higher in schools having a large number of students who came from feeder schools which adopted the Positive Action program, as evidenced by such measures as standardized writing tests and substance use incidents. Using randomized matched-pair experimental designs, follow-up studies by Beets et al. (2009) and by Li et al. (2011) showed that elementary school children attending schools for which the Positive Action program was implemented had more positive outcomes than control children, as reflected on such indices as reduced substance abuse and violence. More generally, *positive youth development* programs aimed at competence enhancement have received considerable support (for a recent review, see McWhinnie et al. 2008).

5.4.2   Well-Being Therapy

Well-being therapy was developed by Fava and Ruini (2003) as an intervention aimed at boosting levels of well-being by addressing areas of deficit among facets of Ryff's (1989) psychological well-being dimensions, such as deficits in autonomy or in environmental mastery. Albieri et al. (2009) present the cases of four boys (aged 8–11) treated with well-being therapy for disorders such as attention deficit hyperactivity disorder, generalized anxiety disorder, and oppositional defiant disorder. The therapy explicitly addressed positive personality characteristics, autonomy, purpose in life, and happiness. Positive outcomes were described on both diagnostic status and a global rating of functioning. Ruini et al. (2006) applied well-being therapy in a group format to non-clinic-referred students, which generated improvements in well-being and decreases in anxiety. More recently, Tomba et al. (2010) conducted a randomized comparison study of well-being therapy and anxiety management with 162 non-disordered students with a mean age of 11.41 years. Pretest and 6-month follow-up measures included psychological well-being scales and symptom measures. Students in the anxiety management condition showed greater improvement on an anxiety symptom measure, whereas students in the well-being therapy condition showed greater improvement on a measure of friendliness. However, the two groups did not differ on psychological well-being subscales.

5.4.3   Positive Psychotherapy

As described by Rashid and Anjum (2008), positive psychotherapy is an 8-week group-administered intervention aimed at bolstering pleasure, engagement, and meaning. Components of the therapy include making use of character strengths, expressing gratitude, and savoring positive experiences. In a pilot study, 22 children (mean age = 12) were randomized to an intervention or control group. Treated children obtained higher scores than control children on a measure of happiness.

5.4.4   Strengths-Based Interventions

C. Proctor et al. (2011) describe the development and testing of the *Strengths Gym* program among 218 students aged 12–14. Students received a strengths-based exercise intervention, identified their own character strengths, and received instruction on how to further develop them. Results showed that students who received the intervention had higher life satisfaction compared to those who did not. Similarly, Madden et al. (2011) tested a strengths-based coaching program applied to 38 male children, aged 10–11. The program emphasized identification of children's strengths, and the setting of goals that maximized use of signature strengths. Compared to pretest scores, posttest scores were enhanced on measures of engagement and hope. Finally, Vohra (2006) developed and tested an intervention for adolescents that promoted development of such strengths and values as altruism, forgiveness, and self-analysis.

5.4.5   Mindfulness-Based Interventions

Another form of intervention for boosting the well-being of youth is mindfulness-based interventions. Mindfulness is the process of maintaining an attentional focus upon the present while adopting a nonjudgmental, accepting attitude (Cardaciotto et al. 2008). A review of 16 studies concerning mindfulness and other meditative practices among youth suggested replicable effects on measures of both psychological and physiological outcomes for a number of conditions (Black et al. 2009). Mindfulness-based interventions are now being employed to foster positive mental health among non-clinic-referred children and adolescents, with significant effects. For example, Schonert-Reichl and Lawlor (2010) showed a significant increase in optimism from pre- to posttest among 246 4th through 7th graders undergoing a mindfulness education program. Adolescents in a wait-list control condition did not show similar increases. Similarly, Joyce et al. (2010) assessed 109 students aged 10–13 before and after participation in a mindfulness program consisting of ten 45-min modules. Results revealed that children experienced both a reduction of problems (e.g., hyperactivity/inattention and conduct problems) and gains in prosocial behaviors.

5.4.6   Hope-Oriented Interventions

Lopez et al. (2004) describe a hope-oriented intervention called *Making Hope Happen*, which was validated with 4th and 7th graders. The program, conducted in a group format over 5 weeks, teaches children to identify (via the use of age-appropriate games, stories, and activities) important goals, pathways towards those goals, and means of maintaining motivation in working toward the goals. Examination of changes from pre-intervention to post-intervention revealed significant gains in hope as measured with the Children's Hope Scale. With the older age group, changes in hope scores were not observed among a control group of children, and gains in the intervention group were shown to persist at a 6-month follow-up. In a recent meta-analysis, Weis and Speridakos (2011) reported a reliable but small effect on hope scores across six studies applying hope-focused interventions to youth.

5.4.7 Gratitude Expression

Froh and Bono (2008) summarize the small literature supporting gratitude interventions as a means of boosting well-being among youth. For example, Froh et al. (2008) randomly assigned students to either identify (on a daily basis for 2 weeks) things for which they were grateful, to identify things they found annoying, or to do nothing. Expressing gratitude was related to outcomes such as optimism and life satisfaction, and was also shown to boost satisfaction with school.

A number of interventions aimed at boosting scores on the mental health dimension of functioning have thus received support, although additional research on a number of these approaches is needed to provide additional validation. Moreover, these interventions target variables identified previously as significantly predictive of well-being in youth, such as hope, engagement, meaning in life, gratitude, and strengths of character.

5.5 Discussion and Future Directions

Significant progress has been made toward better understanding and fostering well-being in youth. Here, we address or raise a number of outstanding issues in the area.

The dual-factor or complete state mental health models have not been closely associated with the development of well-being interventions for youth. Perhaps interventions would be optimized to the extent that they are tailored to the particular characterization of individuals along the mental health and mental disorder dimensions (Eklund et al. 2011; Greenspoon and Saklofske 2001; Keyes 2005a). Youth low in well-being and high in psychopathology may especially benefit from well-being oriented interventions that are combined with traditional mental disorder treatment, such as combining well-being therapy with cognitive-behavioral therapy. Those low in well-being and low in psychopathology would presumably benefit sufficiently from well-being interventions alone, while those high in well-being and high in psychopathology would presumably benefit sufficiently from mental disorder treatment alone. It would also be reasonable to target the precise nature of the well-being deficit experienced by youth (e.g., employing a hope-focused intervention for those lacking hope). Beyond the treatment context, Suldo and Shaffer

(2008) suggest that psychoeducational and clinical *assessment* would benefit from an explicit consideration of both mental health and mental disorder dimensions (i.e., measuring strengths, assets, and well-being as well as deficits and symptoms).

Beyond the dual-factor and complete state models, additional conceptualizations of the interplay between mental health and mental disorder have also been devised. As an example, Kia-Keating et al. (2011) argue for an integration of work on resilience (i.e., competencies that are brought to bear on mitigating the experience of risk) and positive youth development (i.e., competencies that are used to foster optimal outcomes, regardless of the experience of risk). They conceptualize a *protecting* pathway between risk factors and healthy development, a *promoting* pathway between assets and healthy development, and interactions between the two pathways (e.g., assets can mitigate risks). The framework emphasizes mutual interactions among multiple aspects of youth's social network (e.g., peers, school, family, society, and culture) and evolution and fluctuation in healthy development over time. Kia-Keating et al. (2011) further argue that the two pathways (i.e., resilience and positive youth development) complement each other; for example, assets can mitigate the role of risk experiences in the development of youth. This model argues for eight important developmental domains relevant to the fostering of resilience and/or positive youth development: belongingness, self-efficacy, prosocial activities and having an orientation toward others, strengths of character, emotional self-regulation, hope, school engagement, and adult supervision and monitoring. These are highly overlapping with the factors highlighted previously in this chapter; indeed, each of these factors emerged either as a predictor of well-being or as a target for well-being interventions.

Another recent conceptualization of the interplay between youth mental health and disorder is the concept of *thriving* as studied by Benson and colleague (e.g., Benson and Scales 2009). Thriving youth are identified by the presence of various markers of well-being including positive emotions, passion in a specific domain, a sense of purpose, optimism, a prosocial orientation, and spirituality (Benson and Scales 2009). The attainment of thriving is conceptualized as requiring positive inputs from the environment in the form of support, empowerment, boundaries and expectations, and constructive use of time, and internal assets in the form of commitment to learning, positive values, social competencies, and positive identity (Benson and Scales 2009). Thus, the thriving concept is highly congenial with core factors emphasized herein as characterizing and contributing to youth well-being. The thriving concept also emphasizes the dynamic interplay between the youth and his or her social context; a key role for finding an intrinsically-driven interest or spark in one's life; the inherent potential for positive growth of all youth; the importance of adoption of a prosocial orientation; and the role of thriving in fostering resilience and even growth in the face of adversity (Benson and Scales 2009).

The promoting versus protecting and thriving frameworks are good examples of recent theory development organizing processes and outcomes related to youth mental health and disorder. Future youth well-being research would also potentially profit from a greater utilization of *existing* psychological theories concerning well-being. For example, while self-determination theory has been influential in contributing to understanding of well-being in adults, it has been infrequently applied to youth. Nonetheless, key concepts of self-determination theory are seen in various approaches to the understanding of youth well-being, such as the concepts attached to the thriving construct (i.e., inherent human potential for growth; intrinsic motivation). As another example, Fredrickson's (1998, 2001) broaden-and-build theory argues that positive affective states such as happiness cause mental capacities to be broadened and personal competencies to be developed, and that such states buffer the impact of negative affective states. This theory was applied by Reschly et al. (2008) to students in grades 7–10, showing that frequent positive affect was associated with greater student engagement and adaptive coping. Broaden-and-build theory is also relevant to findings by Suldo and Huebner (2004), who showed that stressful life events could be buffered by high life satisfaction in protecting against externalizing symptoms.

The potential application of self-determination theory or broaden-and-build theory to youth well-being research reflects the fact that youth well-being research has generally benefitted from the consideration of predictors and intervention targets identified as fruitful in research on adults (e.g., hope, gratitude expression). *Negative* findings emerging in the adult literature may also be informative for work in youth well-being. For example, the concepts of benefit finding and post-traumatic growth in the adult literature have proven contentious in some applications (Coyne and Tennen 2010); this might suggest caution with respect to how these concepts apply to youth populations. Indeed, some anomalous findings were described above regarding post-traumatic growth in youth (Levine et al. 2009). As another example, in the domain of positive thinking and optimism, it has been suggested that adaptive optimism among adults falls within the parameters of what is realistic (Schneider 2001); similarly, recent evidence suggests that repeating positive self-statements may be not be advantageous for individuals characterized by low self-esteem (Wood et al. 2009). Research could profitably examine the extent to which levels of optimism or positive thinking among youth are moderated by such additional personal and situational factors. As a final example, recent evidence has suggested that the highest levels of well-being are not always optimal for adults. Oishi et al. (2007) showed that the optimal level of happiness or life satisfaction related to achievement was a *moderately high* level, perhaps reflecting the fact that motivation toward accomplishment is highest if one's well-being is not yet maximized (Oishi et al. 2007). Again, the extent to which findings such as these may also apply to youth well-being could be a useful focus of future research.

This latter example raises two additional issues. First, distinctions between *hedonic* and *eudaimonic* conceptualizations of well-being in research on youth may be important. Hedonic conceptualizations emphasize positive emotions and life satisfaction, whereas eudaimonic notions emphasize positive growth and fulfillment (e.g., Keyes and Annas 2009). Few studies have examined this distinction in youth well-being research, but it may be highly relevant. For example, perhaps moderate levels of hedonic well-being, but maximum levels of eudaimonic well-being, are optimal when it comes to achievement striving. Second, to what extent do we focus on child well-being as an end in itself or, conversely, as a means to an end, such as success later in life? Here, a distinction has been made between *child well-becoming* and *child well-being,* with the former emphasizing the future benefits of childhood mental health and the latter emphasizing the here-and-now functioning of the child (Moore and Lippman 2005). Bradshaw and Richardson (2009), for example, argue that one should give "priority to indicators of child well-being now, rather than indicators of well-becoming – how a child might do in adulthood – on the grounds that childhood is a life stage to be valued in its own terms" (p. 321). Child well-being and child well-becoming are not, however, exclusive concepts. Measures can be developed that aim to predict both present and future outcomes (Moore and Lippman 2005), while efforts can be made to "improve the quality of life for the child *during childhood* and for that child's *later* adulthood" (Roberts et al. 2002, p. 671; see also Benson and Scales 2009).

The issue of child well-being versus child well-becoming can also be illustrated with the example of play. In the midst of research aimed at developing programs to increase child and youth well-being, the importance of play – that "simple joy that is a cherished part of childhood" (Ginsburg 2007, p. 183) – must not be forgotten. In addition to being pleasurable, and therefore contributing to child well-being, child-driven play enables children and youth to develop essential problem solving skills (Kashdan 2009; National Institute for Play 2009), to learn "the interpersonal skills needed to become effective social beings" (Elkind 2007, p. 145), and allows "children to become secure and self-confident on their own" (Brown and Vaughan 2009, p. 108), thereby contributing to child well-becoming. Broaden-and-build theory also emphasizes that joyful, exuberant affective states promote play, which in turn promote the development of personal and social resources that can be called upon in the future (e.g., friendships, specific physical abilities). Self-determination theory might also be applicable to play, in that play may oftentimes provide nutriments for the meeting of the basic needs of autonomy, competence, and relatedness. Engaging in spontaneous, self-directed play driven by curiosity also allows children to become attuned with their own passions and inner motivations for activities (Brown and Vaughan 2009; Kashdan 2009), some of which may "later blossom into a motive force for life" (Brown and Vaughan 2009, p. 105). Therefore, the youthful activity of play may be an exemplar of activities conducive to both well-being and well-becoming.

Another area that would benefit from additional consideration is developmental changes in well-being suggested by several findings mentioned herein. C. L. Proctor et al. (2009) and Keyes (2006) showed that adolescents reported lower well-being than younger children. And, Park and Peterson (2006b) showed that some strengths are lower among adolescents than among younger children, possibly suggesting "that adolescence can take a toll on good character" (p. 905). These changes could be examined through a general developmental perspective (e.g., reflecting the unique stage of adolescence in comparison to childhood) or through the perspective of specific theories, such as self-determination theory. Regarding the latter, for example, it may be that basic psychological needs (i.e., of autonomy, competence, and relatedness) are less likely to be met during adolescence than during early stages. These changes could also be examined from the perspective of hedonic versus eudaimonic conceptualizations of well-being; for example, perhaps the former but not the latter is lower in adolescence relative to childhood. Keyes' (2006) finding that youth experience more emotional (i.e., hedonic) well-being than psychological and social (i.e., eudaimonic) well-being also requires further exploration and explanation.

The research and interventions presented in this chapter show that we have moved far beyond the traditional deficit framework and pathology model in our approach to mental health in children and adolescents. Indeed, the benefits of many of the interventions described in this chapter begin to address what Kahn (2011) has described as *unfulfilled flourishing*: "… physical, material, or psychological benefits that do not occur but could have and sometimes rightly should have" (p. 199). Imagine the child, and the adult that child will become, who has never known the joy of close friendships; who has never experienced the rewards of a mindful, grateful, and hope-oriented approach to daily life; who does not celebrate their strengths; or who does not engage in creative play. Such a person may or may not remain free of mental disorder, but they will necessarily remain free of a life of flourishing.

References

Albieri, E., Visani, D., Offidani, E., Ottolini, F., & Ruini, C. (2009). Well-being therapy in children with emotional and behavioral disturbances: A pilot investigation. *Psychotherapy and Psychosomatics, 78*, 387–390.

Beets, M. W., Flay, B. R., Vuchinich, S., Snyder, F. J., Acock, A., Li, K.-K., Burns, K., Washburn, I. J., & Durlak, J. (2009). Use of a social and character development program to prevent substance abuse, violent behaviors, and sexual activity among elementary-school students in Hawaii. *American Journal of Public Health, 99*, 1438–1445.

Benson, P. L., & Scales, P. C. (2009). The definition and preliminary measurement of thriving in adolescence. *The Journal of Positive Psychology, 4*, 85–104.

Black, D. S., Milam, J., & Sussman, S. (2009). Sitting-meditation interventions among youth: A review of treatment efficacy. *Pediatrics, 124*, e532–e541.

Bradburn, N. M. (1969). *The structure of psychological well-being*. Chicago: Aldine.

Bradshaw, J., & Richardson, D. (2009). An index of child well-being in Europe. *Child Indicators Research, 2*, 319–351.

Brown, S., & Vaughan, C. (2009). *Play: How it shapes the brain, opens the imagination, and invigorates the soul*. New York: Penguin.

Cardaciotto, L. A., Herbert, J. D., Forman, E. M., Moitra, E., & Farrow, V. (2008). Assessment of present-moment awareness and acceptance: The Philadelphia Mindfulness Scale. *Assessment, 15*, 204–223.

Coyne, J. C., & Tennen, H. (2010). Positive psychology in cancer care: Bad science, exaggerated claims, and unproven medicine. *Annual Review of Behavioral Medicine, 39*, 16–26.

Dowling, E. M., Gestsdottir, S., Anderson, P. M., von Eye, A., Almerigi, J., & Lerner, R. M. (2004). Structural relations among spirituality, religiosity, and thriving in adolescence. *Applied Developmental Science, 8*, 7–16.

Eklund, K., Dowdy, E., Jones, C., & Furlong, M. J. (2011). Applicability of the dual-factor model of mental health for college students. *Journal of College Student Psychotherapy, 25*, 79–92.

Elkind, D. (2007). *The power of play: Learning what comes naturally*. Berkeley: Perseus Book Group.

Eryilmaz, A. (2012). A model of subjective well-being for adolescents in high school. *Journal of Happiness Studies, 13*(2), 275–289.

Fava, G. A., & Ruini, C. (2003). Development and characteristics of a well-being enhancing psychotherapeutic strategy: Well-being therapy. *Journal of Behavior Therapy and Experimental Psychiatry, 34*, 45–63.

Flay, B. R., & Allred, C. G. (2003). Long-term effects of the Positive Action program. *American Journal of Health Behavior, 27*, S6–S21.

Fredrickson, B. L. (1998). What good are positive emotions? *Review of General Psychology, 2*, 300–319.

Fredrickson, B. L. (2001). The role of positive emotions in positive psychology: The broaden-and-build theory of positive emotions. *American Psychologist, 56*, 218–226.

Froh, J. J., & Bono, G. (2008). The gratitude of youth. In S. J. Lopez (Ed.), *Positive psychology: Exploring the best in people* (Vol. 2, pp. 55–78). London: Praeger.

Froh, J. J., Sefick, W. J., & Emmons, R. A. (2008). Counting blessings in early adolescents: An experimental study of gratitude and subjective well-being. *Journal of School Psychology, 46*, 213–233.

Froh, J. J., Kashdan, T. B., Yurkewicz, C., Fan, J., Allen, J., & Glowacki, J. (2010). The benefits of passion and absorption in activities: Engaged living in adolescents and its role in psychological well-being. *The Journal of Positive Psychology, 5*, 311–332.

Froh, J. J., Emmons, R. A., Card, N. A., Bono, G., & Wilson, J. (2011). Gratitude and the reduced costs of materialism in adolescents. *Journal of Happiness Studies, 12*, 289–302.

Gallagher, M. W., Lopez, S. J., & Preacher, K. J. (2009). The hierarchical structure of well-being. *Journal of Personality, 77*, 1025–1049.

Gillham, J. E., Reivich, K., & Shatte, A. (2002). Positive youth development, prevention, and positive psychology: Commentary on "Positive youth development in the United States". *Prevention and Treatment, 5*, Article 18.

Gillham, J., Adams-Deutsch, Z., Werner, J., Reivich, K., Coulter-Heindl, V., Links, M., Winder, B., Peterson, C., Park, N., Abenavoli, R., Contero, A., & Seligman, M. E. P. (2011). Character strengths predict subjective well-being during adolescence. *The Journal of Positive Psychology, 6*, 31–44.

Gilman, R., & Huebner, E. S. (2006). Characteristics of adolescents who report very high life satisfaction. *Journal of Youth and Adolescence, 35*, 311–319.

Ginsburg, K. R. (2007). The importance of play in promoting health child development and maintaining strong parent-child bonds. *Pediatrics, 119*, 182–191.

Greenspoon, P. J., & Saklofske, D. H. (2001). Toward an integration of subjective well-being and psychopathology. *Social Indicators Research, 54*, 81–108.

Halle, T. G. (2003). Emotional development and well-being. In M. H. Bornstein, C. L. M. Keyes, & K. A. Moore (Eds.), *Well-being: Positive development across the life course* (pp. 125–138). Mahwah: Lawrence Erlbaum Associates Inc., Publishers.

Han, K.-T. (2009). Influence of limitedly visible leafy indoor plants on the psychology, behavior, and health of students at a junior high school in Taiwan. *Environment and Behavior, 41*, 658–692.

Holder, M. D., Coleman, B., & Wallace, J. M. (2010). Spirituality, religiousness, and happiness in children aged 8–12 years. *Journal of Happiness Studies, 11*, 131–150.

Joyce, A., Etty-Leal, J., Zazryn, T., Hamilton, A., & Hassed, C. (2010). Exploring a mindfulness meditation program on the mental health of upper primary children: A pilot study. *Advances in School Mental Health Promotion, 3*, 17–25.

Kahn, P. H. (2011). *Technological nature: Adaptation and the future of human life*. Cambridge, MA: MIT Press.

Kashdan, T. (2009). *Curious? Discover the missing ingredient to a fulfilling life*. New York: Harper-Collins Publishers.

Kellert, S. R. (2005). *Building for life: Designing and understanding the human-nature connection*. Washington, DC: Island Press.

Kelley, B. S., & Miller, L. (2007). Life satisfaction and spirituality in adolescents. *Research in the Social Scientific Study of Religion, 18*, 233–261.

Keyes, C. L. M. (1998). Social well-being. *Social Psychology Quarterly, 61*, 121–140.

Keyes, C. L. M. (2002). The mental health continuum: From languishing to flourishing in life. *Journal of Health and Social Behavior, 43*, 207–222.

Keyes, C. L. M. (2005a). Mental illness and/or mental health? Investigating axioms of the complete state model of health. *Journal of Consulting and Clinical Psychology, 73*, 539–548.

Keyes, C. L. M. (2005b). The subjective well-being of America's youth: Toward a comprehensive assessment. *Adolescent and Family Health, 4*, 3–11.

Keyes, C. L. M. (2006). Mental health in adolescence: Is America's youth flourishing? *The American Journal of Orthopsychiatry, 76*, 395–402.

Keyes, C. L. M. (2007). Promoting and protecting mental health as flourishing: A complementary strategy for improving national mental health. *American Psychologist, 62*, 95–108.

Keyes, C. L. M. (2009). The nature and importance of mental health in youth. In R. Gilman, M. Furlong, & E. S. Huebner (Eds.), *Promoting wellness in children and youth: Handbook of positive psychology in the schools* (pp. 9–23). New York: Routledge.

Keyes, C. L. M., & Annas, J. (2009). Feeling good and functioning well: Distinctive concepts in ancient philosophy and contemporary science. *The Journal of Positive Psychology, 4*, 197–201.

Keyes, C. L. M., Wissing, M., Potgieter, J. P., Temane, M., Kruger, A., & van Rooy, S. (2008). Evaluation of the Mental Health Continuum Short Form (MHC-SF) in Setswana speaking South Africans. *Clinical Psychology & Psychotherapy, 15*, 181–192.

Kia-Keating, M., Dowdy, E., Morgan, M. L., & Noam, G. G. (2011). Protecting and promoting: An integrative conceptual model for healthy development of adolescents. *The Journal of Adolescent Health, 48*, 220–228.

Lamers, S. M. A., Westerhof, G. J., Bohlmeijer, E. T., ten Klooster, P. M., & Keyes, C. L. M. (2010). Evaluating the psychometric properties of the Mental Health Continuum-Short Form (MHC-SF). *Journal of Clinical Psychology, 67*, 99–110.

Lamers, S. M. A., Glas, C. A. W., Westerhof, G. J., & Bohlmeijer, E. T. (2012). Longitudinal evaluation of the mental health continuum-short form (MHC-SF): Measurement invariance across demographics, physical illness, and mental illness. *European Journal of Psychological Assessment*. doi:10.1027/1015-5759/a000109.

Land, K. C., Lamb, V. L., & Mustillo, S. K. (2001). Child and youth well-being in the United States, 1975–1998: Some findings from a new index. *Social Indicators Research, 56*, 241–320.

Land, K. C., Lamb, V. L., & Zheng, H. (2011). How are the kids doing? How do we know? Recent trends in child and youth well-being in the United States and some international comparisons. *Social Indicators Research, 100*, 463–477.

Lerner, R. M. (2009). The positive youth development perspective: theoretical and empirical bases of a strengths-based approach to adolescent development. In S. J. Lopez & C. R. Snyder (Eds.), *Oxford handbook of positive psychology* (pp. 133–148). New York: University Press, Inc.

Levine, S. Z., Laufer, A., Hamama-Raz, Y., Stein, E., & Solomon, Z. (2008). Posttraumatic growth in adolescence: Examining its components and relationship with PTSD. *Journal of Traumatic Stress, 21*, 492–496.

Levine, S. Z., Laufer, A., Stein, E., Hamama-Raz, Y., & Solomon, Z. (2009). Examining the relationship between resilience and posttraumatic growth. *Journal of Traumatic Stress, 22*, 282–286.

Li, K.-K., Washburn, I., DuBois, D. L., Vuchinich, S., Ji, P., Brechling, V., Day, J., Beets, M. W., Acock, A. C., Berbaum, M., Snyder, F., & Flay, B. R. (2011). Effects of the Positive Action programme on problem behaviours in elementary school students: A matched-pair randomized control trial in Chicago. *Psychology and Health, 26*, 187–204.

Lopez, S. J., Snyder, C. R., Magyar-Moe, J. L., Edwards, L. M., Pedrotti, J. T., Janowski, K., Turner, J. L., & Pressgrove, C. (2004). Strategies for accentuating hope. In P. A. Linley & S. Joseph (Eds.), *Positive psychology in practice* (pp. 388–404). Hoboken: Wiley.

Madden, W., Green, L. S., & Grant, A. M. (2011). A pilot study evaluating strengths-based coaching for primary school students: Enhancing engagement and hope. *International Coaching Psychology Review, 7*, 71–83.

McWhinnie, C., Abela, J. R. Z., Hilmy, N., & Ferrer, I. (2008). Positive youth development programs: an alternative approach to the prevention of depression in children and adolescents.

In J. R. Z. Abela & B. L. Hankin (Eds.), *Handbook of depression in children and adolescents* (pp. 354–373). New York: Guilford Press.

Michel, G., Taylor, N., Absolom, K., & Eiser, C. (2010). Benefit finding in survivors of childhood cancer and their parents: Further empirical support for the Benefit Finding Scale for Children. *Child: Care, Health and Development, 36,* 123–129.

Milyavskaya, M., Gingras, I., Mageau, G. A., Koestner, R., Gagnon, H., Fang, J., & Boiché, J. (2009). Balance across contexts: Importance of balanced need satisfaction across various life domains. *Personality and Social Psychology Bulletin, 35,* 1031–1045.

Moore, K. A., & Keyes, C. L. M. (2003). A brief history of the study of well-being in children and adults. In M. H. Bornstein, C. L. M. Keyes, & K. A. Moore (Eds.), *Well-being: Positive development across the life course* (pp. 1–12). Mahwah: Lawrence Erlbaum Associates Inc., Publishers.

Moore, K. A., & Lippman, L. H. (2005). Introduction and conceptual framework. In K. A. Moore & L. H. Lippman (Eds.), *What do children need to flourish? Conceptualizing and measuring indicators of positive development* (pp. 1–12). New York: Springer.

National Institute for Play. (2009). *Play science: The patterns of play.* Retrieved January 15, 2012, from http://nifplay.org/states_play.html

Oishi, S., Diener, E., & Lucas, R. E. (2007). The optimum level of well-being: Can people be too happy? *Perspectives on Psychological Science, 2,* 346–360.

Park, N., & Peterson, C. (2006a). Character strengths and happiness among young children: Content analysis of parental descriptions. *Journal of Happiness Studies, 7,* 323–341.

Park, N., & Peterson, C. (2006b). Moral competence and character strengths among adolescents: The development and validation of the Values in Action Inventory of Strengths for Youth. *Journal of Adolescence, 29,* 891–900.

Peter, T., Roberts, L. W., & Dengate, J. (2011). Flourishing in life: An empirical test of the dual continua model of mental health and mental illness among Canadian university students. *International Journal of Mental Health Promotion, 13,* 13–22.

Peterson, C., & Seligman, M. E. P. (2004). *Character strengths and virtues: A classification and handbook.* New York/Washington, DC: Oxford University Press/American Psychological Association.

Phipps, S., Long, A. M., & Ogden, J. (2007). Benefit finding scale for children: Preliminary findings from a childhood cancer population. *Journal of Pediatric Psychology, 32,* 1264–1271.

Proctor, C. L., Linley, P. A., & Maltby, J. (2009). Youth life satisfaction: A review of the literature. *Journal of Happiness Studies, 10,* 583–630.

Proctor, C., Linley, P. A., & Maltby, J. (2010). Very happy youths: Benefits of very high life satisfaction among adolescents. *Social Indicators Research, 98,* 519–532.

Proctor, C., Tsukayama, E., Wood, A. M., Maltby, J., Eades, J. F., & Linley, P. A. (2011). Strengths Gym: The impact of a character strengths-based intervention on the life satisfaction and well-being of adolescents. *The Journal of Positive Psychology, 6,* 377–388.

Rashid, T., & Anjum, A. (2008). Positive psychotherapy for young adults and children. In J. R. Z. Abela & B. L. Hankin (Eds.), *Handbook of depression in children and adolescents* (pp. 250–287). New York: Guilford Press.

Reschly, A. L., Huebner, E. S., Appleton, J. J., & Antaramian, S. (2008). Engagement as flourishing: The contribution of affect and coping to adolescents' engagement at school and with learning. *Psychology in the Schools, 45,* 419–431.

Roberts, M. C., Brown, K. J., Johnson, R. J., & Renke, J. (2002). Positive psychology for children: development, prevention, and promotion. In S. J. Lopez & C. R. Snyder (Eds.), *Handbook of positive psychology* (pp. 663–675). New York: University Press, Inc.

Robitschek, C., & Keyes, C. L. M. (2009). The structure of Keyes' model of mental health and the role of personal growth initiative as a parsimonious predictor. *Journal of Counseling Psychology, 56,* 321–329.

Ruini, C., Belaise, C., Brombin, C., Caffo, E., & Fava, G. A. (2006). Well-being therapy in school settings: A pilot study. *Psychotherapy and Psychosomatics, 75,* 331–336.

Ryan, R. M., & Deci, E. L. (2000). Self-determination theory and the facilitation of intrinsic motivation, social development and well-being. *American Psychologist, 55,* 54–67.

Ryff, C. D. (1989). Happiness is everything, or is it? Explorations on the meaning of psychological well-being. *Journal of Personality and Social Psychology, 57*, 1069–1081.

Ryff, C. D., & Keyes, C. L. M. (1995). The structure of psychological well-being revisited. *Journal of Personality and Social Psychology, 69*, 719–727.

Schneider, S. L. (2001). In search of realistic optimism: Meaning, knowledge, and warm fuzziness. *American Psychologist, 56*, 250–263.

Schonert-Reichel, K. A., & Lawlor, M. S. (2010). The effects of a mindfulness-based education program on pre- and early adolescents' well-being and emotional competence. *Mindfulness, 1*, 137–151.

Shaffer-Hudkins, E., Suldo, S., March, A., & Loker, T. (2010). How adolescents' mental health predicts their physical health: Unique contributions of subjective well-being and psychopathology. *Applied Research in Quality of Life, 5*, 203–217.

Soenens, B., & Vansteenkiste, M. (2005). Antecedents and outcomes of self-determination in three life domains: The role of parents' and teachers' autonomy support. *Journal of Youth and Adolescence, 34*, 589–604.

Suldo, S. M., & Huebner, E. S. (2004). Does life satisfaction moderate the effects of stressful life events on psychopathological behavior during adolescence? *School Psychology Quarterly, 19*, 93–105.

Suldo, S. M., & Huebner, E. S. (2006). Is extremely high satisfaction during adolescence advantageous? *Social Indicators Research, 78*, 179–203.

Suldo, S. M., & Shaffer, E. J. (2008). Looking beyond psychopathology: The dual-factor model of mental health in youth. *School Psychology Review, 37*, 52–68.

Suldo, S., Thalji, A., & Ferron, J. (2011). Longitudinal academic outcomes predicted by early adolescents' subjective well-being, psychopathology, and mental health status yielded from a dual factor model. *The Journal of Positive Psychology, 6*, 17–30.

Taylor, A. F., Kuo, F. E., & Sullivan, W. C. (2002). Views of nature and self-discipline: Evidence from inner city children. *Journal of Environmental Psychology, 22*, 49–63.

Tomba, E., Belaise, C., Ottolini, F., Ruini, C., Bravi, A., Albieri, E., Rafanelli, C., Caffo, E., & Fava, G. A. (2010). Differential effects of well-being promoting and anxiety-management strategies in a non-clinical school setting. *Journal of Anxiety Disorders, 24*, 326–333.

VanderVen, K. (2008). *Promoting positive development in early childhood: Building blocks for a successful start*. Pittsburgh: Springer.

Veronneau, M.-H., Koestner, R. F., & Abela, J. R. Z. (2005). Intrinsic need satisfaction and well-being in children and adolescents: An application of the self-determination theory. *Journal of Social and Clinical Psychology, 24*, 280–292.

Vohra, S. S. (2006). Sowing seeds of happiness through value inculcation in adolescents. *Psychological Studies, 51*, 183–186.

Weis, R., & Speridakos, E. C. (2011). A meta-analysis of hope enhancement strategies in clinical and community settings. *Psychology of Well-Being, 1*, 5.

Wells, N. M., & Evans, G. W. (2003). Nearby nature: A buffer of life stress among rural children. *Environment and Behavior, 35*, 311–330.

Westerhof, G. J., & Keyes, C. L. M. (2010). Mental illness and mental health: The two continua model across the life span. *Journal of Adult Development, 17*, 110–119.

Wood, J. V., Perunovic, W. Q. E., & Lee, J. W. (2009). Positive self-statements: Power for some, peril for others. *Psychological Science, 20*, 860–866.

Chapter 6
Assessment of Character Strengths in Children and Adolescents

Tayyab Rashid, Afroze Anjum, Carolyn Lennox, Denise Quinlan, Ryan M. Niemiec, Donna Mayerson, and Fahim Kazemi

6.1 Introduction

For more than a century, psychology has been fascinated with the clichéd question "*what is wrong with you, Johnny?*" Since the dawn of this millennium, positive psychology has seriously urged psychologists to also probe into a much deeper and a loftier question, "*what are you good at, Johnny?*" Psychologists have been asking the former question in copious ways through formal and informal, objective and subjective, and normative and ipsative psychological assessments. The latter question has unfortunately remained unasked, leaving the positive aspects of Johnny largely unpacked and underexplored. A bibliographic database search (as of July 2, 2012) of PsycINFO and ERIC (accessed through CSA Illumina[1]) with scoping search using descriptors *assessment* and *psychopathology* and *children* and *adolescents* covering the period of 2000 through 2012, yielded 24,129 peer reviewed journals

---

[1]CSA Illumina can be accessed at: http://www.csa.com

T. Rashid (✉) • F. Kazemi
Health and Wellness Centre, University of Toronto Scarborough, SL-270,
1265 Military Trail, Toronto, ON M1C 1A4, Canada
e-mail: trashid@utsc.utoronto.ca; f.kazemi@mail.utoronto.ca

A. Anjum • C. Lennox
Psychological Services, South-West Education Office, Toronto District School Board,
1 Civic Centre Court, Toronto, ON M9C 2B3, Canada
e-mail: Afroze.Anjum@tdsb.on.ca; Carolyn.Lennox@tdsb.on.ca

D. Quinlan
Department of Psychology, University of Otago, P.O. Box 56, Dunedin 9054, New Zealand
e-mail: denise.quinlan@otago.ac.nz

R.M. Niemiec • D. Mayerson
VIA Institute on Character, 312 Walnut Street, Suite 3600, Cincinnati, OH 45202, USA
e-mail: ryan@viacharacter.org; donnam@viacharacter.org

C. Proctor and P.A. Linley (eds.), *Research, Applications, and Interventions for Children and Adolescents: A Positive Psychology Perspective*, DOI 10.1007/978-94-007-6398-2_6,
© Springer Science+Business Media Dordrecht 2013

article whereas only 3,330 articles were found when the descriptor *psychopathology* was replaced with *strengths*. This clearly suggests that we have just started exploring the intact aspects of Johnny and we have a long way to go in understanding what is wrong with Johnny as well as what is strong about him. Our central point, in this chapter, is to underscore the importance of exploring the positive aspects of Johnny without dismissing, minimizing, or avoiding weakness. To make our case, we underscore the shortcomings of a deficit model of assessment for children and adolescents, and define a strength-based assessment and the benefits of exploring strengths. Positive psychology posits that the use of signature strengths – the highest strengths that individuals believe are most core to who they are – is associated with greater well-being and less psychological distress. This notion has been well tested with adults (e.g., Linley et al. 2010; Rust et al. 2009; Mongrain and Anselmo-Matthews 2012; Seligman et al. 2005). However, this assertion has not been widely tested with children and adolescents. Major shortcoming of these studies is that signature strengths, almost exclusively are determined by one self-report measure, (usually VIA-IS [Values in Action – Inventory of Strengths], explained later in the chapter) which ranks top five strengths. We find determination of signature strengths, based on one self-report measure, limiting. Signature strengths of children and adolescents should be assessed considering their context which inherently includes a number of adults including their parents, teachers, coaches, siblings, peers, friends…etc.

We present a new and comprehensive model of assessing signature strengths and evaluate the impact of strengths identification and development on boosting student life satisfaction, well-being, and social skills. Furthermore, practical strategies to use strength in solving problems are also illustrated. We conclude the chapter with applied strategies to assess and build signature strengths of children and adolescents.

6.1.1 What Is a Strength-Based Assessment?

Strengths-based assessment, according to M. H. Epstein (2004), is a measurement of the emotional and behavioral skills, competencies, and characteristics that foster a sense of personal accomplishment, contribute to supportive and satisfying relationships with family members, peers, and adults, enhance one's ability to cope with challenges and stress, and promote one's personal, social, and academic development. Although strengths-based assessment finds a convenient thrust in the contemporary positive psychology movement, it has been part of humanistic psychology tradition (Friedman and MacDonal 2006). Moreover, school psychologists and social workers have long emphasized assessing and working with strengths (Rhee et al. 2001; Laursen 2003; Rapp 1997).

In promoting strength-based assessment we ought to keep in mind that our brains have evolved in such a way that we are better at attending, selecting, discerning, and remembering grudges than expressions of gratitude; criticism than compliments; conflict than cooperation; and hubris than humility (Rashid and Ostermann 2009).

Evidence supports that negatives weigh more heavily than positives of equal value and impact (Kahneman and Tversky 1984; Cottrell and Neuberg 2005). Educational settings from classrooms to playgrounds are not immune from this. Consider the following mini experiment. Below are two vignettes. Approach each one in a particular way: read the description twice, close your eyes and visualize the student, and write down a few descriptors of the student described in numbers 1 and 2:

1. Joey is an 8th grade student and is in his fourth school in 6 years. Joey's concentration is poor, he is described as disruptive and as a procrastinator by most of his teachers.
2. Consider Joseph, also an 8th grade student who is also attending his fourth school in 6 years. Joseph has good personal hygiene, and although he is not very social, he has two consistent friends who describe him as loyal and fun to hang around with. Joseph doesn't particularly enjoy academics but occasionally he is able to focus and complete his assignments without much difficulty. He is a good basketball player and is considered an important member of the school team. Joseph is very good with digital equipment and often helps teachers when they are technologically challenged.

Compare your notes. Your descriptors for these decontextualized vignettes may differ with the former carrying more negatives than the latter. Ironically, these vignette descriptions are of the same student. The vignettes were taken from two psychoeducational evaluations. The first was completed by a school psychologist, trained in a traditional psychopathology model of assessment while the second was completed by the first author. Both assessments were completed within a year. These contrasting vignettes offer important considerations for the assessment of children and adolescents and subsequent interventions. Descriptors organize and simplify the information. If the information is negatively labeled for the most part, the perception of the individual is likely to be formed in an unfavorable way. If a practitioner only perceives the negative traits described in the former vignette (e.g., distraction, procrastination…etc.), this may overshadow several positive traits (e.g., curiosity, loyalty, self-regulation…etc.) of Joey/Joseph – offering a skewed and limited impression of him. Furthermore, negative traits are more likely to reinforce the notion that weaknesses reside inside Joey – minimizing the role of risks and resources embedded within the environment.

A deficit-oriented assessment reduces children and adolescents into synthetic labels and categories of psychopathology. Sophisticated objective and projective measures are used to validate the existence of these categories. These labels have become so pervasive that adolescents may readily fit themselves in these categories before seeking professional help. While labeling may help categorize and organize the world, at the same time, it may oversimplify the rich, nuanced, and idiosyncratic complexities of children and adolescents. In worst-case scenarios, vulnerable adolescents may perceive themselves from an early age as disturbed, anxious, or depressed.

The traditional deficit-oriented assessment is based on the assumption that weaknesses, if remediated, will make children and adolescents happy. Challenging this assumption, Corey Keyes (2009) posits that the absence of symptoms does not necessarily mean the presence of mental health. Keyes terms the presence of mental health as flourishing, and the absence of mental health as languishing. He has examined the flourishing and languishing of more than 1,200 nationally representative adolescents between the ages of 12 and 18 and has found that approximately 38 % of adolescents are flourishing, 56 % are moderately mentally healthy, and 6 % are languishing. The languishing adolescents report more conduct problems (arrests, truancy, alcohol use, cigarette smoking, and marijuana use) while the flourishing adolescents report better psychosocial functioning (global self-concept, self-determination, closeness to others, and school integration). Independent lines of research support Keyes' (2009) findings. Wood and Joseph (2010) recently demonstrated that after controlling for negative characteristics, individuals who score low on positive characteristics will still be at a two-fold risk of developing depression compared to individuals who score high on positive characteristics. Similarly, even after controlling for neuroticism, the prospective relationship between depression and gratitude remains significant (Wood et al. 2008). Positive traits can also act as a buffer between negative life events and psychopathology. For example, Johnson and colleagues (2010) found that positive beliefs about relationship support and coping ability ("resilience appraisals") buffer against suicidality. For people with low positive beliefs, more negative life events lead to greater suicidality. Jane Gillham and colleagues (2011) recently studied the character strengths and depression of 149 adolescents as part of a positive psychology intervention. They found that other-directed strengths (e.g., forgiveness, kindness, teamwork) and self-regulation predicted fewer symptoms of depression through the end of Grade 10. Furthermore, higher life satisfaction was associated with hope, gratitude, curiosity and love of learning. Therefore, the assumption that fixing weaknesses will ensure well-being has been seriously challenged and will continue to be scrutinized in years to come. With that being said, in order to make children and adolescents feel good and worthwhile, hundreds of interventions in educational and community settings are delivered every year. Many of these interventions are based on external validation of the self, which can foster unhealthy levels of self-esteem. Some research has found that externally validated self-esteem tends to be more detrimental than beneficial (Crocker et al. 2003; Lyubomirsky et al. 2006). Rather than seeking external validation, developing character strengths and other strengths, such as talents/abilities, skills, and assets, boosts both subjective and psychological well-being, even when controlling for the effects of self-efficacy and self-esteem (Govindji and Linley 2007). Finally, Bird and colleagues (2012) in a recent systematic review of strength-based assessment noted that use of a strengths-based assessment fosters a positive relationship between the client and the clinician. Therefore, any assessment and intervention that largely rests on deficits presents a skewed picture of children and adolescents. Furthermore, deficit-oriented assessment limits the role of the professional to diagnose and treat symptoms and disorders, and expands the power differential between children and adolescents and the professional.

Assessment, especially a formal one, is conducted to make important decisions including screening, diagnosing, placing children and adolescents in specialized programs, and providing them with accommodations and modifications. When such important decisions are at stake, the need for a balanced assessment including symptoms and strengths becomes critical. Therefore, we argue that assessment of children and adolescents should always be a hybrid exercise, exploring strengths as well as weakness. Furthermore with children and adolescents, merely assessing strengths could be considered a positive intervention in its own right (Poston and Hanson 2010).

Positive Psychology, for well over a decade now, has made concerted empirical efforts to advance the science that integrates both strengths and weaknesses. In order to do so, positive psychology researchers realized that unlike the *Diagnostic and Statistical Manual of Mental Disorders* (*DSM*; American Psychiatric Association 2000), which numerates a sophisticated classification of disorder, there lacked a common language to describe strengths. Spearheading the first effort to describe a systematic classification of core human strengths were C. Peterson and Seligman (2004), who published the VIA (formerly called the "Values in Action") Classification of strengths. C. Peterson and Seligman (2004) define character strengths as capacities of cognition, affect, volition, and behavior, which constitute the basic psychological ingredients that enable us to act in ways that contribute to our well-being and the well-being of others. They acknowledge that character strengths are morally desired traits of human existence, which are valued in every culture. However, the VIA Classification is descriptive rather than prescriptive, thus character strengths are open to empirical examination. The character of human beings is plural in nature, meaning that character strengths are expressed in combinations (rather than singularly), and are expressed in degrees relative to context. The 24 character strengths in the VIA Classification are subsumed under six broader categories called virtues. Table 6.1 presents the language of character, that is, the 24 core character strengths and virtues, and corresponding descriptions.

6.1.2   Character Strengths and Talents/Abilities

It is also important to distinguish character strengths from talents and abilities. According to Chris Peterson (2006), talents and abilities, such as dexterity, aptitude, athletic ability, or musical talent, are more genetically influenced than character strengths, such as humility and social intelligence. Talents and abilities are also more likely to be associated with concrete consequences (fame, wealth) than character strengths, and people may waste them. In contrast, C. Peterson (2006) argues that character strengths are rarely wasted, that is, kindness, social intelligence, or spirituality are either used or not, but rarely wasted. Character strengths, are morally desirable traits. These are aligned with values but at the same time are somewhat distinct from them. Values are largely located on religious, cultural, and political spectrums whereas character strengths are descriptive traits. Their utility, context, and content is being increasingly informed and constrained by scientific knowledge, as discussed next.

Table 6.1 VIA classification of character strengths

Wisdom and knowledge – strengths that involve acquiring and using knowledge
  Creativity [Ingenuity; Originality]: Thinking of novel and productive ways to do things
  Curiosity [Interest; Novelty-seeking; Openness to experience]: Taking an interest in all of
    ongoing experience
  Judgment [Critical thinking]: Thinking things through and examining them from all sides
  Love of learning: Mastering new skills, topics, and bodies of knowledge
  Perspective [Wisdom]: Being able to provide wise counsel to others; taking the "big picture"
    view
Courage – emotional strengths that involve exercise of will to accomplish goals in the face of
    opposition, external or internal
  Bravery [Valor]: Not shrinking from threat, challenge, or pain
  Perseverance [Persistence; Industry; Diligence]: Finishing what one starts, completing a
    course of action in spite of obstacles
  Honesty [Authenticity and integrity]: Speaking the truth and presenting oneself in a genuine
    way
  Zest [Vitality]: Approaching life with excitement and energy; not doing things halfway or
    halfheartedly, living life as an adventure, feeling alive and activated
Humanity – interpersonal strengths that involve tending and befriending others
  Love [Capacity to give/Receive love]: Valuing close relations with others, in particular those in
    which sharing and caring are reciprocated; being close to people
  Kindness [Compassion; Altruism; Generosity; Care]: Doing favors and good deeds for others;
    helping them; taking care of them
  Social intelligence: Being aware of the motives and feelings of self and others; knowing what
    to do to fit into different social situations; knowing what makes other people tick
Justice – strengths that underlie healthy community life
  Teamwork [Citizenship; Social responsibility; Loyalty]: Working well as member of a group
    or team; being loyal to the group; doing one's share
  Fairness [Equity]: Treating all people the same according to notions of fairness and justice; not
    letting personal feelings bias decisions about others; giving everyone a fair chance
  Leadership: Encouraging a group of which one is a member to get things done and at the same
    time maintain good relations within the group; organizing group activities and seeing that
    they happen
Temperance – strengths that protect against excess and vices
  Forgiveness [Mercy]: Forgiving those who have done wrong; accepting the shortcomings of
    others; giving people a second chance; not being vengeful
  Humility [Modesty]: Letting one's accomplishments speak for themselves; not seeking the
    spotlight; not regarding oneself as more special than one is
  Prudence: Being careful about one's choices; not taking undue risks; not saying or doing
    things that might later be regretted
  Self-regulation [Self-control]: Regulating what one feels and does; being disciplined;
    controlling one's appetites and emotions
Transcendence – strengths that forge connections to the larger universe and provide meaning
  Appreciation of beauty and excellence [Awe; Wonder; Elevation]: Noticing and appreciating
    beauty, excellence, and/or skilled performance in all domains of life, from nature to arts to
    mathematics to science
  Gratitude: Being aware of and thankful for the good things; taking time to express thanks
  Hope [Optimism; Future-mindedness]: Expecting the best in the future and working to achieve
    it; believing that a good future is something that can be brought about

(continued)

Table 6.1   (continued)

Humor [Playfulness]: Liking to laugh and tease; bringing smiles to other people, seeing the light side; making (not necessarily telling) jokes

Spirituality [Sense of Purpose; Faith; Meaning; Religiousness]: Knowing where one fits within the larger scheme; having coherent beliefs about the higher purpose and meaning of life that shape conduct and provide comfort

Peterson and Seligman (2004)

6.1.3   What Good Are Character Strengths?

Good character is what parents look for in their children, what teachers look for in their students, what siblings look for in their brothers and sisters, and what friends look for in their peers (Park and Peterson 2009). Character is critical for lifelong optimal human development. Good character is not simply the absence of deficits, problems, and pathology but rather a well-developed cluster of positive personality traits. In recent years, under the rubric of "character education", *good character* is a set of distinct strengths that a person possesses to varying degrees and more importantly they are malleable across the lifespan. For example, among children and adolescents, character strengths of appreciation of beauty and excellence, forgiveness, modesty, and judgment appear to have a developmental trajectory; being least common in youth and increasing over time through cognitive maturation (Park and Peterson 2006a). However, the malleability of character strengths is also dependent upon a number of contextual factors.

Character strengths are strongly associated with several indicators of well-being and inversely related with symptoms of psychopathology. Wood and colleagues (2011) have found that using strengths was associated with decreased stress, increased vitality and positive affect (but not reduced negative affect). Huta and Hawley (2010) have shown that the strengths of zest, spirituality, and appreciation of beauty/excellence are inversely related to cognitive vulnerability; and strengths play a predictive role in improving depressive symptoms. Using character strengths has also been shown to decrease depression and increase well-being in certain samples (Rust et al. 2009; Seligman et al. 2006; Proctor et al. 2011a). Furthermore, using strengths is also associated with better therapeutic outcome (Flückiger and Grosse Holtforth 2008; Larsen and Stege 2010).

Increased use of specific character strengths are associated with fewer symptoms of depression and anxiety (Gillham et al. 2011; Park and Peterson 2008), greater life satisfaction (Gillham et al. 2011), fewer externalizing problems (Park and Peterson 2008), and lower internalizing problems (Beaver 2008). The strength of leadership contributes to helping others and also predicts fewer symptoms of depression (Schmid et al. 2011). Similarly, Bundick (2011) conducted a longitudinal study, which has shown that leadership is positively related to purpose in life and optimism. Richards and Huppert (2011) analyzed data from a 1964 British birth cohort, which began with 563 teens. Children rated as "positive" by their teachers at age 13 or 14 were significantly more likely than those who received no positive rating to report satisfaction with their work, midlife, and to have stronger social ties. Prosocial behavior, such as volunteering, buffered against emotional exhaustion, while positive emotions increased helping and citizenship.

Character strengths are not only associated with favorable psychosocial outcomes, they also predict well-being, over and above IQ scores. Park and Peterson (2008) found that after controlling for IQ, the character strengths of perseverance, fairness, honesty, hope, and perspective/wisdom predicted grade point average (GPA). In a longitudinal study of 140 eighth grade students, Duckworth and Seligman (2005) found that perseverance and self-discipline, measured by self-report, parent report, and teacher report accounted for more than twice as much variance as IQ in final grades, high school selection, school attendance, hours spent doing homework, hours spent watching television (inversely), and the time of day students began their homework. These findings underscore the importance of character strengths in conjunction with intellectual potential. Corroborating this finding, Lounsbury and colleagues (2009) found that perseverance, along with love of learning, fairness, and kindness predicted college GPA.

In a study of more than 1,200 children, the most curious children ($n=207$) were compared to the least curious or bored children ($n=207$). The curious children were more optimistic, hopeful, confident, and had a higher sense of self-determination and self-efficacy believing they were in control of their actions and decisions than the bored children who felt like pawns with no control of their destiny (Hunter and Csikszentmihalyi 2003). These lines of research suggest that character strengths help individuals to build personal resources which help individuals to attain other desirable outcomes (Xanthopoulou et al. 2007).

But how? One hypothesis is that the use of character strengths engenders positive emotions, which broaden thought-action repertoires promoting exploratory behavior that helps individuals create opportunities and goal-directed actions. The mechanisms through which character strengths produce their effects have not yet been identified although it is expected that a number of mechanisms will be involved.

Finally, Seligman (2011), advocating the notion of *positive education* (Seligman et al. 2009), contends that positive traits and states ought to be integrated in the school curriculum because these traits can act as a buffer to prevent depression and many other forms of psychopathologies.

6.2   Assessing Strengths

A number of assessment scales, inventories, and interviews have been developed to assess positive emotions, strengths, meaning, and a host of strengths related constructs. Professionals working with children and adolescents can choose empirically validated instruments to assess specific positive constructs. The most comprehensive positive psychology assessment tool for children and adolescents to date is the VIA Inventory of Strengths for Youth (VIA Youth Survey). This survey uses 198 items to measure the 24 character strengths and provides children between 10 and 17 with feedback about their top character strengths, also known as signature strengths. The VIA Youth Survey has established good psychometrics with positive convergence between parent and self-ratings of the 24 character strengths (Park and Peterson 2006a). Table 6.2 presents an overview of some salient strength-based measures. Most measures of psychopathology are expensive and require specific qualification and credentials to administer. In contrast, most strength-based measures, developed by practitioners and researchers of positive psychology, are readily available online without charge. A number of these measures and their respective theoretical frameworks are discussed in detail in books, such as the *Handbook of Positive Psychology in Schools* (Gilman et al. 2009), *Celebrating Strengths: Building Strength-based Schools* (Fox Eades 2008), *Positive Psychological Assessment: A Handbook of Models and Measures* (Lopez and Snyder 2003), and the *Oxford Handbook of Methods in Positive Psychology* (Ong and van Dulmen 2006).

The assessment of character strengths in very young children has also been attempted by use of parent ratings. Park and Peterson (2006b) conducted a content analysis of parents' written descriptions of their children between the ages of 3 and 10 ($n = 680$). The parents' descriptions had an average of three VIA character strengths mentioned in each description. They explain that prior to this study, there were no investigations of character as a multidimensional construct among young children (below age 10). Another component of this study was to investigate correlations with happiness. The researchers framed the parents' instructions to note the child's personal characteristics and individual qualities (e.g., "What can you tell us so that we might know your child well?"), and encouraged parents to tell a story that captures what the child is all about. The prevalence of character strengths were as follows (highest prevalence listed first): love, kindness, creativity, humor, curiosity, love of learning, perseverance. Some character strengths were significantly correlated with happiness; these strengths included love, zest, and hope.

6.3 Building Strengths

There are a very limited number of interventions that build character strengths in a comprehensive way. Most interventions target one or two specific strengths, for example, gratitude (Froh et al. 2009; Flinchbaugh et al. 2012), optimism (Gillham et al. 1995), and hope (Pedrotti et al. 2008). Few systematic interventions have been completed that have explicitly attempted to build positive traits in children and adolescents. Proctor, Tsukayama and colleagues (2011) examined the impact of *Strengths Gym*, a character strength-based positive psychological intervention program, on adolescent life satisfaction, positive and negative affect, and character strength-based exercises in the school curriculum. Adolescents ($n = 208$) who participated in the program experienced significant increases in life satisfaction compared to adolescents ($n = 101$) who did not participate.

Table 6.2 Salient strength-based measures

Measure	Strength-based subscales	Psychometrics		Concurrent validity
		Internal consistency		
Behavior Assessment System for Children (BASC; Reynolds and Kamphaus 1992, 2004)	Respondent: Parent, Teacher, Self	Alpha coefficients ranged from .80 to .90		Correlations between the BASC Teacher form and the Teacher Report Form (TRF) competence subscales ranged from .52 to .82
	Parent and Teacher forms: Adaptive scale, items that measure Adaptability, Leadership, Social Skills, and Study Skills			Correlation between the BASC Parent form and the Child Behaviour Checklist (CBCL; Achenbach 1992) competence subscales ranged from .40 to .68
	Self-report form: Adaptive scale includes items that measure Relations with Parents, Interpersonal Relations, Self-Esteem, and Self-Reliance			Correlations between the BASC Self form and the Youth Self report competence subscales ranged from .15 to .39
Behavioral and Emotional Rating Scale (BERS; M. H. Epstein and Sharma 1998)	Respondent: Primary Caregiver, Self (BERS-2; M. H. Epstein 2004)	Alpha coefficient = .98		Correlations between BERS subscales and the TRF competence subscales ranged from .29 to .73
	All forms: Interpersonal Strengths, Affective Strengths, Family Involvement, School Functioning, Interpersonal Strengths	Test-retest = .99 Inter-rater reliability ranged from .83 to .98		Correlations between BERS and SSRS (Gresham and Elliot 1990) Social Skills correlations ranged from .46 to .73 and Academic Competence ranged from .50 to .72
California Healthy Kids Survey-Resilience Youth Development Module (RYDM; Constantine et al. 1999)	Respondent: Self	Alpha coefficients ranged from .55 to .88		Correlations between RYDM and the Multidimensional Students' Life Satisfaction Scale (Huebner 1994) ranged from .43 to .66

Instrument	Description	Reliability	Validity
	Externally-situated strengths (e.g., the presence of caring relationships, high expectations, and opportunities to participate in meaningful activities) and internally situated strengths (e.g., social competence, autonomy, sense of meaning, and purpose)	The exception to this was the Meaningful Participation in the Community subscale, which had "low reliability and new items were [subsequently] written to be assessed in the next phase of the field test" (Constantine et al. 1999, p. 7)	Correlations between RYDM and the Extended Life Orientation Test (Scheier et al. 1994) were .56
Multidimensional Students' Life Satisfaction Scale (MSLSS; Huebner 1994)	Respondent: Self Satisfaction in multiple domains; Family, Friends, School, Living Environment, and Self	Coefficients between .72 and .85 2 and 4-week test-retest ranged from .70 to .90	Family domain correlated .62 with BASC Parent scale. Friends domain correlated .56 with Loneliness and Social Dissatisfaction Scale (Cassidy and Asher 1992). School domain correlated .68 with Quality of School Life Scale (Epstein and McPartland 1976). Self domain correlated .62 with General Self-Esteem scale of Self Description Questionnaire-I (Marsh 1992)
School Social Behavior Scale-2 (SSBS-2; Merrell 2002)	Respondent: Self Social Competence included items that measure Peer Relations, Self-Management/Compliance, and Academic Behavior	Alpha and split-half reliability coefficients ranged from .96 to .98	Moderate correlation between SSBS-2, CBCL, and TRF

(continued)

Table 6.2 (continued)

Measure	Strength-based subscales	Psychometrics		Concurrent validity
		Internal consistency		
Social Skills Rating System (SSRS; Gresham and Elliott 1990)	Respondent: Parent, Teacher, Self. All forms: Social Skills Scale includes items that measure Cooperation, Assertion, Responsibility, Empathy, and Self-Control Teacher form: Academic Competence Scale measures reading and mathematics performance, general cognitive functioning, as well as motivation and parental support	Alpha coefficient ranged from .75 to .94`		Moderate to high correlations between SSRS and SSBS-2, BASC (Teacher, Parent, and Student Self-Report forms), Teacher Rating Scale (Harter 1985), Piers-Harris Self-Concept Scale (Piers and Harris 1984), Walker-McConnell Scale of Social Competence and School Adjustment (Walker and McConnell 1995)
Children's Hope Scale (CHS: Snyder et al. 1997)	Respondent: Self. Assesses children's dispositional hope. Measures problem solving and decision-making abilities.	Alpha coefficient ranged from .77 to .88		
Gratitude Questionnaire-6 (GQ-6; McCullough et al. 2002)	Respondent: Self. Measures the disposition to experience gratitude.	Alpha coefficients ranged from .82 and .87		Positively related to optimism, life satisfaction, hope, spirituality and religiousness, forgiveness, empathy, and prosocial behavior. Negatively associated with depression, anxiety, materialism, and envy

Short Grit Scale (Grit-S; Duckworth and Quinn 2009)	Respondent: Self	Alpha coefficient ranged from .73 to .83. Alphas for consistency of interest subscale ranged from .73 to .79. For Perseverance of Effort subscale, alphas ranged from .60 to .78.
Positive and Negative Affect Schedule for Children (PANAS-C; Ebesutani et al. 2011)	Respondent: Parents. Yields Positive Affect (PA) and Negative Affect (NA) scales that are used to identify children with anxiety and mood problems	Alpha coefficient was .85 for reduced 5-item PA scale and .88 for original 12-item PA scale. For NA, alpha coefficients were .82 and .90 for 5- and 12-item scales, respectively.
Clifton StrengthsFinder 2.0 (StrengthsFinder 2.0; Asplund et al. 2007)	Respondent: Self and Informant Report. Yields top five "Signature Themes", and "action items" for development and suggestions about how subject can use their talents.	Satisfactory test-retest reliability values.
Child and Youth Resilience Measure-28 (CYRM-28; Ungar and Leibenberg 2009)	Respondent: Self. Used as a screening tool to explore the resources available to youth that may bolster their resilience.	Alpha coefficient ranged from .65 to .91 for 28-item test.

(continued)

Table 6.2 (continued)

Measure	Strength-based subscales	Psychometrics	
		Internal consistency	Concurrent validity
VIA Inventory of Strengths for Youth (VIA Youth Survey; Park and Peterson 2006a)	Respondent: Self Measures 24, universal character strengths and provides a rank-order of strengths from most to least endorsed.	Alpha coefficients ranged from .72 to .91 for each of the 24 character strengths.	Results converged with teacher ratings of the 24 character strengths. There was agreement between self-reported behaviors (the 24 strengths) and abstract judgments (summary self-ratings). Four strengths (hope, love, zest, and gratitude) were robustly linked with life satisfaction. End of year GPA (grade point average) was predicted by the strengths of perseverance, fairness, gratitude, honesty, hope, and perspective. Student popularity was connected with leadership, fairness, self-regulation, prudence, and forgiveness. In terms of the four subscales of the SSRS, cooperation was most linked with fairness, gratitude, honesty, social intelligence, teamwork, and perspective; assertion with the strengths of leadership and zest; empathy with the strengths of love and kindness; and self-control with the strengths of perseverance, prudence, and self-regulation. For the CBCL, the strengths of hope, zest and leadership correlated with less internalizing problems; and the strengths of perseverance, honesty, prudence, and love correlated with fewer externalizing problems

Over the past 5 years, we (Rashid and Anjum) along with our graduate students have devised and refined three strength-based interventions, which first assess and then systematically attempt to build strengths in children and adolescents.

6.3.1   Signature Strengths

According to Seligman (2002), each person possesses several signature strengths. These are strengths of character that one owns, celebrates, and (if he or she can arrange life successfully) exercises every day in school, work, play, and recreation. Seligman suggests the following possible criteria for a signature strength:

- A sense of authenticity ("this is the real me").
- A feeling of excitement while displaying it.
- A rapid learning curve as themes are attached to the strength and practiced.
- Continuous learning of new ways to enact the strength.
- A sense of yearning to act in accordance with the strength.
- A feeling of inevitability in using the strength, as if one cannot be stopped or dissuaded from its display.
- Invigoration rather than exhaustion when using the strength.
- The creation and pursuit of fundamental projects that revolve around the strength.
- Intrinsic motivation to use the strength.

Seligman's formulation of a good life entails using your signature strengths daily in the main realms of one's life, such as work, love, and play in order to achieve an authentic sense of well-being and happiness (Seligman 2002). Seligman's formulation has been empirically tested. T. D. Peterson and E. W. Peterson (2008) found using one's signature strengths leads to decreased likelihood of depression and stress and an increase in satisfaction. Linley and colleagues (2010) have also found that using signature strengths helps in making progress towards goals and meeting basic needs for independence, relatedness, and competence. Seligman et al. (2006) found using signature strengths among young adults decreased symptoms of depression and increased life satisfaction. Mongrain and Anselmo-Matthews (2012) have found similar results. However, the use of signature strengths to improve well-being or decrease psychological distress has only recently begun to be explored among adolescents (e.g., Proctor, Tsukayama et al. 2011).

In the non-adolescent studies noted above, the individual's signature strengths were determined by their top five scores on the *VIA Inventory of Strengths* (VIA-IS; Peterson and Seligman 2004). Replicating these studies with children and adolescents in a school setting, we explored another way of determining one's signature strengths.

Next, we will briefly discuss three intervention studies, which identified signature strengths of children and adolescents. For these studies, we used the following measures:

- **VIA Inventory of Strengths for Youth** (VIA Youth Survey; Park and Peterson 2006a) is a 198-item self-report inventory of strengths that measures the 24 VIA strengths on a Likert Scale ranging from 1 ("Not like me at all") to 5 ("Very much like me"). The VIA-Youth scales have demonstrated good internal consistency (with alpha's ranging from 0.72 to 0.91).
- **Children's Depression Inventory** (CDI; Kovacs 1992) is a 27-item self-report measure that assesses the affective, cognitive, and behavioral symptoms of depression with a score range of 0–52.
- **Social Skills Rating System (SSRS) or Social Skills Improvement System (SSIS)** (Gresham and Elliot 1990, 2008) contains 79–83 items and has teacher, parent, and self-report versions. It has a Social Skills Composite score with the following subscales: cooperation, assertion, responsibility, and self-control, and a Problem Behavior Composite, which includes subscales of: externalizing, internalizing, and hyperactivity. For study one, we used SSRS and for study three we used SSIS. For both studies, we used parent and teacher report.
- **Conners 3** (self-report version; Conners 2008) is a widely used measure to assess hyperactivity and attention deficit. Only positive and negative impression scales were used for intervention two.
- **Students' Life Satisfaction Scale** (SLSS; Huebner 1991) is a 7-item self-report measure that assesses students' overall life satisfaction.
- **Positive Psychotherapy Inventory – Children Version** (PPTI; Rashid and Anjum 2007) is an 18-item self-report measure that assesses positive emotions, engagement, and meaning.

6.3.1.1 Intervention One

In our first study,[2] we randomly assigned Grade 6 students to a strength-based well-being group or to a control group. Our sample was 41 % female with a mean age of 11.77 ($SD = .68$). The intervention group, after the orientation session, completed the VIA Youth Survey (Park and Peterson 2006a) in a group format. The subsequent eight sessions focused on how to use signature strengths in various domains, and a description of these exercises is given in Table 6.3. Students also undertook a personal project in which they were asked to think of becoming a better person, that is, nicer, kinder, more socially attuned, more curious, more creative, more grateful, more industrious and so forth (see examples for several character strengths in Appendix 6.1). The students' parents and teachers in both groups were provided the feedback about their signature strengths and were asked to notice and record any behavior changes they notice weekly on a sheet provided. In addition, they also completed the SSRS at the beginning and end of the intervention.

---

[2]Conducted in compliance with the Research Services of the Toronto District School Board.

Table 6.3 Strength-based assessment and intervention

Topic	Description
One	Students introduce themselves through a concrete story/narrative, which depicts them at their best. Facilitator guides them by modeling and personal narrative. Students identify their two problem areas to work through this group
You at your best	**Homework**: Students write or express "You at your best" through art, story…etc
Two	The 24 character strengths are introduced through film clips, narratives, and stories; problem areas are further refined in concrete terms
Character strengths	**Homework**: Parents/Guardians are asked to identify the student's top five signature strengths
Three	Students complete VIA Youth survey online
Signature strengths	**Homework**: Students discuss their strengths and identified problems with parents/guardians
Four	Students are coached in use of signature strengths in solving problems and design a Signature Strength Action Plan on paper through narratives, graphics, or pictures
Signature strengths in action	**Homework**: Student draw a solution map connecting each identified problem with a strength, ways to use it and its consequences
Five	Students are taught how to recognize character strengths of others in the school including peers, teachers, support staff, and also at home with their family members, friends and significant others
Signature strengths of others	**Homework**: Students draw a family map of strengths
Six	Students are coached in depth about the use of character strengths in solving problems
Signature strengths in problem solving	**Homework**: Progress on signature strength action plan with emphasis on solving problem initially identified
Seven	Students are given examples and discuss the overuse and underuse of their signature strengths
Overuse and underuse of strengths	**Homework**: Progress on signature strength action plan
Eight	Students do a brief presentation about progress, outcome of their signature strengths project; feedback from parents and teachers is incorporated
Signature strength action plan presentation	Parents are invited to come in person to support their child's presentation or are asked to send their feedback about progress/ changes they noticed. Ways to maintain positive behavioral gains are discussed

After the first orientation session, the children completed the VIA Youth Survey online in a group format. Some students experienced difficulty in completing the 198-item measure, finding it long and repetitive. However, eventually, students in both groups were able to complete the online measure in the school's computer lab. Each participant was encouraged to imagine himself or herself as a better person at the end of the intervention by undertaking a signature strength project. In the following three sessions, the children were extensively coached about ways of using their top strengths, also known as *signature strengths* and devised a practical behavioral project. Legends, real-life narratives, and popular films, such as *Pay It*

Forward, Billy Elliot, Forest Gump, Life Is Beautiful, and My Left Foot, illustrated the use of strengths. Movies have been shown to offer powerful exemplars of each of the 24 character strengths in action (Niemiec and Wedding 2008). Parents and teachers in both groups were requested to complete the SSIS before and after the treatment. From sessions three to seven, participants were extensively taught about a strength-based, problem-solving approach which entailed understanding and appreciating the context and fit between situation and intended use of the character strength. Table 6.4 presents some sample strategies of using strengths in solving specific problems. In the final session, each of the 11 participants described their experience using their signature strengths. One participant, who had experienced bullying, utilized her social intelligence to team up with a friend and perform a small skit illustrating the impact of bullying. The skit was so well done that the school principal asked the student to perform the skit at a school assembly. Another student, who constantly argued with her mother, utilized her gratitude and started expressing her thanks towards her mother – even for small favors. Another student whose signature strength was not self-regulation, nonetheless, used it to stop saying impolite and unkind words towards his younger sibling. As children discussed their use of signature strengths within the group, we noticed a synergistic contagion, which motivated other group members.

Furthermore, gratitude and savoring were addressed through specific exercises. Overall, this was an 8-week intervention with each session lasting 1 and 1/2 h. The control group completed pre- and post-intervention measures and also completed the VIA Youth Survey online. At the end of the intervention, both groups did not change on measures of depression and student satisfaction but significant differences were found on the well-being measure (PPTI) with a large effect size (Cohen's $d=0.90$) and the social skills measure (SSRS), on the parent version, but not on the teacher version (Cohen's $d=1.88$). This is consistent with the results of the individualized positive psychotherapy pilot (Seligman et al. 2006). At a 6-month follow-up the gains were maintained on the well-being measure with slight but not statistically significant decline. However, the two groups did not differ on the social skills measure (SSRS) (parent version).

6.3.1.2 Intervention Two

The promising results of the first intervention encouraged us to replicate the intervention. However, in order to assess the experimenter bias (first and second author being closely affiliated with the development of the Positive Psychology Center, University of Pennsylvania, during their postdoctoral residency), we decided to train two graduate students to run a similar intervention at an inner city neighborhood. This presented an elevated level of behavioral and emotional challenges. To address these, we slightly changed the exercises in the intervention (Table 6.3) adding an exercise called Negativity Bias. Among the measures, we dropped CDI, as it was expected to be a nonclinical sample, but given the behavioral challenges, added two subscales of the Conners 3 (positive and negative impressions),

Table 6.4 Using strengths in challenges and in solving problems – some illustrations

Character strength	Challenge	Strategy
Zest, vitality, enthusiasm: Student is energetic, cheerful, and full of life	Student does not show interest with other students (e.g., does not talk much, share or participate much in group activities, has few friends)	Encourage student to do at least one outdoor activity weekly such as hiking, biking, mountain biking, mountain climbing, brisk walking or jogging
Persistence, industry, diligence and perseverance: Student finishes most things, even when distracted, and is able to refocus to complete task	Student gives up easily, has difficulty finishing tasks and performs assignments carelessly	Help student identify factors that diminish their interest in the assignment, and help students monitor their progress to incrementally overcome difficulties
Self-regulation and self-control: Students gladly follows rules and routines	Student behaves impulsively, without self-control, lacks time-management skills, and is disorganized	Help student be aware of the time of day when they are most productive. Ask them to remove distractions and utilize this time in tasks requiring mental and physical organization rather than mundane tasks
Forgiveness and mercy: Student does not hold a grudge and forgives easily those who offend him/her	Student holds grudges, exaggerates minor offenses of others, and does not accept sincere apologies	Identify how holding a grudge affects student emotionally. Help student picture themself as offender and remember times when they offended someone and were forgiven
Hope and optimism: Student hopes and believes that more good things will happen than bad ones	Student is preoccupied with their failures and shortcomings, and is overly negative	Coach student to focus on their strengths, and find positive aspects of bad things that have happened to them
Humor and playfulness: Students is playful, funny, and uses humor to connect with others	Student responds inappropriately to friendly teasing (e.g., jokes, name calling)	Encourage student to engage in light-hearted gestures and playful activities with a good-natured attitude
Social and emotional intelligence: Student manages themselves well in social situations and has good interpersonal skills	Student does not socialize appropriately with peers and does not respond appropriately to nonverbal cues from others	Encourage student to watch others how they make and maintain connections, rather than seeking friends, student can seek experience which bring together like-minded people together
Teamwork and citizenship: Student relates well with teammates or group members and contributes to the success of the group	Student is very competitive, will not let others take turns, and cannot stand to lose in a game	Help student identify their motivation for completion and help create a motivational climate focused on doing their best, not to achieve external rewards. Coach student to cultivate reciprocity and to promote cooperation

(continued)

Table 6.4 (continued)

Character strength	Challenge	Strategy
Open-mindedness: Student thinks through and examines all sides before making a decision. Is not reluctant to change mind	Student is rigid, and inflexible. Does not adjust well to changes such as new settings, teachers, peers and situations	Ask student to adopt the perspective of the "other side" in an argument in which they are inflexible or have strong opinions
Gratitude: Student expresses thankfulness for good things through words and actions	Student takes good things in life and well-intentioned acts of others for granted	Encourage student to reflect on the positive things that have happened throughout their day before going to bed. Discuss with student some of the things they are most grateful for
Modesty and humility: Student does not like to be the center of attention and prefers others to shine	Student lacks modesty, draws attention unnecessarily, and overrates one's qualities and achievements	Coach student to an accurate, realistic estimate of their abilities and achievements. Have student write statements acknowledging their imperfections and how they make them human
Perspective/Wisdom: Student often is the source of advice for peers and often settles disputes among peers	Student does not learn from mistakes and often repeats them. Lacks deeper understanding of moral and ethical issues. Is unable to apply knowledge to practical problems	Help student become open to experience. Encourage students to be adventurous, curious and inquisitive about different things. Encourage students to find the purpose and motivations of their past decisions
Capacity to love and be loved: Student shows genuine love and affection through actions	Student withdraws by isolating himself or herself or appearing uninterested. Other student do not accept student	Help student communicate care in small ways to those who are interested in them and to be honest and transparent with their friends
Fairness, equity and justice: Student stands up for others when they are treated unfairly, bullied or ridiculed	Student behaves inappropriately in specific situations and does not demonstrate sensitivity or care towards those who are different	Encourage student to reflect how she/he would like to be treated, in situations he treats others unfairly

along with the PPTI, and the SLSS. The participants were a convenience sample of students in Grade 6, an intervention group ($n=21$) and a control group ($n=22$). The intervention was administered by two graduate students in school psychology. Both students were trained and supervised by the first author. The classroom teacher was present during eight, weekly (60 min) sessions. Some students have had difficulty completing the 198-item VIA Youth Survey, and since this population was an inner city school with students with academic and behavioral challenges, this concern was heightened. One student, a proficient reader at her grade level, gave up at item 181 stating that she didn't care about exploring her strengths. Unfortunately, the online server didn't save the results. She was eventually able to complete the measure at her home. Similar challenges were experienced with other students who lost concentration as the test progressed and some became disruptive. Given the experience of the intervention group, we altered the intervention and the control group was not administered the VIA Youth Survey. They only completed the remaining measures aforementioned. Both groups did not differ on any of the outcome measures. However, participants' degree of enjoyment in the intervention group was significantly related to how much they perceived what they learned from the group ($r = .63$, $p < .001$). A 6-month follow-up showed similar trends. However, by teacher anecdotal report, several students in the intervention group started discussing strengths and their problem-solving skills improved.

We compiled several findings from our first two interventions. First, an 8-week long, stand-alone intervention of character strengths-based well-being, when delivered by experienced professionals, yields better results. Second, an 8-week period might be too short to produce a significant and meaningful impact. Third, teachers' active involvement in both of our first interventions was missing. Classroom teachers needed to play an important role in these interventions. Fourth, outcome measures needed to include impact of intervention on teacher reported academic performance and the intervention needed more integration within the school curriculum. Fifth, it was felt that more active parental involvement was needed to help children ascertain and use their character strengths at home. Finally, and most importantly, the VIA Youth Survey's length of 198 items posed a challenge to disengaged students at the onset of intervention.

6.3.1.3 Intervention Three

Part One: Development and Validation of a Brief Measure to Assess Signature Strengths

To address the aforementioned challenges, we made the classroom teacher the focal point of the intervention. The teacher was first trained on the VIA Classification through a detailed manual which included detailed descriptions of the 24 character strengths, their links with well-being, and behavioral methods to build character strengths in school settings. The classroom teacher was then asked to establish links between character strengths and the curriculum, and he offered useful tips in this regard. For the third intervention, we did not use any structured exercises as done in interventions one and two (Table 6.5). Given the challenges we faced in having students complete the VIA Youth Survey, we decided to use a shorter measure of character strengths, still based on the VIA Classification model. This measure is referred to as the Signature Strengths Assessment of Youth (SSAY). Our goal was to create a shorter measure, using the VIA Classification that could distinguish a young person's signature strengths from his/her non-signature strengths. Therefore,

Table 6.5 Integration of character strengths in the curriculum (Intervention Three)

	Description	Frequency
Phase one	Explicit instruction on character strengths, their correlates, benefits, overuse and underuse	Once a week
	Character strengths discussed in community circles	Twice a week
	Student brought up scenarios from their lives, which included conflicts, dilemmas, or a problem that needed a solution. Students were asked to think of someone with the character strengths of kindness or prudence, and consider how that person would solve the problem using one of those strengths. Students also discussed how someone who lacks these strengths would deal with these problems?	
Phase two	Integration of character strengths in the curriculum	Classroom discussion as needed
	An illustration: Students read four novels	
	Discussed character strengths mentioned	
	Homework was done through blogging	
	Students were asked to identify character guided	
	By specific character strengths and how character	
	Strengths of character impacted others	
	Novels: "*Misfits*" (Howe), "*Homeless bird*" (Gloria Whelan), "*Sacred Leaf*" (Deborah Ellis)	
	Community circles continued, students kept on discussing a real life problem and a solution utilizing character strengths	Weekly

we decided to capture each of the 24 signature strengths through three items. The first item, referred as the *signature strength item* was written keeping the aforementioned signature strength criteria in mind so that if it is a person's signature strength, he/she is able to endorse it strongly. For example the signature strength item for love of learning was, "I love spending a lot of time learning from other people (parents, teachers, friends) as well as through books and/or educational media (television, internet, radio)". The second item, referred as the *middle item*, was deliberately written as if it was not a person's signature strength (e.g., love of learning, "I like to learn new things in school and at home"). Whereas the *third item* was a reverse item with the intention that the person reading the item with a specific signature strength such as love of learning, would not endorse it highly (e.g., love of learning, "I learn new things because I have to, not because I love it").

Along with the intervention study, we ran a validation study to explore the psychometrics of the SSAY. The data was collected from three schools in Toronto and from more than 15 schools in Australia, the United Kingdom, and the United States. All students completed the SSAY online, along with the PPTI (children's version) and the SLSS. A total of 2,435 elementary and high school students completed the measure online. Of these, 161 students completed both the VIA Youth Survey and the SSAY. The correlation of 20 of 24 character strengths was significant for spirituality ($r = .66$, $p < .001$), love of learning ($r = .50$, $p < .001$), and forgiveness ($r = .54$, $p < .001$) demonstrating medium to high correlation, whereas self-regulation ($r=.24$, $p<.001$) and prudence ($r=.27$, $p<.001$) showed small correlations. We also gathered data from a subset of students ($n=963$) on their self-reported behaviors through single item questions and correlated it with the average of 24 SSAY scores. We found that a high average SSAY is significantly correlated with self-reported academic performance[3] ($r=.35$, $p<.001$). We also found that a low average SSAY score was correlated with watching more television ($r=.20$, $p<.001$), spending more time on the Internet for non-academic purposes ($r=.16$, $p<.001$), and also playing more video games ($r=.16$, $p<.001$). We also found that those who on average ate more meals with their family had more friends ($r=.38$, $p<.001$). In summary, SSAY's psychometrics were mixed, by traditional consistency standards, we found low alphas due to the discrepant nature of item content within each strength scale. However, the measure yielded satisfactory construct validity.

Part Two: Administration of Intervention Three

The participants in intervention three were 59 Grade 6 students from two Toronto elementary schools with a mean age of 11.76 years ($SD=1.5$). Females comprised 53 % of the entire sample with 42 % Caucasian, 21 % Asian, and 19 % from a Chinese background. One school served as the intervention group while the other served as the control group and only completed pre- and post-measures.

   Parents in the intervention group received two workshops on character strengths of children and their role in their child's well-being. In identifying children's signature strengths, we adopted a dynamic assessment approach, which had the following two steps: (1) children completed SSAY online; and (2) their parents, teacher, and one peer (a classmate but not the best friend to control for favorability bias) identified their top five strengths, from descriptions of the 24 VIA character strengths (Table 6.1). This description did not include names of the strengths. A composite was calculated which assigned differential weight to scores, such as the top five SSAY score received a score of 1, five strengths identified by parents and teacher were assigned a weight of .75, whereas strengths identified by a peer were assigned a weight of .5. These scores were computed and the top five scores were regarded as signature strengths. In cases of ties, strengths identified by SSAY were given preference. A detailed five-page feedback report was provided to the teacher and parents (See Appendix 6.1 for a sample feedback report). This feedback was provided prior to the winter break, and children were invited to use their signature strengths as part of a New Year's resolution project. Parents were asked to consult with the first and second author about signature strengths and to be active participants in helping their children devise a personalized Signature Strength Action Project (see Appendix 6.2). Evening workshops and individual consultations after the winter break offered parents the opportunity to discuss their child's

---

[3] Students were asked compared to their peers, how would they rate their academic performance in general on a scale of 1 = weak to 5 = excellent.

signature strengths. Parents were provided with practical strategies to share with their children the anecdotes, memories, experiences, real life stories, accomplishments and skills, which illustrated their and their child's strengths. This process was overwhelmingly positive as most parents were pleasantly surprised to name a positive trait as a strength. The process was infectious enough that initially 29 of 33 parents in the intervention group consented to participate in the project. However, as the strengths assessments were taking place, three of the four who did not consent initially, requested to join the project.

In the classroom, instead of doing structured exercises that we completed in the first two interventions, the classroom teacher was focused on integrating the strengths in the Grade 6 curriculum, especially in language and arts. The teacher heavily emphasized using character strengths in solving problems. Integration into the curriculum was not a challenge, as the Ministry of Education requires character education in schools.

6.3.1.4   Results

On our primary outcome measures, the SSIS, we found that use of signature strengths improved social skills (the overall composite score), as reported by the teacher, from pre- to post-intervention level with a large effect size (Cohen's $d = 1.12$). In the parent report, the Problem Behavior (overall composite score) also improved from pre- to post-intervention level. We also found significant teacher-reported changes in academic performance, from pre- to post-intervention level. Caution is warranted in interpreting these results – because of logistic limitations, we only administered the social skills questionnaire to the intervention group. On the well-being measure (PPTI) and on student life satisfaction, which was administered to both the intervention and control groups, the two groups did not differ at post-intervention level.

Our results showed that, when assessed from multiple perspectives (self-report, parents, teacher, and peer), the most endorsed character strengths were zest, love, hope, curiosity, honesty, appreciation of beauty and excellence, and forgiveness. In contrast, spirituality, self-regulation, and perspective/wisdom were the least endorsed. Of these strengths, large to medium size correlations were found for love ($r = .57$**[4]), zest ($r = .43$**), and hope ($r = .46$**) and gratitude ($r = .43$**), also were among the top five strengths associated with life satisfaction. Our finding is consistent, with previous findings by Park et al. (2004) who found that love, hope, and zest are consistently related to life satisfaction for individuals across all ages. We also found significant correlations between SSAY scores and at least two informant reports (coded as 1 if a character strength was identified as signature strength and 0 if not) for strengths of curiosity, love of learning, perseverance, love, social intelligence, teamwork/citizenship, forgiveness, prudence, hope, and humor. In other words,

---

[4] * $p < .05$; ** $p < .01$.

when the child reported (through SSAY scores) that these were their strengths, his/ her parents, teachers and/or peers also recognized it. These findings suggest that certain strengths are more visible to those around the individual than others.

In this intervention, we incorporated multiple perspectives in determining the signature strengths of students. Furthermore, in order to help children see the integration of character strengths in their school experience, we eliminated structured exercises and relied on an intuitive integration of the teacher in terms of integrating character strengths in two areas: (a) curriculum and (b) problem solving. To incorporate more parental involvement, the first author conducted two after-school workshops to help parents understand character strengths and to help their children build them further. These workshops were well-attended with more than 80 % of the parents of children involved in the intervention actively participating in the workshops, and many regularly corresponded with the teacher and first author about the various phases of the intervention. Finally, we decided that the intervention would last for the whole academic year (September through June).

6.3.1.5 Summary of Our Interventions

Helping children to identify their strengths and teaching them ways to use strengths in problem solving not only makes them efficient problem solvers but also enhances their well-being. Previous research using the 198-item VIA Youth Survey has found substantial correlation between life satisfaction and hope, zest, and love. Our 72-item measure found similar correlations, suggesting that a shorter measure of character strength yields satisfactory construct validity. In our first intervention, which lasted for 8 weeks, we found significant improvement in social skills, but these improvements were not maintained at the 6-month follow-up. However, our third intervention which lasted for a year, integrating character strengths in the curriculum and also involving teacher and parents closely, yielded significant changes in social skills and teacher reported academic performance as well as significant changes in parent reported problem-solving behavior. It appears that the classroom teacher is better suited to deliver strength-based interventions that are embedded within the curriculum rather than outside professionals.

We also found that our second and third intervention studies did not yield significant pre to post changes on measures of well-being and life satisfaction. It could be argued that the baseline scores on both well-being and life satisfaction were at a level where room for improvement in these scores was limited. In other words, these findings could be attributed to the ceiling effect of these constructs; however, further analyses would needed in order to determine this. Moreover, procedural differences in delivery of the interventions and sociocultural environmental effects may have also had an impact on the results. For example, intervention three relied upon a classroom teacher with whom the students and parents already had an established a relationship and the teacher had the opportunity to incorporate strengths in the curriculum.

We conclude with the following strategies in assessing and building strengths extracted from best practices in the literature and also from our experience in working across three different countries with diverse student samples:

- **Integration**: Integrating measures of psychopathology and strengths is perhaps the most efficient strategy to understand children and adolescents in a holistic and balanced way. One illustration of such an integration is by Greenspoon and Saklofske (2001) who employed measures of subjective well-being (i.e., life satisfaction) along with traditional measures of psychopathology (i.e., self-reported internalizing and teacher-reported externalizing behavior scores on the BASC; Reynolds and Kamphaus 1992). They showed that students with low subjective well-being had significantly lower functioning across psychosocial, academic, and physical health domains. Since most measures of psychopathology have good psychometrics, establishing a relationship with strength-based measures will make the assessment of children and adolescent more comprehensive and will help professionals appreciate the incremental validity of their conclusions by adding these measures.

- **Reinterpreting existing measures**: Given the pervasive use of psychometrically sound measures which assess weaknesses and deficits of children, Wood and Joseph (2010) suggest that one way to assess strengths is to reinterpret these existing measures that contain positive items (often reverse coded). For example, the Conners 3 (2008) is widely used to assess symptoms related to attention-deficit/hyperactivity disorder, executive dysfunction, learning problems, aggression, and family relationships. The longer version, also contain items such as telling the truth, not telling white lies, fun to be around, sharing feelings, personal interests and achievement with others. Similarly, the BASC-2 (Reynolds and Kamphaus 2004) has items such as paying attention, encouraging others to do their best, communicating clearly, offering help to others, being well organized, making friends easily, working well under pressure, recovering well under pressure, adjusting well to changes, volunteering to help others, setting realistic goals, etc. These items are often reverse-coded. One strategy is to keep positive items as positive suggesting the presence of positive states and traits, rather than their absence. Rather than regarding negatives and positive as separate dimensions, common states such as depression and anxiety could be considered on a continuum with happiness and relaxation or these could form two separate continua.

- **Interview**: Interviews guided by research can also be used to assess strengths. If a professional prefers not to use formal assessment, he/she can use questions during informal assessments or formal psycho-educational evaluations that elicit strengths, positive emotions, and meaning. For example, discuss with children and adolescents what they consider satisfying, their goals, their wishes, their attainable goals, and what they are particularly good at. Other questions to consider include: What activities, tasks, and challenges do they find intrinsically motivating and absorbing? Which accomplishment are they most proud of? Which relationships in school, at home, and elsewhere do they find trustworthy?

Discussing positive aspects openly, explicitly and consciously lays a motivational foundation, which can later be changed into concrete, achievable, and favorable goals.

- **Paragons**: To help children and adolescents discern and identify their own strengths, professionals can use paragons of certain strengths (e.g., Gandhi, Mother Theresa, Nelson Mandela, Martin Luther King, Albert Einstein, Aung San Suu Kyi, Ken Saro Wiwa), real-life narratives, and popular films (e.g., *Pay it Forward, Forest Gump, My Left Foot*). A professional can use strengths displayed by specific paragons and film characters and discuss with students whether they partly or fully identify with them, which conditions seem to display these strengths maximally, and what might be the consequences of displaying these strengths. A comprehensive list of over 1,000 films from around the world illustrating each of the 24 character strengths can be found in Niemiec and Wedding (2008).
- **Collateral data**: Collateral information from family members, teachers, and peers about the strengths of the child or adolescent can be very useful, as we found in our interventions. It is particularly helpful to assess and identify social and communal buffers for children and adolescents living in neighborhoods ridden with social problems. For example, in addition to inquiring about problems with family members, professionals can also assess attachment, love, and nurturance from the primary support group. Instead of looking for problems related to the social environment, a child or adolescent can be asked to describe humor and playful interactions, connectedness, and empathetic relationships at work.
- **Informal assessment**: Standardized tests may often overlook or hide individuality. While there are advantages of establishing normative common denominators, individuality in this process is compromised. Therefore one strategy is to integrate both standardized as well as informal ways of assessing strengths. For example, inquiring about strengths displayed during challenges and setbacks can provide rich information that may not be captured by a standardized measure. For example, we have asked questions such as: *"Tell me about a challenge you handled adaptively?"* or *"What have you done to overcome a serious difficulty?"* or *"Tell me about a setback from which you learned a lot about yourself."* These lines of inquiry can be customized to adapt to the cognitive and academic level of children and adolescents. Furthermore, standardized questionnaires, which assess resilience can be adapted to an interview format and critical items can be used to initiate discussion. This will also help to conceptualize the cultural context of strengths, which is difficult to capture within standardized measures.
- **Formal evaluations**: Assessment of strengths should be an important part of formal psychoeducational assessment and should be creatively integrated into Individualized Educational Plans (IEPs). Following is an excerpt from one of the psychoeducational assessments completed by the first author, which integrates strengths in a formal evaluation of an 11-year-old boy who was referred for having math difficulties.

Tyron has good verbal skills including vocabulary, reading comprehension, and decoding. In addition, he is resilient, a good leader, athletic, and playful. His intellectual and character strengths have to be harnessed efficiently to help him overcome significant behavioral challenges and cognitive difficulties posed by his weak visual and non-verbal skills. Tyron's deductive and inductive reasoning skills – key for acquiring new information – are weak, especially when information is non-verbal such as mathematical calculations, figures, illustrations, and graphs. Therefore, he will benefit from an instructional approach that is explicit and systematic rather than one which is based on a discovery learning type approach. When teaching Tyron any new process or skills, provide slow and step-by-step instructions. Use manipulative and concrete objects to supplement verbal instructions so that he can comprehend concepts thoroughly. Use Tyron's leadership skills to pair him with someone who could benefit from Tyron verbal skills, and in turn, can offer help to Tyron in non-verbal communication. This will likely enhance Tyron's self-confidence and positive interaction with others.

- **Integrating strengths into academic performance**: Character strengths can also be incorporated in meaningful ways in existing measures of psychopathology. A school in the New York area has started to do so. School's admiration posits that if you are a parent, wouldn't you want to know how your son or daughter stacked up next to the rest of class in character as well as reading ability.
- **Narratives**: Relatedly, another strategy to elicit and build strengths in children and adolescents is to ask them to share a real story that shows their strengths. This strategy, due to its personalized narrative appeal can connect the professional and the child or adolescent and can build rapport promptly as well as a powerful therapeutic alliance. If children or adolescents cannot come up with a story, they can tell a favorite story which they find inspiring or motivating. Stories can be replaced with poems, songs, fictional characters, metaphors, living exemplars, or paragons.
- **Strengths translated into actions and habits**: The professional should assess whether children and adolescents are able to translate abstract strengths into concrete actions, behaviors, and habits. This assessment is important because in real life challenges rarely come in neat packages with labeled instructions such as, "When feeling down, use zest and vitality." Challenges and hassles often occur amidst a dizzying jumble of emotions, actions, and their effects. The role of the strengths-based professional is to gently guide the student to use their strengths adaptively, to solve their problems adaptively, and to come to know themselves better.
- **Building self-efficacy**: Some children and adolescents, especially those with behavioral concerns may be reluctant to explore or believe their strengths because they have been conditioned to associate negatives about themselves. In such cases, the professional may first work on building the self-efficacy of children and adolescents by using evidence-based strategies such as cognitive-behavioral programs that can help them to believe that they have the ability to change. Once they focus and spend more time on what they are capable off, they will automatically spend less time in thinking about their shortcomings.
- **Family life**: It is of critical importance that strengths are built within the family context. If the adults in children's lives are not aware of the children's strengths, they will not able to coalesce resources to build strengths, skills, and competence. As observed by Seligman and Csikszentmihalyi (2000), "promoting competence in children is more than fixing what is wrong with them. It is about identifying and

nurturing their strongest qualities, what they own and are best at, and helping them find niches in which they can best live out these strengths" (p. 6). Another way to assess strengths in children and adolescents is to explore how they spend time with their immediate and extended family, including time doing recreation (indoor and outdoor games; art and sports activities), household chores, caregiving to a sibling or grandparent, play with neighborhood peers, and time with volunteering.

- **Teacher**: Importantly, strength-based assessment and intervention cannot succeed if the classroom teacher does not believe in it. If the teacher's focus is primarily remedial focused on correcting weakness, he/she will have a mindset that looks for and discovers problems. Teachers serve as role models, if they don't demonstrate acknowledgement and cultivation of strengths, students are unlikely to do so. Working from a strength-based perspective can help teachers to have a huge impact on students, in inspiring them and motivating them because teachers not only teach curriculum but also implicitly teach emotional and psychological well-being. Furthermore, enhancing strengths of students will help teachers to refine their own.

Appendices

Appendix 6.1

Sample feedback report: Signature strengths of your child

1. **Zest, Enthusiasm, and Vitality**: You are an energetic, cheerful, and full-of-life person. You approach most things with excitement and enthusiasm. Nothing is done half-way or half-heartedly for you. You wake up most mornings feeling energized and happy. The enthusiasm and passion you bring to activities often attract others to join you. When you experience something well done, you feel inspired and motivated.

    Balance: Too much zest and enthusiasm can make you overactive and can cause social challenges with peers who may experience you as "intense". On the other hand, if you do not use this signature strength, you will come across as passive and inhibited, maybe even withdrawn.

2. **Love of Learning**: You love to learn new things – in school or on your own. You make very good use of opportunities where you can gain knowledge about skills, concepts, ideas, and facts. You have always enjoyed school and reading. When it comes to learning, you are persistent; even if you get frustrated or distracted, you refocus and don't give up until you have mastered the topic or skill.

    Balance: Too much use of this signature strength may result in less participation in fun extra-curricular activities. Also, overuse of this strength could compromise your social interactions – you could be considered a geek who knows everything but isn't much fun to hang out with. Then again, a lack of "love of learning" may keep you naively uninformed and unaware of many facts of life.

3. **Humor and Playfulness**: It is very easy for you to find opportunities to laugh, be witty, playful, and humorous in most situations. You are known for bringing smiles to other people and making them comfortable. You are also very good at seeing the lighter side of most situations and therefore use humor to take the edge off a stressful situation. Your sense of humor bonds you with others.

   Balance: An overuse of this signature strength may find you expressing playfulness and humor in some situations that require demonstration of other strengths – such as self-regulation or caution. Moreover, use of playfulness and humor during classroom activities may distract you and others, and you may not be able to attend specific details of a challenging assignment. On the other hand, a lack of playfulness and humor may make you too serious and inhibited and it may impact your interpersonal relationships.

4. **Leadership**: You excel at leadership tasks and activities. You are very good at organizing group activities and seeing that they happen. That is why you are the one children like to follow or often prefer that you take the lead. You also make everyone feel included. As a leader, whenever differences or conflicts occur, you are able to resolve these amicably and keep the harmony of the group intact. In fact, you are often able to bring best out of every member.

   Balance: An overuse of this strength may show you as bossy or dominating. A lack of this strength may show overly compliant behavior or lack of necessary independence.

5. **Appreciation of Beauty and Excellence**: You are very good at perceiving and appreciating beauty and excellence in many areas of life, from nature to art to mathematics to science. Display of excellence inspires you. You love to incorporate things of beauty in your surroundings. You feel at ease when you are amid art or watching a great performance.

   Balance: An overuse of this strength may not let you be sensitive to those who do not have access to great art or performances and are more concerned with meeting basic needs of everyday living. Also, an overuse of this strength may give other people the impression at times that you are bit snobbish and have an elitist attitude. An underuse of this strength may manifest in naïve ignorance or disrespect of great performances (including in sports) or pieces of art.

Appendix 6.2

Signature strength action project – Years resolution: Using my signature

> **Dear Child**: Visualize what kind of person you would like to be in 2011? Perhaps nicer, kinder, more social, inquisitive, spiritual, courageous, playful, knowledgeable, modest, cheerful and perhaps more engaged…etc. Think and consult with your parents and friends; how you could use your signature strengths to become that person? Briefly describe your plan below. What

(continued)

(continued)
exactly you would like to do? How frequently? What kind of support you
would like from your parents and friends in making this plan a success? We
would like you to complete this by June 2011. What are some timelines and
phases of this plan (beginning, middle and ending)? What would happen if
you become that person?

_____

_____

_____

_____

_____

_____

Three things you like (or dislike) about your signature strength profile?
1._____
2._____
3._____

Acknowledgements We are deeply thankful to Carolyn Lennox, Ruth Baumal, Joy Reiter, James
Bowen, Tamara Kornaki, Aarti Kumar, Nina Vitopolous, Peter Chang, and Neal Mayerson for their
support in the running of the intervention studies.

References

Achenbach, T. M. (1992). *Manual for the child behavior checklist/2-3 and 1992 profile*. Burlington:
    University of Vermont Department of Psychiatry.
American Psychiatric Association. (2000). *Diagnostic and statistical manual of mental disorders*
    (4th ed., text rev.). Washington, DC: American Psychiatric Association.
Asplund, J., Lopez, S. J., Hodges, T., & Harter, J. (2007). *The Clifton StrengthsFinder® 2.0 techni-
    cal report: Development and validation*. Princeton: The Gallup Organization.
Beaver, B. R. (2008). A positive approach to children's internalizing problems. *Professional
    Psychology: Research and Practice, 39*, 129–136.
Bird, V. J., Le Boutillier, C., Leamy, M., Larsen, J., Oades, L. G., Williams, J., & Slade, M. (2012).
    Assessing the strengths of mental health consumers: A systematic review. *Psychological
    Assessment, 24*, 1024–1033. doi:10.1037/a0028983.
Bundick, M. J. (2011). Extracurricular activities, positive youth development, and the role of
    meaningfulness of engagement. *The Journal of Positive Psychology, 6*, 57–74. doi:10.1080/
    17439760.2010.536775.
Cassidy, J., & Asher, S. (1992). Loneliness and peer relations in young children. *Child Development,
    63*, 350–365.
Conners, K. C. (2008). *Conners* (3rd ed.). Toronto: Multi-Health Systems.
Constantine, N., Benard, B., & Diaz, M. (1999). *Measuring protective factors and resilience traits
    in youth: The Healthy Kids Resilience assessment*. Paper presented at the Seventh Annual
    Meeting of the Society for Prevention Research, New Orleans, LA.

Cottrell, C. A., & Neuberg, S. L. (2005). Different emotional reactions to different groups: A sociofunctional threat-based approach to "prejudice". *Journal of Personality and Social Psychology, 88*(5), 770–789. doi:10.1037/0022-3514.88.5.770.

Crocker, J., Luhtanen, R. K., Cooper, M. L., & Bouvrette, A. (2003). Contingencies of self-worth in college students: Theory and measurement. *Journal of Personality and Social Psychology, 85*, 894–908. doi:10.1037/0022-3514.85.5.894.

Duckworth, A. L., Steen, T. A., & Seligman, M. E. P. (2005). Positive Psychology in clinical practice. *Annual Review of Clinical Psychology, 1*(1), 629–651.

Duckworth, A. L., & Quinn, P. D. (2009). Development and validation of the Short Grit Scale (Grit-S). *Journal of Personality Assessment, 91*, 166–174.

Duckworth, A. L., & Seligman, M. E. P. (2005). Self-discipline outdoes IQ in predicting academic performance of adolescents. *Psychological Science, 16*(12), 939–944. doi:10.1111/j.1467-9280.2005.01641.x.

Ebesutani, C., Okamura, K., Higa-McMillan, C., & Chorpita, B. F. (2011). A psychometric analysis of the positive and negative affect schedule for children – Parent version in a school sample. *Psychological Assessment, 33*, 406–416.

Epstein, M. H. (2004). *Behavioral and emotional rating scale* (2nd ed.). Austin: PRO-ED.

Epstein, J. L., & McPartland, J. M. (1976). The concept and measurement of the quality of school life. *American Educational Research Journal, 13*(1), 15–30.

Epstein, M. H., & Sharma, J. (1998). *Behavioral and emotional rating scale: A strength-based approach to assessment*. Austin: PRO-ED.

Flinchbaugh, C. L., Moore, E. W. G., Chang, Y. K., & May, D. R. (2012). Student well-being interventions: The effects of stress management techniques and gratitude journaling in the management education classroom. *Journal of Management Education, 36*, 191–219. doi:10.1177/1052562911430062.

Flückiger, C., & Grosse Holtforth, M. (2008). Focusing the therapist's attention on the patient's strengths: A preliminary study to foster a mechanism of change in outpatient psychotherapy. *Journal of Clinical Psychology, 64*(7), 876–890. doi:10.1002/jclp.20493.

Fox Eades, J. M. (2008). *Celebrating strengths: Building strength-based schools*. Coventry: CAPP Press.

Friedman, H. L., & MacDonal, D. A. (2006). Humanistic testing and assessment. *Journal of Humanistic Psychology, 46*, 510–529.

Froh, J. J., Kashdan, T. B., Ozimkowski, K. M., & Miller, N. (2009). Who benefits the most from a gratitude intervention in children and adolescents? Examining positive affect as a moderator. *The Journal of Positive Psychology, 4*, 408–422.

Gillham, J. E., Reivich, K. J., Jaycox, L. H., & Seligman, M. E. P. (1995). Prevention of depressive symptoms in school children: Two-year follow-up. *Psychological Science, 6*, 343–351.

Gillham, J., Adams-Deutsch, Z., Werner, J., Reivich, K., Coulter-Heindl, V., Linkins, M., & Seligman, M. E. P. (2011). Character strengths predict subjective well-being during adolescence. *The Journal of Positive Psychology, 6*, 31–44. doi:10.1080/17439760.2010.536773.

Gilman, R., Huebner, S., & Furlong, M. (2009). *Handbook of positive psychology in schools*. New York: Rutledge.

Govindji, R., & Linley, P. A. (2007). Strengths use, self-concordance and well-being: Implications for strengths coaching and coaching psychologists. *International Coaching Psychology Review, 2*, 143–153.

Greenspoon, P. J., & Saklofske, D. H. (2001). Toward an integration of subjective well-being and psychopathology. *Social Indicators Research, 54*, 81–108.

Gresham, F. M., & Elliot, S. N. (1990). *Social skills rating system manual*. Circle Pines: American Guidance Service.

Gresham, F. M., & Elliot, S. N. (2008). *Social skills improvement system manual*. Circle Pines: Pearson Assessment.

Harter, S. (1985). *Manual for the self-perception profile for adolescents*. Denver: University of Denver.

Huebner, E. (1991). Further validation of the students' life satisfaction scale: The independence of satisfaction and affect ratings. *Journal of Psychoeducational Assessment, 9,* 363–368. doi:10.1177/073428299100900408.

Huebner, E. S. (1994). Preliminary development and validation of a multidimensional life satisfaction scale for children. *Psychological Assessment, 6,* 149–158.

Hunter, J. P., & Csikszentmihalyi, M. (2003). The positive psychology of interested adolescents. *Journal of Youth and Adolescence, 32*(1), 27–35.

Huta, V., & Hawley, L. (2010). Psychological strengths and cognitive vulnerabilities: Are they two ends of the same continuum or do they have independent relationships with well-being and ill-being? *Journal of Happiness Studies, 11,* 71–93. doi:10.1007/s10902-008-9123-4.

Johnson, J., Gooding, P., Wood, A. M., & Tarrier, N. (2010). Resilience as positive coping appraisals: Testing the schematic appraisals model of suicide (SAMS). *Behaviour Research and Therapy, 48,* 179–186.

Kahneman, D., & Tversky, A. (1984). Choices, values, and frames. *American Psychologist, 39,* 341–350.

Keyes, C. L. M. (2009). The Black–White paradox in health: Flourishing in the face of social inequality and discrimination. *Journal of Personality, 77,* 1677–1706. doi:10.1111/j.1467-6494.2009.00597.x.

Kovacs, M. (1992). *Children depression inventory: Manual.* New York: Multi Health System.

Larsen, D., & Stege, R. (2010). Hope-focused practices during early psychotherapy sessions: Part I: Implicit approaches. *Journal of Psychotherapy Integration, 20*(3), 271–292.

Laursen, E. K. (2003). Frontiers in strength-based treatment. *Reclaiming Children and Youth, 12,* 12–17.

Linley, P. A., Nielsen, K. M., Gillett, R., & Biswas-Diener, R. (2010). Using signature strengths in pursuit of goals: Effects on goal progress, need satisfaction, and well-being, and implications for coaching psychologists. *International Coaching Psychology Review, 5,* 6–15.

Lopez, S. J., & Snyder, C. R. (2003). *Positive psychological assessment: A handbook of models and measures.* Washington, DC: American Psychological Association.

Lounsbury, J. W., Fisher, L. A., Levy, J. J., & Welsh, D. P. (2009). An investigation of character strengths in relation to the academic success of college students. *Individual Differences Research, 7,* 52–69.

Lyubomirsky, S., Tkach, C., & DiMatteo, M. R. (2006). What are the differences between happiness and self-esteem. *Social Indicators Research, 78*(3), 363–404. doi:10.1007/s11205-005-0213-y.

Marsh, H. W. (1992). *Self Description Questionnaire (SDQ) I: A theoretical and empirical basis for the measurement of multiple dimensions of preadolescent self-concept. An interim test manual and research monograph.* Macarthur: University of Western Sydney, Faculty of Education.

McCullough, M. E., Emmons, R. A., & Tsang, J.-A. (2002). The grateful disposition: A conceptual and empirical topography. *Journal of Personality and Social Psychology, 82,* 112–127.

Merrell, K. W. (2002). *School social behavior scales* (2nd ed.). Eugene: Assessment-Intervention Resources.

Mongrain, M., & Anselmo-Matthews, T. (2012, March). Do positive psychology exercises work? A replication of Seligman et al. (2005). *Journal of Clinical Psychology, 68,* 382–389.

Niemiec, R. M., & Wedding, D. (2008). *Positive psychology at the movies: Using films to build virtues and character strengths.* Cambridge, MA: Hogrefe.

Ong, A. D., & van Dulmen, M. (Eds.). (2006). *Handbook of methods in positive psychology.* New York: Oxford University Press.

Park, N., & Peterson, C. (2006a). Moral competence and character strengths among adolescents: The development and validation of the values in action inventory of strengths for youth. *Journal of Adolescence, 29*(6), 891–909.

Park, N., & Peterson, C. (2006b). Character strengths and happiness among young children: Content analysis of parental descriptions. *Journal of Happiness Studies, 7,* 323–341.

Park, N., & Peterson, C. (2008). Positive psychology and character strengths: Application to strengths-based school counseling. *Professional School Counseling, 12*(2), 85–92.

Park, N., & Peterson, C. (2009). Strengths of character in schools. In R. Gilman, E. S. Huebner, & M. J. Furlong (Eds.), *Handbook of positive psychology in schools* (pp. 65–76). New York: Routledge.

Park, N., Peterson, C., & Seligman, M. E. P. (2004). Strengths of character and well-being. *Journal of Social and Clinical Psychology, 23*, 603–619.

Pedrotti, J., Edwards, L., & Lopez, S. (2008). Promoting hope: Suggestions for school counselors. *Professional School Counseling, 12*, 100–107.

Peterson, C. (2006). *A primer in positive psychology*. New York: Oxford University Press.

Peterson, T. D., & Peterson, E. W. (2008). Stemming the tide of law student depression: What law schools need to learn from the science of positive psychology. *Yale Journal of Health Policy, Law, and Ethics, 9*(2), 357. Available at: http://ssrn.com/abstract=1277303

Peterson, C., & Seligman, M. E. P. (2004). *Character strengths and virtues: A handbook and classification*. New York/Washington, DC: Oxford University Press/American Psychological Association.

Piers, E. V., & Harris, D. B. (1984). *Piers-Harris children's self-concept scale*. Los Angeles: Western Psychological Service.

Poston, J. M., & Hanson, W. E. (2010). Meta-analysis of psychological assessment as a therapeutic intervention. *Psychological Assessment, 22*, 203–212. doi:10.1037/a0018679.

Proctor, C., Maltby, J., & Linley, P. (2011a). Strengths use as a predictor of well-being and health-related quality of life. *Journal of Happiness Studies, 12*, 153–169. doi:10.1007/s10902-009-9181-2.

Proctor, C., Tsukayama, E., Wood, A. M., Maltby, J., Fox Eades, J. M., & Linley, P. A. (2011b). Strengths gym: The impact of a character strengths-based intervention on the life satisfaction and well-being of adolescents. *The Journal of Positive Psychology, 6*, 377–388.

Rapp, C. A. (1997). Preface. In D. Saleeby (Ed.), *The strengths perspective in social work practice*. New York: Longman.

Rashid, T., & Anjum, A. (2007). Positive psychotherapy for children and adolescents. In J. R. Z. Abela & B. L. Hankin (Eds.), *Depression in children and adolescents: Causes, treatment and prevention*. New York: Guilford Press.

Rashid, T., & Ostermann, R. F. (2009). Strength-based assessment in clinical practice. *Journal of Clinical Psychology, 65*(5), 488–498. doi:10.1002/jclp. 20595.

Reynolds, C. R., & Kamphaus, R. W. (1992). *Behavior assessment system for children*. Circle Pines: American Guidance Service.

Reynolds, C. R., & Kamphaus, R. W. (2004). *Behavior assessment system for children* (2nd ed.). Circle Pines: American Guidance Service.

Rhee, S., Furlong, M., Turner, J., & Harari, I. (2001). Integrating strength-based perspectives in psychoeducational evaluations. *The California School Psychologist, 6*, 5–17.

Richards, M., & Huppert, F. (2011). Do positive children become positive adults: Evidence from a longitudinal birth cohort study. *The Journal of Positive Psychology, 6*, 75–87.

Rust, T., Diessner, R., & Reade, L. (2009). Strengths only or strengths and relative weaknesses? A preliminary study. *Journal of Psychology, 143*, 465–476.

Scheier, M. F., Carver, C. S., & Bridges, M. W. (1994). Distinguishing optimism from neuroticism (and trait anxiety, self-mastery, and self-esteem): A re-evaluation of the life orientation test. *Journal of Personality and Social Psychology, 67*, 1063–1078.

Schmid, K. L., Phelps, E. M., Kiely, M. K., Napolitano, C. M., Boyd, M. J., & Lerner, R. M. (2011). The role of adolescents' hopeful futures in predicting positive and negative developmental trajectories: Findings from the 4-H Study of Positive Youth Development. *The Journal of Positive Psychology, 6*, 45–56.

Seligman, M. E. P. (2002). *Authentic happiness: Using the new positive psychology to realize your potential for lasting fulfillment*. Toronto: Free Press.

Seligman, M. E. P. (2011). *Flourish: A visionary new understanding of happiness and well-being*. New York: Free Press.

Seligman, M., & Csikszentmihalyi, M. (2000). Positive psychology: An introduction. *American Psychologist, 55*, 5–14.

Seligman, M. E. P., Steen, T. A., Park, N., & Peterson, C. (2005). Positive psychology progress: Empirical validation of interventions. *American Psychologist, 60*, 410–421.

Seligman, M. E. P., Rashid, T., & Parks, A. C. (2006). Positive psychotherapy. *American Psychologist, 61*(8), 774–788. doi:10.1037/0003-066X.61.8.774.

Seligman, M. E. P., Ernst, R. M., Gillham, J., Reivich, K., & Linkins, M. (2009). Positive education: Positive psychology and classroom interventions. *Oxford Review of Education, 35*, 293–311. doi:10.1080/03054980902934563.

Snyder, C. R., Hoza, B., Pelham, W. E., Rapoff, M., Ware, L., Danovsky, M., et al. (1997). The development and validation of the Children's Hope Scale. *Journal of Pediatric Psychology, 22*(3), 399–421.

Ungar, M., & Liebenberg, L. (2009). *The Child and Youth Resilience Measure (CYRM) – 28*. Halifax: Resilience Research Center.

Walker, H. M., & McConnell, S. R. (1995). *Walker-McConnell scale of social competence and school adjustment*. Belmont: Cengage Learning.

Wood, A. M., & Joseph, S. (2010). The absence of positive psychological (eudemonic) well-being as a risk factor for depression: A ten year cohort study. *Journal of Affective Disorder, 122*, 213–217.

Wood, A. M., Maltby, J., Gillett, R., Linley, P. A., & Joseph, S. (2008). The role of gratitude in the development of social support, stress, and depression: Two longitudinal studies. *Journal of Research in Personality, 42*, 854–871. doi:10.1016/j.jrp. 2007.11.003.

Wood, A. M., Linley, P. A., Maltby, J., Kashdan, T. B., & Hurling, R. (2011). Using personal and psychological strengths leads to increases in well-being over time: A longitudinal study and the development of the strengths use questionnaire. *Personality and Individual Differences, 50*, 15–19. doi:10.1016/j.paid.2010.08.004.

Xanthopoulou, D., Bakker, A. B., Demerouti, E., & Schaufeli, W. B. (2007). The role of personal resources in the job demands-resources model. *International Journal of Stress Management, 14*, 121–141.

Chapter 7
Gratitude Intervention in Adolescence and Young Adulthood

Nathaniel M. Lambert and Amanda Veldorale-Brogan

7.1 Introduction

Gratitude is a positive emotion of joy or thankfulness in response to receiving a gift or the perception of having benefitted from an intentional, costly, and voluntary action of another person (McCullough et al. 2008). Gratitude can also be conceptualized more broadly to include both the emotion resulting from a specific benefit received (benefit-triggered gratitude), as well as a more general appreciation for the people and blessings of one's life (generalized gratitude; Lambert et al. 2009a). What are the effects of experiencing gratitude from perceived benefits of others and perceived blessings of life?

Gratitude has been associated with many intrapersonal benefits including psychological well-being (Froh et al. 2009b; Wood et al. 2009), enhanced life satisfaction (Froh et al. 2008), greater sense of coherence (i.e., the perception of life as comprehensible, meaningful, and manageable; Lambert et al. 2009c), more optimism, less negative affect (Froh et al. 2008), lower materialism (Lambert et al. 2009b), and less behavioral disengagement, self-blame, substance use, and denial (Wood et al. 2007).

In addition, gratitude yields many interpersonal benefits including creating and sustaining positive social bonds and friendships (Algoe et al. 2008; Bartlett and DeSteno 2006; Emmons and Shelton 2002; Harpham 2004; McCullough et al. 2001), improved social support (Algoe and Haidt 2009; Froh et al. 2009b; Wood et al. 2008), cooperation (DeSteno et al. 2010), enhanced communal strength

N.M. Lambert (✉)
School of Family Life, Brigham Young University, 2065 JFSB, Provo, UT 84604, USA
e-mail: natemlambert@gmail.com

A. Veldorale-Brogan
Department of Family and Child Services, College of Human Sciences, The Florida State University, 120 Convocation Way, P.O. Box 3061, Tallahassee, FL 32306-1491, USA
e-mail: amv08c@my.fsu.edu

C. Proctor and P.A. Linley (eds.), *Research, Applications, and Interventions for Children and Adolescents: A Positive Psychology Perspective*, DOI 10.1007/978-94-007-6398-2_7,
© Springer Science+Business Media Dordrecht 2013

(Lambert et al. 2010), more comfort in voicing relationship concerns (Lambert et al. 2011b), and higher levels of forgiveness (Neto 2007).

7.2 Gratitude Research Among Children and Adolescents

Despite the burgeoning literature on gratitude, little research has been conducted on gratitude in children and adolescents. The extensive gratitude literature and intervention studies among children and adolescents to this point have focused on mental health, academic outcomes, and social integration and have been conducted almost exclusively by Froh and his colleagues.

7.2.1 Gratitude and Mental Health

Froh et al. (2009a) examined the impact of positive affect on the experience of gratitude expression with students aged 8–19. The students were randomly assigned to either a gratitude intervention group or the control group. Those in the gratitude intervention group were directed to write a letter to a benefactor to whom they had never given proper thanks and then read it aloud to that person. The students in the control group wrote about their previous day's activities and how they felt doing them. Students completed these tasks in class for 5 days over a 2-week period. Data were collected at four time points, immediately prior to the students beginning the intervention (T1), at the end of the intervention (T2), and twice more at 1-month intervals (T3 and T4). The authors conducted three hierarchical regressions to determine if T1 positive affect moderated the effects of condition on gratitude, positive affect, and negative affect at T2, T3, and T4. They found that positive affect moderated the effects of the experimental condition on well-being, such that students low in T1 positive affect who received the gratitude intervention reported more T2 gratitude and T2 and T4 positive affect compared with those low in T1 positive affect in the control group.

Aside from positive affect, gratitude has been related to several other mental health outcomes in adolescence. In a cross-sectional study of 1,035 high school students, ages 14–19, Froh et al. (2011) found that gratitude predicts life satisfaction, absorption, social integration, envy, and depression.

7.2.2 Gratitude Predicts Satisfaction with School and Grades

Some research has begun to examine how gratitude may affect satisfaction with school and academic performance. Satisfaction with school is an important outcome among adolescents. In fact, satisfaction with school predicts a number of school-related factors, such as engagement in or withdrawal from school (Elmore and Huebner 2010), grade point average (GPA; Huebner and Gillman 2006), as well as non-school related factors, such as self-esteem, anxiety (Huebner and Gilman 2006), and marijuana use (Hoff et al. 2010). Some intervention research indicates that gratitude can boost satisfaction with school. In a study of 6th and 7th grade students, Froh et al. (2008) examined the impact of gratitude on school satisfaction, psychological, physical, and social well-being. Eleven classes of students were randomly assigned to one of three conditions (gratitude, hassles, or control). Those in the gratitude condition were asked to list up to five things for which they were grateful since the previous day. Those in the hassles condition were instructed to list up to five hassles they had experienced the previous day. The control group had no assignment.

Participants in all three groups completed a battery of measures designed to assess affect, school satisfaction, and life satisfaction. Data were collected daily for 2 weeks, and then at a 3-week follow-up. Pretest data were collected also. Findings showed that, at the 3-week follow-up, the gratitude intervention was related to increased school satisfaction, optimism, and overall life satisfaction. The authors' finding that those in the gratitude condition experienced greater school satisfaction may be particularly important in terms of implications for this research.

Aside from school satisfaction, gratitude apparently predicts GPA. In a large study of 1,035 high school students, ages 14–19, Froh et al. (2011) contrasted the effects of gratitude with materialism on academic functioning (calculated by GPA). They found that gratitude predicted higher GPA and that materialism was negatively related to GPA. The authors suggest that encouraging gratitude may be one method of countering the trend towards juvenile materialism.

7.2.3 Gratitude and Social Relationships

Several studies on gratitude in youth have examined the impact of gratitude on social relationships. In a study of 700 middle school students aged 10–14, Froh et al. (2010) explored how gratitude impacts and interacts with social integration. Social integration refers to the extent that people (in this case youth) are engaged in and attached to various social organizations, such as school or religious groups (Youniss et al. 1997). Data were collected at three time points (initial [T1], 3-months post [T2], and 6-months post [T3]). They found that T1 gratitude predicted T2 prosocial behavior, which in turn predicted T3 social integration. T1 gratitude independently predicted T3 social integration as well. Additionally, they found that T1 gratitude predicted T2 life satisfaction, which predicted T3 social integration. They also found that gratitude and social integration build upon one another, such that greater social integration at T1 is related with increased gratitude at T3, which in turn is related with greater social integration at T3. The researchers suggest that increasing children's experiences and expression of gratitude may be an important component in improving their social integration and life satisfaction.

Froh et al. (2009b) examined the relationship among gratitude and subjective well-being, social relationships, prosocial behavior, physical symptoms, and gender with students aged 11–13. Data were collected at one time point. They found that relational fulfillment (defined as family and friend satisfaction and support) mediated the relationship between gratitude and physical symptoms, such that higher levels of gratitude predicted higher levels of relational fulfillment, which in turn predicted lower levels of physical symptoms. The authors also noted some gender differences. Girls tended to have higher levels of gratitude overall as compared to boys. Additionally, gender moderated the relationship between gratitude and family support, such that the relationship was stronger for boys than for girls. For girls, gratitude had little impact on family support. However, boys' gratitude significantly predicted family support. Gratitude also predicted social integration in a large study of 1,035 high school students' aged 14–19 (Froh et al. 2011).

Thus, a great deal of the foundational work has been done in this area, especially in regards to mental health, academic outcomes, and social relationships. However, much more gratitude research is needed on this age group, particularly in the realm of intervention.

7.3 Gratitude Interventions Among Late Adolescents

As with many topics, little research has been done among adolescents, but quite a large amount of research has been conducted on young adult college students. A large proportion of college students are in fact still teenagers and thus it seems important to at least discuss some of the intervention work that has been conducted among late adolescents. We will describe three types of interventions: counting your blessings through gratitude journaling, sharing your grateful experiences, and expressing gratitude to close relationship partners.

7.3.1 Counting Blessings Interventions

As one form of gratitude, some researchers have examined the impact of counting blessings. The effect on psychological and physical well-being of counting one's blessings was examined in three studies of undergraduate students (Emmons and McCullough 2003). In Studies 1 and 2, participants were randomly assigned to one of three experimental conditions (blessings, hassles, or neutral life events/downward social comparison). Participants were then instructed to keep weekly (Study 1) or daily (Study 2) journals of their moods, coping behaviors, health behaviors, physical symptoms, and overall life assessments, including lists of either blessings, hassles, or neutral events (Study 1) or by listing the ways the participant is better off than others (Study 2). In a third study, participants were randomly assigned to either the gratitude condition or to a control condition that included the same general assessments, but no list. The authors found that, across all studies, the blessing/ gratitude groups exhibited heightened well-being across several, though not all, of the outcome measures (i.e., positive and negative affect, coping and health behaviors, physical symptoms, and overall life assessment), relative to the comparison groups. The effect appeared strongest for positive affect.

Other research has examined the motivational predictors and positive emotion outcomes of regularly counting one's blessings. In a 4-week study with entering college freshman, participants were randomly assigned to perform one of three exercises: counting blessings, visualizing best possible selves, or paying increased attention to life details (Sheldon and Lyubomirsky 2006). Participants completed one of the three exercises during Session I and were asked to continue performing it at home until Session II (2 weeks later) and again until Session III (an additional 2 weeks later). The relationship of these interventions to positive affect and initial motivation was examined. Results showed that the practices of counting blessings and visualizing best possible selves boosted immediate positive affect, as compared to the control condition. Additionally, continued performance of these exercises was needed to maintain the increases. Finally, initial motivation to perform the exercise predicted actual performance and moderated the effects of performance on increased mood. These interventions have been the foundation for several other similar interventions among late adolescents.

7.3.2   Sharing Grateful Experiences

Sharing one's positive experiences has been shown to have positive mental health outcomes (Gable et al. 2004; Langston 1994). In a recent study we (Lambert et al. 2013) wanted to test whether regular sharing of grateful experiences would lead to greater gains relative to typical gratitude journaling in happiness, positive affect, and life satisfaction over the course of 4 weeks. Participants initially completed measures of happiness, positive affect, and satisfaction with life, and were then randomly assigned to engage in one of three experimental conditions: a gratitude sharing condition, a sharing of learning condition, or a gratitude journaling condition. Grateful experiences sharing participants were told to journal their grateful experiences and then to share these experiences with a partner of their choice at least twice a week for 4 weeks.

To ensure that gratitude alone was not driving any effect, one group of control participants wrote about the same gratitude topics twice a week for 4 weeks, but were not instructed to share their thoughts or experiences with anyone else. We also ensured that simply having a regular, positive interaction with someone else was not responsible for any outcome of the study by asking another group of control participants to write about things that they were learning in a class and to share it with someone else twice a week for the duration of the study.

At the end of the 4-week study, those who had shared their gratitude experiences with someone else reported significantly more happiness, positive affect, and life satisfaction than participants in either control condition. Thus, it appears that sharing one's grateful experiences has greater potential to positively affect mental health than simply writing about the grateful experiences.

7.3.3   Expression of Gratitude Interventions

Most gratitude interventions have focused on writing about things for which one is grateful. However, expressing gratitude for what someone else has done can reap enormous relational benefits both for the mental health of the person expressing gratitude as well as for the relationship. For instance, Seligman et al. (2005) asked participants to compose and deliver a letter expressing their gratitude to someone important in their life and those who did so reported fewer depressive symptoms than control participants.

In a recent intervention, late adolescent participants were randomly assigned to write about daily events, express gratitude to a partner, think grateful thoughts about a partner twice a week (to ensure that simply thinking grateful thoughts wasn't driving the effect) or discuss a positive memory with a partner (to ensure that simply talking about something positive with a partner was not driving the effect) for 3 weeks. At the end of the 3 weeks, those assigned to the expression of gratitude condition reported higher positive regard for their friend and more comfort voicing relationship concerns than did those in the other two conditions, even when controlling for the initial reported positive regard and comfort in voicing concerns. Also, positive regard mediated the relationship between experimental condition and comfort in voicing relationship concerns (Lambert et al. 2011b). Furthermore, those who expressed gratitude to a friend reported higher levels of willingness to sacrifice and caring (i.e., communal strength) than those individuals any of the control conditions (Lambert et al. 2010). These intervention studies suggest that expressing gratitude to others is an important way by which individuals can make positive relationship deposits (Lambert et al. 2011a).

Thus a great deal of the intervention-focused work in the gratitude field has been conducted with late adolescent college students. These interventions have primarily focused on gratitude lists, sharing grateful experiences, and expressing gratitude to close relationship partners. These studies ought to be replicated in samples of younger adolescents and perhaps older children.

7.4   Future Directions

Significant work has been done in the new field of gratitude research; however, there are many ways in which methodological improvements could be made. Also, there are potentially very fruitful directions for future research that could yield much needed information, especially in regards to gratitude in children and adolescents.

For instance, little is known about how gratitude develops in children and adolescents, which is crucial for designing future interventions. Also, little is known about gratitude in the parent–child relationship. The differences between generalized gratitude and benefit-triggered gratitude have not been explored in adolescent interventions and neither has the role of gratitude to God been explored. All of these provide potentially fruitful avenues for future research.

7.4.1   Methodological Improvements

Gratitude research has made its mark on the positive psychology movement as well as on the social sciences more broadly. However, much of the current gratitude interventions employ weak control conditions, do not extend beyond self-report, and do not examine mediator or moderators of proposed relationships. Such improvements could drastically improve the contribution of gratitude research to science.

7.4.1.1   The Case for Stronger Control Conditions

Initial experimental studies on gratitude were very important for launching the study of gratitude; however, many gratitude researchers have not moved on from some of the initial, weak control conditions. For instance, in the groundbreaking gratitude intervention by Emmons and McCullough (2003) conducted on young adults included a "hassles" condition in which individuals journaled about the hassles they experienced on a daily basis. The study also included a neutral condition. They found that relative to the hassles and neutral conditions, those who journaled about gratitude showed several improvements in mental health and physical health. Many of the subsequent studies on gratitude have followed this general model in their interventions, which limits what can be inferred. For instance, it could be that any positive action would contrast well with a hassles condition or even with a neutral condition. Future research should seek to answer the question, "is gratitude unique from other positive processes?".

7.4.1.2   The Case for Going Beyond Individual Self-Report

The overwhelming majority of research on gratitude has focused exclusively on one member of the relationship, which provides only one piece in the puzzle. The Actor-Partner Interdependence Model can be used to analyze the interactions between individuals nested within couples and uses the dyad as the unit of analysis (Kenny 1990, 1996; Kenny and Cook 1999; Kenny et al. 2006). Oftentimes the other relationship partner's response is left out or analyzed incorrectly, making this type of statistical procedure very important. Gratitude (when expressed) is oftentimes an interpersonal construct and therefore these types of procedures need to be used more regularly.

Furthermore, intervention research ought to focus more on behavioral outcomes. For instance, videotaping how participants respond in certain situations and then coding their behavior could be a fruitful avenue for future research. In addition, asking participants to sign up to donate time in service could be one way to behaviorally assess prosocial behavior (see Lambert et al. 2012). The *Prisoner's Dilemma* (e.g., Komorita et al. 1991) could be used to behaviorally assess cooperative behavior. These types of behavioral measures can help alleviate some of the bias due to social desirability.

7.4.1.3 Mediators and Moderators

Finally, there is a shortage of studies in gratitude research that answer questions of "how" and "why" by using mediators or that address questions of "for whom" or "under what conditions" by examining potential moderators. Once the main effect of gratitude on another variable is demonstrated, more attempts should be made to answer further questions about how or under what circumstances.

In sum, increased rigor points to the need for adding positive control conditions to experiments to test the unique contribution of gratitude on other variables, inclusion of designs that include more than one person's self-report, and increased investigation of mediators and moderators. Making such improvements will significantly raise the bar for research in gratitude research.

7.4.2 What Develops Gratitude in Children and Adolescents

The majority of research has examined the outcomes and correlates associated with gratitude; however, very little research has investigated how gratitude is developed in children and adolescents. This is potentially a very important topic, because many of the attitudes and behaviors that persist throughout adulthood are set in motion during these early formative years. It is not completely clear whether gratitude is a naturally occurring characteristic or whether it is learned and developed. To what degree can gratitude be taught? What are some of the most important factors that can impact the development of gratitude?

Some research has begun to examine predictors of gratitude. For instance, Lambert and colleagues (2012) found that parental valuing of recreational activities predicted changes in adolescent trait gratitude over the course of 2 years. This effect was mediated by parent–child connectedness. These results seem to indicate that engaging in recreational activities as a family may engender trait gratitude insomuch as engaging in these activities fosters connection with parents.

Given all the positive outcomes predicted by gratitude, parents may be keenly interested in what they might be able to do to raise grateful children. Thus, future research should continue to examine what predicts gratitude in children and adolescents and whether this is something that can be developed.

7.4.3   Gratitude to Parents Intervention

A key relationship in the lives of children and adolescents is the parent–child relationship. Despite the salience of this relationship, existing studies and interventions have barely begun to tap the potential effect of gratitude on parent–child relationships. Many parent-adolescent relationships are characterized by conflict and strife. How might interventions focusing on gratitude expression to a parent help to minimize such contention?

7.4.4   Generalized Versus Benefit-Triggered

Lambert et al. (2009c) provided evidence for two types of gratitude: benefit-triggered gratitude and generalized gratitude. Benefit-triggered gratitude reflects a response to an interpersonal benefit transfer described by many gratitude researchers as the primary definition of gratitude (e.g., Emmons 2004; Roberts 2004), and may be characterized as being "grateful to someone" for some specific benefit provided. Lambert et al. (2009c) found that the layperson also acknowledged a second type of gratitude, termed generalized gratitude, as also appreciating what is valuable and meaningful to oneself, characterized by being "grateful for something or someone," which has been described as appreciation (Adler and Fagley 2005) or transpersonal gratefulness (Steindl-Rast 2004). This could include the grateful feelings one experiences when witnessing a beautiful sunset or when reflecting on the blessings one enjoys, such as good health or supportive relationships. The key difference between these gratitude types is that benefit-triggered gratitude is elicited by a *specific* benefit provided by a *specific* person (e.g., one's spouse performed a needed favor), whereas generalized gratitude is triggered by thinking of things one is grateful for, not provided by a specific person in a specific instance (e.g., "I'm grateful for having good friends"). We propose that, due to the focus on a specific benefit from a specific entity, benefit-triggered gratitude would be more strongly related to feelings of indebtedness and hence reciprocity.

   This distinction is an important one to make going forward with gratitude intervention research as some interventions have focused on benefit-triggered gratitude (e.g., doing something extra to express your appreciation to friends or romantic partners; Lambert et al. 2010, 2011a) and some have focused on generalized gratitude by having people write what they are grateful for more generally (e.g., Emmons and McCullough 2003). We propose that benefit-triggered gratitude is likely to provide a greater benefit for interpersonal relationships whereas generalized gratitude is more likely to promote mental health. However, this and other questions relevant to should be tested by future research

7.4.5   Gratitude to God

Most gratitude interventions to date have focused on the school or college setting, but could gratitude be successfully implemented in a church setting? Might there be any unique contribution of gratitude to God as opposed to other types of gratitude? Gratitude is prized across the major religious traditions of the world (McCullough et al. 2001). Emmons and Kneezel (2005) found that daily gratitude correlated with every one of their 10 measures of religion and spirituality, with r's ranging from .25 to .55 (median $r = .40$). Gratitude to God is intertwined with both the lay experience of gratitude, and the practice of prayer. For instance, when they asked participants to describe prototypical experiences of gratitude, Lambert et al. (2009c) found a high prevalence of spontaneously generated statements of gratitude to God. Despite these links, the phenomenon of expressing gratitude to God through prayer remains largely unstudied. We propose that gratitude to God should uniquely contribute to prosocial behavior.

For instance, perceiving that one is the recipient of freely given blessings from God should inspire motivation to help others as a way to return the favor, leading to increased prosocial behavior. As an example, an individual might think about having wealth and prosperity, which could not only lead to generalized gratitude but also a sense of personal pride in one's good fortune. Conversely, shifting the focus to benefit-triggered gratitude by attributing one's prosperity to God through praying to thank God for bestowing this wealth should trigger a desire to repay God for this blessing by using the wealth to help others. In other words, a focus of God as the source of one's received benefits could lead an individual to perceive oneself as an endowed steward of something that actually belongs to God. A steward is one who administers anything as the agent of another. Thus, rather than feeling grateful for one's good fortune, attributing this fortune to God should facilitate perception of oneself as a steward of a sacred trust. Thus, we propose that gratitude to God provides an additional, unique pathway for enhancing well-being and prosocial behaviors. This could be a fertile avenue for future research and intervention.

7.5   Conclusion

Gratitude research is burgeoning and yet research that focuses specifically on children and adolescents is not keeping up. Nonetheless, there is a strong foundation of intervention research that indicates the effect gratitude has on prosocial behaviors and on well-being. Much needs to be done – yet the future looks bright for research on gratitude in children and adolescents.

References

Adler, M., & Fagley, N. (2005). Appreciation: Individual differences in finding value and meaning as a unique predictor of subjective well-being. *Journal of Personality, 73*(1), 79–114.

Algoe, S., & Haidt, J. (2009). Witnessing excellence in action: The other-praising emotions of elevation, admiration, and gratitude. *Journal of Positive Psychology, 4*, 105–127.

Algoe, S., Haidt, J., & Gable, S. (2008). Beyond reciprocity: Gratitude and relationships in everyday life. *Emotion, 8*, 425–429.

Bartlett, M. Y., & DeSteno, D. (2006). Gratitude and prosocial behavior: Helping when it costs you. *Psychological Science, 17*, 319–325.

DeSteno, D., Bartlett, M., Baumann, J., Williams, L., & Dickens, L. (2010). Gratitude as moral sentiment: Emotion-guided cooperation in economic exchange. *Emotion, 10*, 289–293.

Elmore, G., & Huebner, E. S. (2010). Adolescent's satisfaction with school experiences: Relationships with demographics, attachment relationships and school engagement. *Psychology in the Schools, 47*(6), 525–537.

Emmons, R. A. (2004). The psychology of gratitude: An introduction. In R. A. Emmons & M. E. McCullough (Eds.), *The psychology of gratitude* (pp. 3–16). New York: Oxford University Press.

Emmons, R. A., & Kneezel, T. T. (2005). Giving thanks: Spiritual and religious correlates of gratitude. *Journal of Psychology and Christianity, 24*, 140–148.

Emmons, R. A., & McCullough, M. E. (2003). Counting blessings versus burdens: Experimental studies of gratitude and subjective well-being in daily life. *Journal of Personality and Social Psychology, 84*, 377–389.

Emmons, R. A., & Shelton, C. S. (2002). Gratitude and the science of positive psychology. In C. R. Snyder & S. J. Lopez (Eds.), *Handbook of positive psychology* (pp. 459–471). New York: Oxford University Press.

Froh, J. J., Sefick, W. J., & Emmons, R. A. (2008). Counting blessings in early adolescents: An experimental study of gratitude and subjective well-being. *Journal of School Psychology, 46*, 213–233.

Froh, J. J., Kashdan, T. B., Ozimkowski, K. M., & Miller, N. (2009a). Who benefits the most from a gratitude intervention in children and adolescents? Examining positive affect as a moderator. *The Journal of Positive Psychology, 4*, 408–422.

Froh, J. J., Yurkewicz, C., & Kashdan, T. B. (2009b). Gratitude and subjective well-being in early adolescence: Examining gender differences. *Journal of Adolescence, 32*, 633–650.

Froh, J. J., Bono, G., & Emmons, R. A. (2010). Being grateful is beyond good manners: Gratitude and motivation to contribute to society among early adolescents. *Motivation & Emotion, 34*, 144–157.

Froh, J. J., Emmons, R. A., Card, N. A., Bono, G., & Wilson, J. (2011). Gratitude and the reduced costs of materialism in adolescents. *Journal of Happiness Studies, 12*, 289–302.

Gable, S., Reis, H., Impett, E., & Asher, E. (2004). What do you do when things go right? The intrapersonal and interpersonal benefits of sharing positive events. *Journal of Personality and Social Psychology, 87*, 228–245.

Harpham, E. (2004). Gratitude in the history of ideas. In R. A. Emmons & M. E. McCullough (Eds.), *The psychology of gratitude* (pp. 19–36). New York: Oxford University Press.

Hoff, D., Andersen, A., & Holstein, B. (2010). Poor school satisfaction and number of cannabis using peers within school classes as individual risk factors for cannabis use among adolescents. *School Psychology International, 31*(5), 547–556.

Huebner, E. S., & Gilman, R. (2006). Students who like and dislike school. *Applied Research in Quality of Life, 1*, 139–150.

Kenny, D. A. (1990). Design issues in dyadic research. In C. Hendrick & M. S. Clark (Eds.), *Review of personality and social psychology: Research methods in personality and social psychology* (Vol. 11, pp. 164–184). Newbury Park: Sage.

Kenny, D. A. (1996). Models of nonindependence in dyadic research. *Journal of Social and Personal Relationships, 13*, 279–294.

Kenny, D. A., & Cook, W. (1999). Partner effects in relationship research: Conceptual issues, analytic difficulties, and illustrations. *Personal Relationships, 6,* 433–448.

Kenny, D. A., Kashy, D. A., Cook, W. L., & Simpson, J. A. (2006). *Dyadic data analysis.* New York: Guilford Press.

Komorita, S. S., Hilty, J. A., & Parks, C. D. (1991). Reciprocity and cooperation in social dilemmas. *Journal of Conflict Resolution, 48,* 494–518.

Lambert, N. M., Fincham, F. D., Braithwaite, S. R., Graham, S. M., & Beach, S. R. H. (2009a). Can prayer increase gratitude? *Psychology of Religion and Spirituality, 1,* 39–49.

Lambert, N. M., Fincham, F. D., Stillman, T. F., & Dean, L. (2009b). More gratitude, less materialism: The mediating role of life satisfaction. *The Journal of Positive Psychology, 4,* 32–42.

Lambert, N. M., Graham, S. M., & Fincham, F. D. (2009c). A prototype analysis of gratitude: Varieties of gratitude experiences. *Personality and Social Psychology Bulletin, 35,* 1193–1207.

Lambert, N. M., Clarke, M. S., Durtschi, J. A., Fincham, F. D., & Graham, S. M. (2010). Benefits of expressing gratitude for the expresser: An examination of gratitude's contribution to perceived communal strength. *Psychological Science, 21,* 574–580.

Lambert, N. M., Fincham, F. D., & Graham, S. M. (2011a). Feeling comfortable voicing concerns in a relationship: The role of gratitude. *Emotion, 11,* 52–60.

Lambert, N. M., Fincham, F. D., Gwinn, A. M., & Ajayi, C. (2011b). The fourth pillar of positive psychology: Positive relationships. In K. Sheldon, T. Kashdan, & M. Steger (Eds.), *Designing the future of positive psychology: Taking stock and moving forward.* Oxford: Cambridge University Press.

Lambert, N. M., Brown, P., Coyne, Walker. L., & Fincham, F. D. (2012). Family recreation and gratitude. Unpublished Manuscript.

Lambert, N. M., Gwinn, A. M., Baumeister, R. F., Fincham, F. D., Gable, S. L., Stachman, A., & Washburn, I. J. (2013). A boost of positive affect: The perks of sharing positive and grateful experiences. *Journal of Social and Personal Relationships, 30,* 24–43.

Langston, C. A. (1994). Capitalizing on and coping with daily-life events: Expressive responses to positive events. *Journal of Personality and Social Psychology, 67,* 1112–1125.

McCullough, M. E., Kilpatrick, S. D., Emmons, R. A., & Larson, D. B. (2001). Is gratitude a moral affect? *Psychological Bulletin, 127,* 249–266.

McCullough, M. E., Kimeldorf, M. B., & Cohen, A. D. (2008). An adaptation for altruism? The social causes, social effects, and social evolution of gratitude. *Current Directions in Psychological Science, 17,* 281–285.

Neto, F. (2007). Forgiveness, personality and gratitude. *Personality and Individual Differences, 43*(8), 2313–2323.

Roberts, R. (2004). The blessings of gratitude: A conceptual analysis. In R. A. Emmons & M. E. McCullough (Eds.), *The psychology of gratitude* (pp. 282–291). New York: Oxford University Press.

Seligman, M. E. P., Steen, T., Park, N., & Peterson, C. (2005). Positive psychology progress: Empirical validation of interventions. *American Psychologist, 60*(5), 410–421.

Sheldon, K. M., & Lyubomirsky, S. (2006). How to increase and sustain positive emotion: The effects of expressing gratitude and visualizing best possible selves. *The Journal of Positive Psychology, 1,* 73–82.

Steindl-Rast, D. (2004). Gratitude as thankfulness and gratefulness. In R. A. Emmons & M. E. McCullough (Eds.), *The psychology of gratitude* (pp. 282–291). New York: Oxford University Press.

Wood, A. M., Joseph, S., & Linley, P. A. (2007). Coping style as a psychological resource of grateful people. *Journal of Social and Clinical Psychology, 26*(9), 1076–1093.

Wood, A. M., Maltby, J., Gillett, R., Linley, P. A., & Joseph, S. (2008). The role of gratitude in the development of social support, stress, and depression: Two longitudinal studies. *Journal of Research in Personality, 42,* 854–871.

Wood, A. M., Joseph, S., & Maltby, J. (2009). Gratitude predicts psychological well-being above the big five facets. *Personality and Individual Differences, 46,* 443–447.

Youniss, J., Yates, M., & Su, Y. (1997). Social integration: Community service and marijuana use in high school seniors. *Journal of Adolescent Research Special Issue: Adolescent Socialization in Context: Connection, Regulation, and Autonomy in Multiple Contexts, 12*(2), 245–262.

Part III
Family, Friends, and Community

Chapter 8
Parent-Child Relationships and Well-Being

Shannon M. Suldo and Sarah A. Fefer

8.1 Introduction

Modern parenting often entails a seemingly endless cycle of schedules and concerns, complicated by information overload. Parents are pressured to have their children reading and toilet-trained at near impossible ages, to expose their children to novel and enriching situations (while ensuring the children do not disrupt tranquility at restaurants or on airplanes, of course), to develop an impressive array of extracurricular talents in their young sons and daughters, and to buy "necessities" (e.g., college savings plans, summer camps, gifts for teachers) that require a disposable income level most accessible to households with dual earners. While parents are making difficult choices about how to spend their time and what to sacrifice, they are bombarded with media messages replete with statistics and warnings: an alarming number of youth turn to drugs, drop out of high school, commit crimes, lack empathy, fail to marry before starting a family, etcetera. In a quest to protect children from dismal outcomes, successful parenting turns from fostering excellence to preventing despair. This chapter summarizes the growing body of research finding that happy children have parents who express warmth, care, and support, and spend quality time with their children. Particularly in fast-paced and fear-oriented societies, parents seeking insight about how to raise happy children need to hear the value of relatively simple parenting practices that do not require extensive funds or time. After defining well-being as entailing the presence of positive indicators of psychological functioning, this chapter advances applications and interventions from studies that delineate which aspects of the parent-child relationship co-occur with optimal psychological well-being in children and adolescents.

S.M. Suldo (✉) • S.A. Fefer
Department of Psychological and Social Foundations, University of South Florida,
4202 East Fowler Avenue, EDU 105, Tampa, FL 33620, USA
e-mail: suldo@usf.edu; sfefer33@gmail.com

C. Proctor and P.A. Linley (eds.), *Research, Applications, and Interventions for Children*   131
and Adolescents: A Positive Psychology Perspective, DOI 10.1007/978-94-007-6398-2_8,
© Springer Science+Business Media Dordrecht 2013

8.1.1 Defining Well-Being

The bulk of psychological research has focused on remediating deficits or ameliorating mental health problems. In contrast, researchers and clinicians operating from a positive psychology perspective have sought to understand what contributes to states of optimal functioning. Such a perspective intentionally involves striving for complete well-being that is beyond the asymptomatic or neutral point of existence. Well-being outcomes included under the positive psychology umbrella include subjective well-being (Diener et al. 2009) and other indicators of flourishing (Keyes 2009). Diener and colleagues (2009) define high subjective well-being as "experiencing high levels of pleasant emotions and moods, low levels of negative emotions and moods, and high life satisfaction" (p. 187). As such, happy individuals experience more frequent positive affect relative to negative affect, and judge the quality of their lives to be high in relation to their satisfaction with personally-relevant domains of life. More is known about links between parent-child relationships and the cognitive component of subjective well-being in comparison to the affective component. While subjective well-being (and life satisfaction in particular) is a dominant indicator of well-being, other indicators of wellness and flourishing merit consideration. For instance, Seligman (2002) advances that well-being entails positive emotions about one's past (e.g., gratitude) and one's future (e.g., hope, optimism) in addition to contentment with one's present (e.g., positive affect). Keyes (2009) operationalizes positive mental health as including indicators of social well-being (e.g., positive interpersonal relationships, social contribution, community integration) and psychological well-being (e.g., personal growth, purpose in life, self-acceptance) in addition to emotional well-being (akin to the positive affect and life satisfaction components of subjective well-being). This model yields mental health categories that range from languishing (equivalent to mental unhealth) to flourishing – high hedonic/emotional well-being in addition to positive functioning in more than half of the social and psychological domains. Due to the variety of terms currently available for use when defining youth well-being in a positive manner, the subsequent literature review was intentionally comprehensive and specifies how well-being was operationalized in a given study.

8.1.2 Defining Parent-Child Relationships

The parent-child relationship in relation to child outcomes has most often been studied in terms of behavioral dimensions of parenting practices. As summarized by O'Connor (2002), the dimensions of parenting that have been examined the most include: (a) warmth/support/responsiveness; (b) conflict or rejection; (c) level of supervision and [punitive] control techniques; and (d) autonomy promotion. Overarching parental attitudes and patterns of use of specific parenting practices in combination are reflected in parenting styles. An *authoritative* style, characterized by high parental responsiveness in tandem with high control/demandingness (including firm behavioral control and supervision), is most commonly associated with enhanced competence and reduced psychopathology in youth (Baumrind 1991; Steinberg et al. 2006).

Studies on parenting practices in relation to youth well-being are summarized next. Conclusions from this synthesis should be tempered in light of the following limitations in the extant literature: (a) failure to account for method variance (i.e., few studies that assessed the parent-child relationship and youth well-being via different methods or sources); (b) few studies with young children (most samples include older children or adolescents, or even adults who retrospectively recall parenting, largely due to the current lack of means for assessing well-being among children who do not have the cognitive capacity and/or reading ability to complete self-report rating scales); and (c) proliferation of studies that purport to assess youth "well-being" but instead measure psychopathology, and equate well-being with a lack of symptoms. This misuse of terms is contradictory to studies in the positive psychology literature that demonstrate psychopathology and subjective well-being are not synonymous (e.g., Antaramian et al. 2010; Suldo and Shaffer 2008), and instead both an absence of mental health problems and the presence of well-being are needed to attain optimal outcomes.

8.2 Empirical Links Between Parent-Child Relationships and Youth Well-Being

The family context is a central determinant of subjective well-being throughout the lifespan, including the childhood and adolescent years (Diener and Diener McGavran 2008). For example, a cross-sectional study of 587 American middle school students found that in early adolescence, high life satisfaction was much more tied to positive relationships (in terms of attachment [perceptions of trust, support, care]) with parents than with friends (Ma and Huebner 2008). While high attachment to both sources co-occurred with greater life satisfaction, parent attachment explained 19 % of the unique variance in early adolescents' life satisfaction scores, in comparison to 3 % unique variance explained by peer attachment. Further, peer attachment partially mediated the influence of parent attachment on girls' life satisfaction, with greater parent attachment predicting greater peer attachment, which, in turn, linked to higher life satisfaction. Thus, while adolescents' peer relationships take on significant meaning during youth, relationships within the family set the foundation for the potential benefits of strong friendships on youth well-being.

The strong association between youth well-being and parent-child relationships is robust across cultures. This conclusion is illustrated by a study of 1,034 early adolescents (ages 10–14) from 11 cultures ($n=31$–246 children per country) that evaluated the relationships between children's life satisfaction and their peer and parent relationships, while considering average levels of family values in a given culture (e.g., family vs. individuation orientation; Schwarz et al. 2012). Adolescent life satisfaction was assessed by a 5-item measure of global satisfaction and satisfaction with four domains (friendships, family, school, and health). Zero-order bivariate relationships between these variables in the entire sample suggested that higher life satisfaction co-occurred with higher reports of intimacy with parents (i.e., self-disclosure and open communication in parent-child relationships) and peer acceptance, and particularly with admiration from parents (i.e., feelings of warmth and acceptance). Results of multi-level modeling concluded that whereas the strength of the association between peer acceptance and life satisfaction varied by culture (with a weaker association within cultures that placed greater importance on family values), admiration from parents yielded strong, positive associations with life satisfaction across cultural groups and a positive trend between intimacy with parents and life satisfaction was noted across cultures. Findings led Schwarz and colleagues (2012) to conclude that "parental warmth and acceptance are important for early adolescents relatively independent of the respective cultural values" (p. 72).

In light of the robust link between youth subjective well-being and family dynamics, a logical question is which aspects of the parent-child relationship are most important. Some insight was provided by a qualitative study of 19 youth (ages 12–16) in South Finland, in which participants explained what family factors contribute to their happiness (Joronen and Astedt-Kurki 2005). The researchers identified six themes in children's responses, including that family factors associated with high subjective well-being included: (a) a safe, inviting, and comfortable physical home; (b) family interactions that were primarily harmonious and fun in nature; (c) open communication between family members that engendered trust; (d) high levels of parent involvement and supervision; (e) permission for a child to have a life outside of the family; and (f) child's sense that they were a valued and contributing member of the household. A cross-sectional study of 239 youth (ages 12–17) from the same region confirmed significant associations between adolescent life satisfaction and multiple aspects of family dynamics; specifically, adolescents' perceptions of mutuality (i.e., high perceptions of comfort and support by family members in addition to low feelings of isolation) and stability (i.e., low disorganization) in the family predicted 54 % of the variance in adolescents' life satisfaction (e.g., positive attitudes towards, and joy in, life; Rask et al. 2003).

A review of empirical studies with multiple samples of youth in different cultures concluded that the parenting practices linked to high youth subjective well-being are aligned with an authoritative parenting style (e.g., promotion of psychological autonomy, supervision of youth whereabouts), with a particular emphasis on high levels of warmth, care, and emotional support (Suldo 2009). In contrast, low subjective well-being appears to co-occur with parental over control and punishment, as well as parent-child conflict. These conclusions have been confirmed in research published since that review was written. Case in point, among 448 high school students in China, greater life satisfaction and positive affect co-occurred with higher perceptions of fathers' and mothers' care and emotional warmth, and were inversely associated with youth report of punitive parenting (Yang et al. 2008). In a separate sample of Chinese youth (specifically, 625 children ages 10–18 in migrant families), the parent-child relationship accounted for 15 % of the variance in youth life satisfaction (Wong et al. 2010). Aspects of the relationship that drove the effect were parent-child loving exchanges (i.e., "genuine harmonious displays of love, respect, and understanding between parents and children" p. 152) and companionship (i.e., greater time spent together in structured and play activities). These dimensions emerged as more influential than other family relationship factors such as parent-child conflict and the child's perceived contribution to the relationship. The benefits of positive parenting practices may last into the adult years, as suggested by a study of 984 adult women (in England) who reported greater psychological well-being (i.e., environmental mastery, personal growth, purpose in life, self-acceptance) in mid-life when they recalled their mothers and fathers as demonstrating more care and greater autonomy promotion (lower levels of over control) during their childhood (Huppert et al. 2010).

The simplistic hypothesis that parenting behaviors effect youth may not tell the entire story; longitudinal studies suggest that children's well-being may shape their family experiences. This bi-directionality is illustrated by research with a sample of 819 middle and high school students who rated their life satisfaction and parents' levels of authoritative parenting at two time points separated by 1 year (Saha et al. 2010). Findings included that higher levels of authoritative parenting were correlated with greater youth life satisfaction the following year (specifically, small correlations were associated with parental supervision and autonomy promotion; parent support yielded a moderate correlation). These bivariate correlations are in accordance with the bulk of previous research showing that greater life satisfaction is linked to higher levels of authoritative parenting, experienced either concurrently or earlier in life. However, in regression analyses that controlled for baseline (Time 1) levels of life satisfaction, none of the parenting behaviors at Time 1 predicted changes in life satisfaction. Rather than parenting behaviors predicting changes in life satisfaction, the reverse direction was supported, with baseline life satisfaction predicting positive increases in perceived parental support the following year (Time 2). Thus, child characteristics (life satisfaction) appeared to exert an effect on changes in the parent-child relationship (i.e., parental support) rather than the parent-child relationship predicting changes in child well-being.

Such bi-directionality notwithstanding, positive parent-child relationships appear to exert promotive and protective effects on youth subjective well-being, as illustrated by an ongoing study our lab is completing. In an effort to understand the development of subjective well-being in high school students, we are assessing 500 high school students at two time points separated by a year. Preliminary analyses from the first year of data pertain to the extent to which social support from parents and school sources (teachers, classmates) predicts students' subjective well-being (youth self-reports of life satisfaction, positive affect, and negative affect), as well as may protect students who experience peer victimization (relational and overt bullying) from diminished subjective well-being. Results of regression analyses indicated that students who perceived higher social support from their parents reported the greatest happiness, indicative of a promotive effect of parent-child relations among the general sample of youth (Hoy et al. 2012). Moreover, parent support emerged as a protective factor. Specifically, students with high parent support reported high subjective well-being regardless of the frequency with which they were bullied by peers. In contrast, for students with average and low levels of parent support, increased bullying co-occurred with lower happiness. This buffer effect underscores the importance of positive parent-child relationships to youth subjective well-being.

More research is needed to understand associations between parent-child relationships and indicators of youth wellness beyond subjective well-being, such as positive emotions about the past and future, or evidence of flourishing in the social or academic realms. One notable exception is a recent study of children's hope in relation to the family context (Padilla-Walker et al. 2011). Within a sample of 489 children (ages 9–14), higher levels of child hope were associated with higher levels of children's perceived connectedness to their mothers and fathers ($r = .51$ to .54). This link was important in that high hope, in turn, co-occurred with a host of desirable outcomes, including better school engagement, more kind/prosocial behavior, and fewer symptoms of psychopathology.

8.3 Interventions

One of the primary criticisms aimed at the relatively new field of positive psychology is that "applications are outstripping the science" (Diener 2009, p. 9). Given that research on correlates of youth well-being has lagged behind the corresponding literature on well-being in adults, this caution is particularly relevant to those desiring to implement clinical interventions to promote optimal family functioning (i.e., desirable parenting practices) or youth happiness (e.g., indicators of subjective well-being). In the absence of empirically-supported interventions that improve children's *well-being* by systematically improving parent-child relationships, what we offer instead are (a) logical applications of the existing studies on family correlates of youth well-being, including interventions that target parenting practices as a means to reduce children's mental health problems, (b) recommendations for improving child well-being by targeting parent well-being, and (c) theoretical models of family-focused applications of positive psychology.

8.3.1 Targeting Parenting Behaviors That Link to Youth Well-Being

Whether through systematic prevention efforts, targeted interventions for at-risk families, or provision of guidance to families seeking advice, a reasonable strategy for improving youth-well-being involves increasing families' use of positive parenting practices that correlate with youth subjective well-being. The key parenting behaviors suggested as viable targets through empirical research on correlates include the hallmarks of an authoritative parenting style, including support, supervision, and autonomy promotion (Suldo and Huebner 2004). Public health campaigns that describe and strengthen these parenting practices could constitute a form of universal intervention to improve overall family functioning and impact youth well-being. For example, parents should be informed of the strong associations between adolescents' happiness and their perceptions of emotional support from parents. In becoming motivated to increase their expression of care, warmth, and acceptance to their children, parents may be interested to learn relevant research findings, such as that youth who are bullied experience much lower happiness levels when parent support is low, whereas happiness is generally intact among bullied high school students who are fortunate to perceive high levels of parent support (Hoy et al. 2012).

Evidence of the efficacy of universal guidance on parenting practices that strengthen relationships and improve child outcomes is provided by the public health approach evident in the media-based parent information campaign component of the Triple P – Positive Parenting Program (Sanders 2008). Triple P is a multi-tiered continuum of interventions designed to promote positive parenting and caring parent-child relationships via teaching of relationship enhancement skills (e.g., spending quality time together, providing affection) and behavior management strategies to teach desirable behaviors as well as prevent and manage misbehavior. The media component of Triple P entails the dissemination of effective parenting strategies via a 12-episode television series designed to highlight the importance of healthy family relationships, normalize parenting challenges, model effective parenting, and instill hope for positive change in children's behavior. Compared to a wait-list control group, mothers of young children who viewed the TV series incurred statistically and clinically significant improvements in the frequency of their children's behavior problems, as well as reported greater perceptions of parenting competence; positive changes were maintained at a 6-month follow-up (Sanders et al. 2000).

Families in need of more intensive, psychologist-facilitated interventions due to the presence of family risk factors or child behavior problems can be referred to behavioral parent training programs that focus on decreasing child behavior problems by enhancing parenting practices. In general, the focus is to equip parents with effective strategies for managing child behavior by teaching parents: (a) the common functions of child behavior; (b) methods to minimally attend to negative behavior and praise positive behaviors; and (c) effective strategies for discipline and limit setting. Although the overarching goal of the parent training programs is often to decrease child behavior problems, these interventions are relevant to the current discussion because the parenting practices addressed are also linked to youth well-being. One example of a targeted intervention that teaches effective parenting practices as well as purposefully attends to relationship building is Parent-child Interaction Therapy (PCIT; Zisser and Eyberg 2010). PCIT is a two-stage family therapy program that first trains parents to increase nurturance and spend quality time in play in order to establish a more positive family context, and then provides instruction in parenting practices that prevent and reduce child misbehavior. Abundant research shows positive effects of PCIT on positive parenting practices, such as praise and effective discipline, and improvements in negative child behaviors, such as aggression and defiance (Bagner and Eyberg 2007; Matos et al. 2009).

A more informal way for parents to learn parenting practices likely to promote youth well-being involves self-study of books written for parents that offer research-based practical guidance. Two examples include *Raising Happiness* (Carter 2010) and *The Ten Basic Principles of Good Parenting* (Steinberg 2004), focused on applications of positive psychology and authoritative parenting, respectively. Carter (2010) synthesizes research on many positive psychology topics (e.g., benefits of positive emotions, emphasizing youth kindness and gratitude, mindfulness) as well as authoritative parenting into a relaxed and informal self-help book for parents. Steinberg's (2004) classic book summarizes the fundaments of effective parenting practices, as determined by decades of psychological studies (e.g., research conducted by Baumrind, Maccoby, and Steinberg himself; representative works include Baumrind 1989; Collins et al. 2000; and Steinberg 2001). He relays the importance of parental warmth, involvement and interest, developmentally appropriate limit-setting and autonomy promotion, and avoidance of overly harsh punishment techniques. Optimism for the ability of parents to internalize evidence-based practices via self-study is gleaned from a study that compared the efficacy of three forms of Triple P on preschoolers' behavioral outcomes (Sanders et al. 2007). Sanders and colleagues (2007) found that the lasting improvements in children's behaviors that were evidenced by families assigned to two therapist-facilitated forms of Triple P (Enhanced and Standard Behavioral Family Intervention) were as strong and well-maintained as those improvements seen in families who completed the Self-Directed form of Triple P. In Self-Directed Triple P, parents are provided with a self-help manual that includes 10 weeks of structured learning activities independent of contact with a psychologist or other professional.

As aforementioned, the bulk of parent-focused interventions developed and tested in the twentieth century target effective parenting practices as a means to improve child behavior. An exciting development relevant to the field of psychology involves interventions that target parents' positive mindsets and/or assess change in positive indicators of well-being in establishing intervention effectiveness. Specifically, a growing body of research extends the practice of mindfulness into the context of parent-child relationships. In brief, mindfulness involves attending to the present and intentionally focusing attention on the here and now. As given by Langer (2009), "the mindful individual is likely to choose to be positive and will experience both the advantages of positivity and the advantages of perceived control for well-being" (p. 279). Increased mindfulness in parenting is likely to help parents focus on the present and become attune to their child's emotions, reduce negative (over) reactivity to challenging child behaviors, and enable parents to select more desirable methods of communicating with their children. Mindful parenting entails five key components which overlap with features of effective parenting, including: listening, acceptance of self as a parent and of the child, emotional awareness of self and child, self-regulated parenting, and compassion (Duncan et al. 2009).

Duncan and colleagues (2009) propose that mindful parenting positively influences the parent-child relationship, which in turn leads to decreased problem behaviors and increased positive outcomes in youth.

Regarding empirical support for this model, Singh and colleagues have used single-subject methodology to investigate the impact of training in mindful parenting among families of three children with autism (Singh et al. 2006), four children with developmental delays (Singh et al. 2007), and two children with Attention-Deficit/ Hyperactivity Disorder (Singh et al. 2010). Findings suggest that mothers who participated in 12 weeks of training in mindful parenting reported reduced parenting stress (Singh et al. 2007), as well as increased satisfaction with parenting and parent-child interactions (Singh et al. 2006, 2007, 2010). Although child behavior was not directly targeted, mindful parenting was linked to less child aggression and more appropriate child social interactions with siblings (Singh et al. 2007), as well as increased child compliance with parents' directives (Singh et al. 2010). These authors suggest that training in mindfulness is a wellness-focused alternative to typical behavioral interventions that focus on decreasing challenging behavior (Singh et al. 2007, 2010). Replication of this mindfulness training is encouraged by the developers who provide a detailed intervention outline in an appendix (Singh et al. 2007).

Promising outcomes (including positive indicators of youth wellness) have also been evidenced in mindfulness interventions delivered separately to both adolescents and their parents (Bogels et al. 2008). Specifically, following eight sessions of mindfulness-based cognitive therapy delivered to the families of 14 youth with externalizing behavior problems, parent ratings showed increases in children's self-control and attunement to others, as well as decreased child behavior problems. Adolescents reported increases in happiness and mindful awareness, and fewer externalizing and internalizing problems (Bogels et al. 2008). These effects were maintained at an 8-week follow-up. Because parents and youth both received training in mindfulness, it is unknown whether increased child happiness and other positive gains were an indirect result of mindful parenting or a direct effect of the youth training in mindfulness.

Perhaps the strongest empirical support for the value of increasing mindful parenting practices is provided by a pilot randomized trial investigating a modified version of the Strengthening Families Program for Parent and Youth 10–14 (SFP 10–14; Molgaard et al. 2001) that incorporated brief training in mindful parenting (Coatsworth et al. 2010). A community sample of 65 families with children in 5th through 7th grade were randomly assigned either to traditional SFP 10–14, SFP 10–14 with mindfulness components, or a wait-list control group. The two SFP 10–14 intervention conditions yielded comparable effects on positive parenting practices, including monitoring and rules communication. In line with the model proposed by Duncan and colleagues (2009), SFP 10–14 with mindfulness yielded the greatest influence on indicators of positive parent-youth relationship, and mindful parenting practices mediated this relationship (Coatsworth et al. 2010). The encouraging results of this preventative study with typically-developing early adolescents provide support for the utility of mindful parenting interventions beyond populations of youth with challenging behaviors.

8.3.2   Targeting Parent Well-Being in Light of Links with Child Well-Being

Well-designed studies have established that mental health problems in adults, ranging from maternal depression to parental externalizing behaviors, predict greater psychopathology in their offspring during childhood and adolescence (e.g., Bornovalova et al. 2010; Campbell et al. 2009). A reasonable extension of this research on familial transmission of psychopathology is that parents' and children's well-being is also likely linked. Support for this notion comes from recent studies with children (ages 9–12; Hoy et al. in press) and adolescents (ages 12–17; Casas et al. 2008) that yielded statistically significant, positive associations between children's and parents' levels of life satisfaction. Specifically, Hoy and colleagues (in press) assessed life satisfaction within 150 American families, using psychometrically-sound measures of global life satisfaction appropriate for the developmental levels of the participating children and parents. Children's global life satisfaction was correlated with both fathers' and mothers' life satisfaction ($r = .29$ and .26, respectively). These findings suggesting happier children have happier parents are consistent with findings from Casas and colleagues' (2008) study of 266 Spanish families, in which both parents and children rated their level of satisfaction with the same seven domains of life (e.g., health, relationships, community connection, safety). Children's sum score on this personal well-being index yielded a .19 correlation with their parents' personal well-being index.

In addition to these studies that establish modest but reliable associations between parents' and children's life satisfaction, research on the affective component of subjective well-being affirms that associations between parents' well-being and their children's behavior and well-being are significant and reciprocal. In a community sample of 944 mothers of 2- to 16-year-olds, maternal levels of positive affect linked to child behavior problems indirectly, through maladaptive parenting (Karazsia and Wildman 2009). Specifically, lower levels of positive affect were associated with increases in maladaptive parenting behaviors (i.e., discipline styles that were overly permissive or angry/authoritarian discipline), which in turn predicted higher levels of child behavior problems. A logical, albeit untested, application of these findings is that improvements in mothers' positive affect may result in enhanced parenting, which would be highly desirable in light of the established links between youth subjective well-being and parenting practices characterized by consistent and caring guidance. The associations between parents' happiness and their children's behavior and well-being are likely bi-directional; for example, among parents of children with intellectual disabilities, mothers reported higher levels of positive affect when their children had fewer behavior problems (Lloyd and Hastings 2009). Weis and Ash's (2009) study on parent characteristics associated with improvements in child outcomes further augments the small but growing body of research that supports the value of attending to parents' positive emotions as a viable mechanism for increasing children's well-being. Specifically, among youth in therapy, adolescents' behavioral improvements were in part predicted by caregivers' levels of hopeful-ness and optimism about their child's treatment prognosis. These findings led Weis (2010) to recommend clinicians incorporate hope-focused interventions for parents of child clients. Durand and Hieneman (2008) have also suggested that targeting parent optimism throughout family-based behavioral interventions increases inter-vention effectiveness and leads to greater change in child challenging behavior.

In light of the positive associations between parents' and their children's subjec-tive well-being, attempting to increase parents' happiness may be a logical strategy for improving children's well-being. In contrast to the paucity of empirical support for systematically improving youth happiness, there is a larger body of literature on the efficacy of happiness-increasing strategies for adults. Optimism for a momentous effect of such interventions is tempered in line with such realities as the genetic set-point (i.e., approximately 50 % of happiness is genetically determined and unlikely to change over time, as summarized by Nes 2010) and the hedonic treadmill (i.e., most individuals eventually acclimate to positive changes in their circumstance by returning to their baseline level of happiness; Diener et al. 2006). Nevertheless, a growing number of systematic experiments prove that lasting changes in adults' happiness can be achieved through their active participation in happiness-increasing interventions targeting increased kindness (Buchanan and Bardi 2010), gratitude (Emmons and McCullough 2003), private reflection on past positive events (Burton and King 2008; Lyubomirsky et al. 2006), and visualizing a positive future (King 2001; Sheldon and Lyubomirsky 2006). Given that increased levels of happi-ness as a result of positive activities are tied to higher levels of personal motivation to become happier (Lyubomirsky et al. 2011), clinicians working to improve families' well-being by targeting adults should inform parents of the many benefits of happiness (Lyubomirsky et al. 2005) as well as the links between parents' and children's levels of well-being (Casas et al. 2008; Hoy et al. in press).

8.3.3   Theoretical Models of Family-Focused Applications of Positive Psychology

A hallmark of the positive psychology perspective involves a strengths-based approach to assessment and intervention in clinical contexts. In addition to develop-ing clinical interventions for improving parenting practices and parents' positive emotions, in recent years psychologists have advanced conceptual models for applying a strengths-based approach to work with family units (as opposed to, or in addition to, individual clients). One relevant model is the ecological Family-Centered Positive Psychology (FCPP) approach, as advanced by Sheridan and colleagues (2004; Sheridan and Burt 2009). FCPP merges ideas from positive psychology with ecological and systems theories (Sheridan et al. 2004). Within an ecological perspective, the family context is recognized as a central domain in which children learn and grow. FCPP focuses on enhancing child outcomes by focusing on family strengths and assets, and building family competence. Sheridan and Burt (2009) assert that family members are motivated to work towards the goals that they value and prioritize, thus the FCPP service delivery model addresses family-developed (rather than clinician-created) goals. Key tenets of FCPP include building upon existing family strengths, empowering parents to play a central role in the intervention process, helping families to acquire skills and competencies related to problem-solving, and promoting child and family social supports. A central assumption of FCPP is that families continue to build capacity, grow, and work towards positive change, even after professional consultation has ended, because family members generalize skills gained during intervention to future endeavors (Sheridan et al. 2004). In accord with its positive psychology roots, the FCPP framework acknowledges that it is not adequate to address or solve problems, but rather the focus is on acting proactively to build family assets that can be applied to a variety of future challenges (Sheridan et al. 2004). Sheridan and colleagues (2004; Sheridan and Burt 2009) offer Conjoint Behavior Consultation (CBC) as an example intervention that helps professionals to collaborate and work *with* families rather than *treat* families, as is traditionally emphasized in models of behavior intervention. CBC focuses on collaborating across key developmental contexts for children (home and school) and engaging in problem-solving, intervention implementation, and data collection to address parent and teacher developed goals; caregivers are empowered to promote change within a family while minimizing dependence on outside professionals (Sheridan et al. 2004; Sheridan and Burt 2009). Empirical studies demonstrate that CBC decreases students' challenging behaviors (Sheridan et al. 2001) and empowers parents and teachers (Sheridan et al. 2006). Research is needed to support the viability of FCPP to improve child well-being in general samples.

Conoley and Conoley (2009) propose a model of family therapy that merges positive psychology research, humanistic and solution-focused therapy orientations, and systemic family therapy into an integrated model termed Positive Family Therapy. This model emphasizes that each individual family member influences overall family development, with a focus on moving towards family goals rather than ameliorating problems within the family context. Specific therapeutic techniques emphasized include: finding the strengths of each individual and the family as a whole, linking existing strengths to family goals, circular questioning, therapist as a neutral individual exhibiting unconditional positive regard, parent modeling of positive behaviors, reframing and finding exceptions, the miracle question, as well as paraphrasing and summarizing (Conoley and Conoley 2009). Other positive psychology strategies, such as practicing gratitude, creating closeness through sharing positive aspects of yourself and celebrating successes of others, and practicing acceptance and awareness (in line with mindfulness practices), are suggested as homework for the therapist to assign to families between therapy sessions. The end goal of Positive Family Therapy is to increase happiness among all members of a family. Research is needed to demonstrate successful outcomes of this approach.

8.4 Conclusions

Information summarized in this chapter illustrates the importance of the family context to youth well-being. Given the resources spent preventing maladaptive youth outcomes, it seems possible and prudent to provide parents with the level of support they need to raise children who flourish. Families with high levels of conflict or children with challenging behaviors may need intensive interventions to achieve harmony and wellness. In contrast, families with a healthier foundation may simply need guidance regarding effective, authoritative parenting practices and the importance of attending to all family members' positive emotions. Virtually all families would benefit from encouragement to limit coercive discipline strategies that may appear to achieve immediate results but at the cost of the affection and emotional support that facilitates youth well-being. As such, applied recommendations for psychologists include:

1. Provide information to all families (via summaries of the literature, recommendations for evidence-based self-help books) regarding the importance of positive parent-child relationships and healthy parenting practices.
2. In individual work with youth clients, encourage children and adolescents to invest time and energy into sustaining and improving family relationships, point out ways that parents demonstrate support and warmth, empower youth to seek autonomy in healthy ways, and discuss youth behaviors that elicit positive parenting.
3. When clinically indicated, enroll families in behavioral parent training programs to strengthen the parent-child relationship, shape parenting practices, and improve child behavior; parent-focused interventions that address mothers' and fathers' hope or optimism for change may be particularly effective.
4. Keeping in mind familial links in happiness, aim to improve adults' positive emotions, including via happiness interventions and mindful parenting.
5. Adopt a strength-based approach to child service provision that includes the entire family, empowers parents, and targets goals relevant to the family.

In many ways, the field of positive psychology and the literature specific to healthy families has come a long way in only a few years. But given the fragmented state of the literature and the gaps in existing knowledge, there are many opportunities for seminal contributions to the research base. Recommendations for future research include:

1. Develop a means to reliably assess positive indicators of well-being in young children, in part to permit the extension of research on happy families to include children in preschool and the early elementary school grades.
2. Identify the family correlates of the full range of youth positive emotions, including gratitude, hope, and indicators of psychological flourishing.
3. Through longitudinal studies, determine the contributions of parent and child behaviors, and the wellness levels of each party, to subsequent parent-child relationship quality and well-being levels in parents and children.

4. Empirically illustrate the superiority, or at least the equivalence, of a strength-based approach to youth clinical services with regard to improving well-being and enhancing family functioning, in addition to remediating psychopathology.
5. Develop and evaluate universal interventions that educate parents on effective parenting practices, the value of conveying emotional social support to their offspring, and the short-sightedness of prioritizing risk prevention over wellness promotion when raising children.

References

Antaramian, S. P., Huebner, E. S., Hills, K. J., & Valois, R. F. (2010). A dual-factor model of mental health: Toward a more comprehensive understanding of youth functioning. *American Journal of Orthopsychiatry, 80*, 462–472.

Bagner, D. M., & Eyberg, S. M. (2007). Parent-child Interaction therapy for disruptive behavior in children with mental retardation: A randomized controlled trial. *Journal of Clinical Child and Adolescent Psychology, 36*, 418–429.

Baumrind, D. (1989). Rearing competent children. In W. Damon (Ed.), *Child development today and tomorrow* (pp. 349–378). San Francisco: Jossey-Bass.

Baumrind, D. (1991). The influence of parenting style on adolescent competence and substance use. *The Journal of Early Adolescence, 11*, 56–95.

Bogels, S., Hoogstad, B., van Dun, L., de Schutter, S., & Restifo, K. (2008). Mindfulness training for adolescents with externalizing disorders and their parents. *Behavioural and Cognitive Psychotherapy, 36*, 193–209.

Bornovalova, M. A., Hicks, B. M., Iacono, W. G., & McGue, M. (2010). Familial transmission and heritability of childhood disruptive disorders. *The American Journal of Psychiatry, 167*, 1066–1074.

Buchanan, K. E., & Bardi, A. (2010). Acts of kindness and acts of novelty affect life satisfaction. *The Journal of Social Psychology, 150*, 235–237.

Burton, C. M., & King, L. A. (2008). Effective of (very) brief writing on health: The two-minute miracle. *British Journal of Health Psychology, 13*, 9–14.

Campbell, S. B., Morgan-Lopez, A. A., Cox, M. J., McLoyd, V. C., & National Institute of Child Health and Human Development Early Child Care Research Network. (2009). A latent class analysis of maternal depressive symptoms over 12 years and offspring adjustment in adolescence. *Journal of Abnormal Psychology, 118*, 479–493.

Carter, C. C. (2010). *Raising happiness: Ten simple steps for more joyful kids and happier parents.* New York: Ballantine Books.

Casas, F., Coenders, G., Cummins, R. A., Gonzalez, M., Figuer, C., & Malo, S. (2008). Does subjective well-being show a relationship between parents and their children? *Journal of Happiness Studies, 9*, 197–205.

Coatsworth, J. D., Duncan, L. G., Greenberg, M. T., & Nix, R. L. (2010). Changing parent's mindfulness, child management skills and relationship quality with their youth: Results from a randomized pilot intervention trial. *Journal of Child and Family Studies, 19*, 203–217.

Collins, W. A., Maccoby, E. E., Steinberg, L., Hetherington, E. M., & Bornstein, M. H. (2000). Contemporary research on parenting: The case for nature and *nurture. American Psychologist, 55*, 218–232.

Conoley, C. W., & Conoley, J. C. (2009). *Positive psychology and family therapy: Creative techniques and practical tools for guiding change and enhance growth.* Hoboken: Wiley.

Diener, E. (2009). Positive psychology: Past, present, and future. In S. J. Lopez & C. R. Snyder (Eds.), *Oxford handbook of positive psychology* (2nd ed., pp. 7–11). New York: Oxford University Press.

Diener, M. L., & Diener McGavran, M. B. (2008). What makes people happy? A developmental approach to the literature on family relationships and well-being. In M. Eid & R. J. Larsen (Eds.), *The science of subjective well-being* (pp. 347–375). New York: Guilford.

Diener, E., Lucas, R. E., & Scollon, C. N. (2006). Beyond the hedonic treadmill: Revising the adaptation theory of well-being. *American Psychologist, 61*, 305–314.

Diener, E., Oishi, S., & Lucas, R. E. (2009). Subjective well-being: The science of happiness and life satisfaction. In S. J. Lopez & C. R. Snyder (Eds.), *Oxford handbook of positive psychology* (2nd ed., pp. 187–194). New York: Oxford University Press.

Duncan, L. G., Coatsworth, J. D., & Greenberg, M. T. (2009). A model of mindful parenting: Implications for parent-child relationships and prevention research. *Clinical Child and Family Psychology Review, 12*, 255–270.

Durand, V. M., & Hieneman, M. (2008). *Helping parents with challenging children: Positive family intervention, facilitator's guide*. New York: Oxford University Press.

Emmons, R. A., & McCullough, M. E. (2003). Counting blessings versus burdens: An experimental investigation of gratitude and subjective well-being in daily life. *Journal of Personality and Social Psychology, 84*, 377–389.

Hoy, B., Thalji, A., Frey, M., Kuzia, K., & Suldo, S. M. (2012, February). *Bullying and students' happiness: Social support as a protective factor*. Poster session presented at the National Association of School Psychologists Annual Conference, Philadelphia.

Hoy, B. D., Suldo, S. M., & Raffaele Mendez, L. (in press). Link between parents' and children's levels of gratitude, life satisfaction, and hope. *Journal of Happiness Studies*.

Huppert, F. A., Abbott, R. A., Ploubidis, G. B., Richards, M., & Kuh, D. (2010). Parental practices predict psychological well-being in midlife: Life-course associations among women in the 1946 British birth cohort. *Psychological Medicine, 40*, 1507–1518.

Joronen, K., & Astedt-Kurki, P. (2005). Familial contribution to adolescent subjective well-being. *International Journal of Nursing Practice, 11*, 125–133.

Karazsia, B. T., & Wildman, B. G. (2009). The mediating effects of parenting behaviors on maternal affect and reports of children's behavior. *Journal of Child and Family Studies, 18*, 342–349.

Keyes, C. L. M. (2009). Towards a science of mental health. In S. J. Lopez & C. R. Snyder (Eds.), *Oxford handbook of positive psychology* (2nd ed., pp. 89–95). New York: Oxford University Press.

King, L. A. (2001). The health benefits of writing about life goals. *Personality and Social Psychology Bulletin, 27*, 798–807.

Langer, E. (2009). Mindfulness versus positive evaluation. In S. J. Lopez & C. R. Snyder (Eds.), *Handbook of positive psychology* (2nd ed., pp. 187–194). New York: Oxford University Press.

Lloyd, T. J., & Hastings, R. (2009). Hope as a psychological resilience factor in mothers and fathers of children with intellectual disabilities. *Journal of Intellectual Disability Research, 53*, 957–968.

Lyubomirsky, S., King, L. A., & Diener, E. (2005). The benefits of frequent positive affect: Does happiness lead to success? *Psychological Bulletin, 131*, 803–855.

Lyubomirsky, S., Sousa, L., & Dickerhoof, R. (2006). The costs and benefits of writing, talking, and thinking about life's triumphs and defeats. *Journal of Personality and Social Psychology, 90*, 692–708.

Lyubomirsky, S., Dickerhoof, R., Boehm, J. K., & Sheldon, K. M. (2011). Becoming happier takes both a will and a proper way: An experimental longitudinal intervention to boost well-being. *Emotion, 11*, 391–402.

Ma, C. Q., & Huebner, E. S. (2008). Attachment relationships and adolescents' life satisfaction: Some relationships matter more to girls than boys. *Psychology in the Schools, 45*, 177–190.

Matos, M., Bauermeister, J. J., & Bernal, G. (2009). Parent-child interaction therapy for Puerto Rican preschool children with ADHD and behavior problems: A pilot efficacy study. *Family Process, 48*, 232–252.

Molgaard, V., Kumpfer, K. L., & Fleming, E. (2001). *The strengthening families program: For parents and youth 10–14*. Ames: Iowa State University Extension.

Nes, R. B. (2010). Happiness in behavior genetics: Findings and Implications. *Journal of Happiness Studies, 11*, 369–381.

O'Connor, T. G. (2002). Annotation: The 'effects' of parenting reconsidered: Findings, challenges, and applications. *Journal of Child Psychology and Psychiatry, 43*, 555–572.

Padilla-Walker, L. M., Hardy, S. A., & Christenson, K. J. (2011). Adolescent hope as a mediator between parent-child connectedness and adolescent outcomes. *Journal of Early Adolescence, 31*, 853–879.

Rask, K., Astedt-Kurki, P., Paavilainen, E., & Laippala, P. (2003). Adolescent subjective well-being and family dynamics. *Scandinavian Journal of Caring Sciences, 17*, 129–138.

Saha, R., Huebner, E. S., Suldo, S. M., & Valois, R. F. (2010). A longitudinal study of adolescent life satisfaction and parenting. *Child Indicators Research, 3*, 149–165.

Sanders, M. R. (2008). Triple P – positive parenting program as a public health approach to strengthening parenting. *Journal of Family Psychology, 22*, 506–517.

Sanders, M. R., Montgomery, D. T., & Brechman-Toussaint, M. L. (2000). The mass media and the prevention of child behavior problems: The evaluation of a television series to promote positive outcome for parents and their children. *Journal of Child Psychology and Psychiatry, 41*, 939–948.

Sanders, M. R., Bor, W., & Morawska, A. (2007). Maintenance of treatment gains: A comparison of enhanced, standard, and self-directed Triple P – positive parenting program. *Journal of Abnormal Child Psychology, 35*, 983–998.

Schwarz, B., Mayer, B., Trommsdorff, G., Ben-Arieh, A., Friedlmeier, M., Lubiewska, K., Mishra, R., & Peltzer, K. (2012). Does the importance of parent and peer relationships for adolescents' life satisfaction vary across cultures? *Journal of Early Adolescence, 32*, 55–80.

Seligman, M. E. P. (2002). *Authentic happiness: Using the new positive psychology to realize your potential for lasting fulfillment*. New York: The Free Press.

Sheldon, K. M., & Lyubomirsky, S. (2006). How to increase and sustain positive emotion: The effects of expressing gratitude and visualizing best possible selves. *Journal of Positive Psychology, 1*, 73–82.

Sheridan, S. M., & Burt, J. D. (2009). Family-centered positive psychology. In S. J. Lopez & C. R. Snyder (Eds.), *Handbook of positive psychology* (2nd ed., pp. 551–559). New York: Oxford University Press.

Sheridan, S. M., Eagler, J. W., Cowan, R. J., & Mickelson, W. (2001). The effects of conjoint behavioral consultation: Results of a four-year investigation. *Journal of School Psychology, 39*, 361–385.

Sheridan, S. M., Warnes, E. D., Cowan, R. J., Schemm, A. V., & Clarke, B. L. (2004). Family-centered positive psychology: Focusing on strengths to build student success. *Psychology in the Schools, 4*, 7–17.

Sheridan, S. M., Clarke, B. L., Knoche, L. L., & Edwards, C. P. (2006). The effects of conjoint behavioral consultation in early childhood settings. *Early Education and Development, 17*, 593–617.

Singh, N. N., Lancioni, G. E., Winton, A. S. W., Fisher, B. C., Walker, R. G., Mcaleavey, K., et al. (2006). Mindful parenting decreases aggression, noncompliance, and self-injury in children with Autism. *Journal of Emotional and Behavioral Disorders, 14*, 169–177.

Singh, N. N., Lancioni, G. E., Winton, A. S. W., Singh, J., Curtis, J., Wahler, R. G., et al. (2007). Mindful parenting decreases aggression and increases social behavior in children with developmental disabilities. *Behavior Modification, 31*, 749–771.

Singh, N. N., Singh, A. N., Lancioni, G. E., Singh, J., Winton, A. S. W., & Adkins, A. D. (2010). Mindfulness training for parents and their children with ADHD increases the children's compliance. *Journal of Child and Family Studies, 19*, 157–166.

Steinberg, L. (2001). We know some things: Parent-child relationships in retrospect and prospect. *Journal of Research on Adolescence, 11*, 1–19.

Steinberg, L. (2004). *The ten basic principles of good parenting*. New York: Simon and Shuster.

Steinberg, L., Blatt-Eisengart, I., & Cauffman, E. (2006). Patterns of competence and adjustment among adolescents from authoritative, authoritarian, indulgent, and neglectful homes: A replication in a sample of serious juvenile offenders. *Journal of Adolescence, 16*, 47–58.

Suldo, S. M. (2009). Parent-child relationships. In R. Gilman, E. S. Huebner, & M. Furlong (Eds.), *Handbook of positive psychology in the schools* (pp. 245–256). New York: Routledge.

Suldo, S. M., & Huebner, E. S. (2004). The role of life satisfaction in the relationship between authoritative parenting dimensions and adolescent problem behavior. *Social Indicators Research, 66,* 165–195.

Suldo, S. M., & Shaffer, E. J. (2008). Looking beyond psychopathology: The dual-factor model of mental health in youth. *School Psychology Review, 37,* 52–68.

Weis, R. (2010). Using evidence-based interventions to instill hope in children. In G. W. Burns (Ed.), *Happiness, healing, enhancement: Your casebook collection for applying positive psychology in therapy* (pp. 64–75). Hoboken: Wiley.

Weis, R., & Ash, S. E. (2009). Changes in adolescent and parent hopefulness in psychotherapy: Effects on adolescent outcomes as evaluated by adolescents, parents, and therapists. *Journal of Positive Psychology, 4,* 356–364.

Wong, D. F. K., Chang, Y., He, X., & Wu, Q. (2010). The protective functions of relationships, social support, and self-esteem in the life satisfaction of child of migrant workers in Shanghai, China. *International Journal of Social Psychiatry, 56,* 143–157.

Yang, A., Wang, D., Li, T., Teng, F., & Ren, Z. (2008). The impact of adult attachment and parental rearing on subjective well-being in Chinese late adolescents. *Social Behavior and Personality, 36,* 1365–1378.

Zisser, A., & Eyberg, S. M. (2010). Treating oppositional behavior in children using parent-child interaction therapy. In A. E. Kazdin & J. R. Weisz (Eds.), *Evidence-based psychotherapies for children and adolescents* (2nd ed., pp. 179–193). New York: Guilford.

Chapter 9
Peer Relations

B. Bradford Brown and Michael T. Braun

9.1 Introduction

From the earliest ages of life young people are drawn into relationships with peers. Given the opportunity, even toddlers are inclined to orient towards age mates. This inclination grows through the rest of childhood to become particularly prominent during adolescence, when many adults express fears that peers will rival or surpass adults in their ability to influence the actions and thoughts of young people. Such concerns have some merit, as researchers routinely report that the strongest correlate of deviant behavior among teenagers is the deviance level of their friends (Elliott and Menard 1996). In such research, however, the capacity for peers to exert positive influences or provide health-enhancing resources is often understated or overlooked. In this chapter we will review evidence of the ways in which peers enhance positive youth development in several domains of young people's lives.

Over the course of childhood the peer social world is dominated by dyadic and small-group relationships. Individual friendships tend to be transient and heavily dependent on continued proximity (e.g., sharing the same school classroom or neighborhood) and involvement in shared activities (Berndt and Hoyle 1985). By middle childhood, larger clusters, or friendship groups, emerge. Throughout childhood, membership in friendship groups fluctuates considerably, even month to month, but slowly grows more stable (Cairns et al. 1995).

B.B. Brown (✉)
Department of Educational Psychology, 880A Educational Sciences,
University of Wisconsin-Madison, 1025 West Johnson Street,
Madison, WI 53706-1796, USA
e-mail: bbbrown@wisc.edu

M.T. Braun
Department of Communication Arts, University of Wisconsin-Madison,
821 University Avenue, Madison, WI 53706, USA
e-mail: michaelbraun@wisc.edu

C. Proctor and P.A. Linley (eds.), *Research, Applications, and Interventions for Children and Adolescents: A Positive Psychology Perspective*, DOI 10.1007/978-94-007-6398-2_9, © Springer Science+Business Media Dordrecht 2013

The advent of adolescence changes peer systems structurally and functionally. Growing concern with reputation or status introduces notions of hierarchy both within and among groups, such that some groups have more prestige or authority than others, and within each group a hierarchy of member status or influence can arise as well (Adler and Adler 1998; Dunphy 1963). Groups may take on identity labels (e.g., jocks, brains, loners, Latinos) reflecting normative activities and values expected of group members (Brown and Larson 2009).

Dyadic relationships are transformed as well. Friendships grow more stable and more intense (Berndt and Hoyle 1985), only to yield some of their authority in time to growing romantic and sexual interests that evolve into emotionally intense romantic relationships (Connolly and Johnson 1996). Occasionally, these two types of dyads are counterbalanced by antipathetic relationships involving an aggressor and victim or joint aggressors (mutual antipathies, Witkow et al. 2005). Sibling relationships also evolve over this period, often emerging as highly influential dyadic ties, although usually with a mix of positive and negative elements (McHale et al. 2006).

Collectively, then, young people must learn to navigate a complex peer social system comprised of several types of dyadic relationships and multiple forms of small group interactions. Suffused within these relationships are issues of identity, status, normative expectations, and social acceptance. Different dynamic forces are at work in these relationships and have varying impacts on a young person's development and behavior. Peers may be a source of modeling appropriate attitudes and activities. They may provide instrumental and emotional support, and they may exert direct and indirect pressures to guide behavior choices. They may also serve as buffers to moderate the influence of other forces, including the demands or expectations of parents or other adults and even other peers.

Assessing or even appreciating the full effect of peers on children and adolescents is an overwhelming task, so it is not surprising that, to date, researchers have focused on a narrow set of issues and outcomes. The bulk of evidence considers peer effects on undesirable behaviors such as delinquency, drug use, or dropping out of school. Some investigators have turned attention to more positive peer influences and effects. Their studies have concentrated on five major domains: academic achievement or school engagement, extracurricular participation, behaviors that promote physical and sexual health, prosocial behavior (or the discouragement of antisocial activity), and positive psychosocial adjustment.

We concentrate attention on these five domains, striving to illustrate the many ways in which and conditions under which peers contribute to positive youth development. Our intent is to illustrate the nature of positive peer dynamics through childhood and adolescence, but this should not be construed as an exhaustive analysis of these dynamics. On the basis of our review we offer suggestions for future research and potential applications and prevention/intervention efforts aimed at fostering positive developmental trajectories of young people.

9.2 Academic Orientations and Achievement

The domain with the most extensive evidence of peers' contributions to positive youth development concerns academic achievement and other school related behaviors. Investigators have explored the types of peer relationships and types of influence processes that are most salient in this setting; there is also some indication of the conditions under which peers promote positive academic behaviors.

Although it is common to find that students who do well in school have friends with high academic achievement levels as well, much of this association may be due to youngsters' selection of friends who share their academic orientations, rather than friend influence. Longitudinal studies, however, indicate that friends are a significant source of influence beyond "selection" effects (Cook et al. 2007; Crosnoe et al. 2003). Friend effects may be contingent on the features of the relationship or the context in which it occurs. Altermatt and Pomerantz (2003), for example, found an effect only for reciprocated best friendships, not for unilateral or less salient friendships. Vaquera (2009) found that, especially for Hispanic youth, who are less likely to have close friendships and especially less likely to share the same school with close friends, the mere presence of a best friend in their school boosted their sense of school belongingness, which in turn enhanced academic performance.

One aspect of the effectiveness of friends is the social support that they provide, either to combat a sense of loneliness and social isolation – again, especially among ethnic minority youth (Benner 2011) – or to bolster a young person's sense of academic competence (Bissell-Havran and Loken 2009). Unlike peer achievement levels, which seem to affect an individual's achievement only when the relationship is close and reciprocated, peer support provides a more general effect. Even measures of general peer support (the amount of support a young person feels from peers in general) are associated with high levels of school engagement (Li et al. 2011) and the pursuit of high achievement levels (Wentzel 1998).

The influence of siblings is more difficult to discern because of the numerous features of this relationship that must be considered, including the age difference between siblings, gender composition of the pair, the quality of their relationship, and whether the younger or older sibling is the target of investigation. In a study of Latino adolescents that considered all of these factors, Alfaro and Umaña-Taylor (2010) found gender differences in influence pathways. For girls, having older siblings was associated with higher quality sibling relationships, which in turn was related to stronger achievement levels. For boys, the presence of older siblings also was related to higher quality sibling relationships, but this was related to academic achievement via the support that siblings provided for achievement. A more puzzling set of findings emerged from a sample of African American and European American early adolescents (Bouchey et al. 2010). Increases in the older sibling's level of academic achievement predicted increasingly levels of achievement for the early adolescent. However, the amount of support the older sibling said they provided predicted *lower* levels of achievement for the target child. Likewise, the level of perceived support from the older sibling was inversely related to achievement levels and academic self-concept – but only for mixed sex dyads.

One clue to these findings may lie in the forms of influence that investigators have suggested are typical in sibling relationships. Whiteman and Christiansen (2008) outlined three different types of sibling influences: emulation, in which a child tried to copy the behavior of a sibling, differentiation, in which the child tried to do something different from the sibling to demonstrate that he or she was a separate and distinct person, and example setting, in which the child consciously behaved in a given way to set a good example for a sibling. A subsequent study (Whiteman et al. 2007) added a fourth process: competition, in which one sibling tried to surpass another's achievements in a given domain or behavior. Although this lexicon of influences has not been applied to studies of achievement related behavior, one can imagine how it might differentiate young people who try to match, surpass, or substantially underperform a sibling's achievement level, depending upon the personality characteristics, family dynamics, and relationship features that characterize a pair of siblings.

Moving beyond dyadic relationships, some investigators have considered the role of broader peer group norms on young people's academic behaviors. Wentzel and Caldwell (1997) found that group membership was a stronger predictor of early adolescent school performance than either being highly accepted by peers or having reciprocated friendships. This group effect can be traced to norms about academic achievement that are common within most adolescent groups. Kindermann (1993) reported that although the membership of early adolescent cliques was unstable, achievement norms persisted over time, even as different young people moved in and out of a group. In other words, the group sets achievement standards that are sustained despite group instability; these standards influence group members beyond the effects of individual dyadic relationships. Nevertheless, the group may not be equally influential in all aspects of academic orientations. Ryan (2001) reported that, controlling for factors affecting young people's selection of group affiliations, their group membership was a strong predictor (from fall to spring of a school year) of changes in members' liking and enjoyment of school and their academic achievement levels, but not of the importance they placed on achievement or their expectancies for success in school.

In sum, investigators have consistently found evidence of potential positive influences that peers can exert on young people's interest in and achievement at school. These influences are rooted in both dyadic relationships and broader group affiliations. The strength and nature of such influences are contingent on features of the peer relationship, individuals' backgrounds (such as ethnicity or gender), and the nature of the social context (e.g., location or ethnic composition of the school). As a result, more extensive and systematic exploration of various peer relationships and affiliations is needed to fully understand the dynamics of peer influence in this domain of youths' behavior.

9.3 Extracurricular Participation

School or community sponsored extracurricular activities are generally regarded as healthy pursuits and contexts that promote positive youth development. In truth, activities vary in the degree to which – or at least the consistency with which – they enhance positive development. Certain sports, for example, seem to be associated with both positive and problematic behavior (Blomfield and Barber 2010; Mays et al. 2010). The preponderance of positive outcomes for extracurricular participants has fueled an interest in factors that encourage youth involvement in these activities (Eccles and Templeton 2002). It is conceivable that peers are instrumental in young people's decision to join extracurricular activities, or that pursuing relationships with co-participants serves as an incentive for involvement. It is also possible that the peer relationships occurring within extracurricular activities foster more positive development than relationships pursued outside these activities. In contrast to academic achievement, the research about peer factors is limited in this domain, both in quantity and sophistication. Our commentary must be regarded as speculative.

Blomfield and Barber (2010) assessed correlations among extracurricular involvement, friend characteristics, and outcomes in a sample of Australian youth. Grouping reports of extracurricular participation into five types of activities, the investigators found different peer profiles depending upon type of activity and different ways in which peer factors might account for associations between extracurricular participation and outcomes. For example, whereas those involved in team sports reported more friends who drank regularly, adolescents in individual sports had an unusually high number of friends who did well in school and encouraged them to excel academically as well, and an unusually low number of friends who skipped school. Friends' level of alcohol use mediated the association between participation in team sports and alcohol use; friends' disinclination to skip school mediated the negative association between individual sports participation and truancy. The study did not determine whether or not friends on whom participants reported were activity co-participants, so it is not entirely clear how the activity context figured into peer influences. This shortcoming is common to studies in this domain. In a sample of early adolescent, predominantly African American youth, Wilson et al. (2010) reported that participants in an after-school program who spent most of their time playing football or basketball were less likely to report positive peer influences toward academic achievement than those who selected other types of sports or non-sport activities, but the authors did not ascertain whether or not friends made the same activity selections in the after-school program.

Some indication of the importance of the social atmosphere established in the extracurricular activity comes from a study of sports team participants by MacDonald et al. (2011). Those who reported positive interaction with peers (among other factors) within the sports team reported stronger personal achievement and enjoyment of the activity than those describing a more competitive atmosphere within their team.

As in the academic domain, sibling influences on extracurricular participation are contingent on whether a young person is attempting to emulate, differentiate from, or set an example for a sibling. In Whiteman et al. (2007) study, modeling was common with regard to all types of extracurricular activities, but differentiation was also a frequent motive behind sports participation. Girls were more interested in sports when their older sibling was and they reported influence from that sibling; but this effect was not apparent among boys. A closer analysis of these sibling effects is clearly warranted.

9.4 Health-Enhancing Behavior

In addition to extracurricular participation, investigators have examined the role of peers in promoting two healthy behavior patterns, namely, physical activity and safe sexual practices.

Physical activity level is a strong concern at adolescence because it tends to decline at this age, which can lead to serious weight gains that, in turn, are correlated with other problematic health conditions (Patrick et al. 2004). Sexual activities also grow more salient in adolescence as young people begin sexual relationships and can establish behavior patterns (unprotected sex, sex with multiple partners) that compromise their health.

9.4.1 Physical Activity

It is not surprising to find that physical activity levels of friends are correlated in adolescence because friends are such central activity companions during this life stage. An important question is whether this correlation arises from the inclination to select friends who share one's level of physical activity or from the tendency to be influenced by a friend's activity level. Evidence from one study suggests that both factors are at play. In a longitudinal study of Australian 8th graders, de la Haye et al. (2011) found that young people tend to select peers who share their activity level as friends; but even controlling for this selection effect, friends have considerable impact on changes in activity level. In fact, the friend influence effect was nearly three times as large as the selection effect.

A major component of the influence effect is the degree of support friends provide for physical activity (Duncan et al. 2005; Raudsepp and Viira 2008). Support may take various forms – from encouraging words to joint participation in activities to instrumental assistance that makes participation possible (e.g., driving a peer to sports practice). The importance of these supportive functions has been found in urban as well as rural youth, in children as well as adolescents.

9.4.2 Safe Sex Practices

The question of whether similarities between friends are a function of selection or influence factors also emerges in research on adolescents' sexual practices. Based on two waves of data from the National Longitudinal Study of Adolescent Health, Henry et al. (2007) found that adolescents tend to befriend peers with similar attitudes, but not necessarily similar behaviors regarding sexual activity. Over time, however, friends tend to grow more alike in terms of both sexual attitudes and practices. This convergence can involve movement towards either safer or riskier sexual behavior. Among a sample of economically disadvantaged Belgian 18-year-olds, most of whom were sexually active, friends' positive attitudes toward safe sex practices were associated with higher rates of condom usage (Hendrickx and Hilde Avonts 2008). Similarly, among a sample of Latino youth, Kapadia et al. (2012) reported that perceived peer norms favoring safe sex were associated with higher rates of condom use and lower likelihood of engaging in sex with multiple partners.

The friendship dynamics related to health behaviors can become complicated. In an intriguing study that followed a set of university students before and after spring break trips that featured major partying in resort settings, Patrick et al. (2011) found that friends sometimes made pacts to depart from their normal behavior patterns and get drunk or have more indiscriminant sexual liaisons. The promise that a friend would watch over these activities and not let a person go "too far" actually enhanced risk taking. On the other hand, undergraduates who placed more emphasis on developing a strong friendship network were less likely to venture into health compromising forms of drug use or sexual activity.

Siblings also can play a role in adolescent sexual behavior. In one longitudinal study of U.S. high school youth, Kowal and Blinn-Pike (2004) found that conversations with older siblings about safe sex practices were correlated with enacting these behaviors in sexual activities. Such discussions were more common among adolescents who reported close relationships with older siblings.

A potentially important source of influence missing from most studies to date is a young person's sexual or romantic partner. Here, again, selection factors (choosing to become involved with someone who shares similar attitudes and experiences with safe or riskier sexual practices) are likely to be important, but as relationships develop and sexual interests become more intense, attitudes may change. Do partner influences supersede those of friends or siblings? Are there gender, ethnic, or age differences in the relative weight given to various peer sources? These are questions that deserve more research attention.

9.5 Prosocial Behavior

Counterbalancing the extensive literature on peer influences on antisocial behavior (especially, various forms of delinquency and drug use) is a modest but growing body of work on prosocial behavior. Operationalized in different ways in different studies, this term encompasses such activities as cooperation, sharing, and helping others, but it also refers to peer efforts to discourage or disavow problem behavior (e.g., Maxwell 2002). Unfortunately, many authors fail to specify the items included in their measure of prosocial behavior.

Prosocial peer influences are not uncommon. In fact, when given an opportunity to describe rates of prosocial as well as antisocial peer pressures, adolescents tend to report that peers encourage constructive pursuits (family and peer involvement, doing well in school) to a greater extent than problem behaviors (Clasen and Brown 1985). Investigators also find that young people resemble each other on prosocial traits, although usually to a lesser extent than their resemblance regarding antisocial behavior (Haselager et al. 1998).

In more basic correlational analyses, investigators have found that young people are at lower risk for problem behavior (drug use or deviant activities) when friends have higher levels of prosocial behavior (Guo et al. 2002; Prinstein et al. 2001). Barry and Wentzel (2006) reported longitudinal evidence that friends' levels of prosocial behavior predicted changes in prosocial behavior among a group of mid-adolescents, especially when the friendships were characterized by high quality and frequent interaction. One peer action that may contribute to these behavior patterns is their inclination to intervene when a friend is gravitating toward deviant activity. One-third of the participants in Smart and Stoduto's (1997) sample of Canadian youth reported that they had intervened when friends were contemplating illicit drug use or reckless (drunk) driving; one-half said they would intervene to stop a friend from smoking. Other evidence suggests that the prosocial behavior that friends display has a stronger impact on an adolescent's activities than more direct efforts to encourage prosocial actions (Padilla-Walker and Bean 2009).

Other aspects of the peer system need to be incorporated into studies of peer influences on prosocial behavior. For example, Ellis and Zarbatany (2007) identified the peer group affiliations of a sample of Canadian youth in grades 5–8, and then calculated the status level of each peer group. Members of higher status peer groups displayed greater short-term (3-month) gains in prosocial behavior than individuals in less central groups. Potential influences of siblings also need broader consideration. Padilla-Walker et al. (2010) found that gains in prosocial behavior were directly associated with levels of sibling affection.

9.6   Psychosocial Assets and Adjustment

A final domain in which investigators have explored positive peer influences concerns peers' actions that promote young people's social adjustment or somehow mitigate circumstances that could lead to victimization or emotional maladjustment.

9.6.1   Bolstering Psychosocial Assets

An important way in which peers can promote positive youth development is to enhance psychological traits or social skills that are instrumental in positive adjustment. For example, Brody et al.'s (2003) longitudinal study of African American youth indicated that older sibling competence not only enhances a younger sibling's self-regulation but also promotes higher quality parenting, both of which increase the younger child's social competence. Aikins et al. (2005) noted that young people's capacity to successfully navigate the transition to middle school was enhanced when they had high quality friendships. It is not clear whether the key to these patterns lies in specific actions of siblings and friends or simply the confidence that can be garnered from knowing that peer resources are available if needed.

9.6.2   Diminishing Emotional Distress

Existing evidence also suggests several ways in which peers may prevent or mitigate emotional distress. One way concerns the quality of peer relationships. In a longitudinal study of youth in middle childhood, Richmond et al. (2005) found that as the quality of sibling relationships improved, rates of depression diminished. Another way is through assets or resources that the relationship partner makes available. Wentzel (1998) found that the amount of social and academic support that 6th-grade students felt from peers was negatively associated with levels of emotional distress, and lower distress levels, in turn, were associated with greater academic engagement. Vance et al. (2002) reported that improvement in levels of serious emotional disturbance within a sample of high-risk adolescents was greater among those who indicated greater involvement with prosocial peers (operationalized as peers who stay out of trouble).

Social network size and structure also may be important factors. Erath et al. (2010) used a sociometric procedure to identify the number of reciprocated close and secondary friends in a sample of early adolescents. The number of reciprocated close friendships attenuated the link between loneliness and anxiety for these young people, whereas the number or reciprocated secondary friendships mitigated the negative association between social anxiety and social self-efficacy.

9.6.3   Protecting Against Victimization

In warding off loneliness, anxiety, or internalizing behaviors, peers diminish young people's susceptibility to bullying or aggression because these traits are often used to target victims. Peers also appear to provide more direct protection against victimization. Some researchers have noted a protective function that peers serve. Young people whose physical attributes or emotional characteristics make them prime targets for bullying may escape victimization if they have friends, especially if these friends have the physical ability or social status to ward off peers' aggressive actions (Fox and Boulton 2006; Hodges et al. 1997, 1999). The protective effects of friends are not always observed, however. Perceived social support from friends did not moderate the association between victimization and depression in a sample of British early adolescents (Rothon et al. 2011).

Peers also may compensate for deficiencies in other facets of young people's social network. Schwartz et al. (2000) found that children who grew up in difficult home circumstances (e.g., exposed to harsh discipline, marital conflict, maternal hostility) later experienced higher rates of victimization by peers, but this association was mitigated by the number of reciprocated friendships they displayed – even if they engaged in relatively high rates of aggression toward peers.

As with academic achievement, peer effects on psychosocial adjustment seem to be complicated and not well evaluated. Friends seem to play bolstering and buffering roles; larger peer collectives can insulate young people from victimization that undermines adjustment. The contributions of siblings and romantic partners remain to be examined.

9.7 An Agenda for Research and Intervention

Peers are such a central feature of childhood and, especially, adolescence that it is not surprising to discover a growing literature documenting their significant impact on positive youth development. Yet, existing information still seems disjointed and inchoate. In an effort to encourage a more systematic exploration of peer effects, we offer four suggestions for future research.

9.7.1 Recommendations to Researchers

9.7.1.1 Moving Beyond Friendships

First, the overwhelming emphasis on friendships and friend characteristics in the studies that we located is understandable, given the centrality of this form of peer relationship to most young people. Nevertheless, examination of other aspects of the peer system must be expanded. Sibling ties and romantic relationships are especially under-represented, and studies of group (clique or crowd) dynamics can be expanded as well. Each of these types of relationships offers challenges to investigators. Romantic affiliations tend to be superficial and fleeting until mid-adolescence. Sibling analyses are complicated by issues of birth order, age differentiation, and gender composition. Peer groups are difficult to identify and track over time; they appear to be affected by the added dimensions of general peer status and group authority structure. Even friend influences may vary according to the closeness or longevity of the relationship. Greater awareness of and attention to the particularly salient dimensions of each segment of the peer system will help to clarify the conditions under which peers provide meaningful positive influences.

9.7.1.2 Multilevel Analyses

As a few investigators have already demonstrated, peer relationships are nested within a complex social system. Friendships and romantic relationships are shaped by the norms of peer groups in which the partners reside. A second need is for more nested designs to determine the extent to which the impact of dyadic relationships is shaped by or differentiated from group level influences. Of course, longitudinal designs are more definitive than data gathered at a single time point. A young person's perceptions of friend or group norms may be more influential than actual group norms, but both types of data ought to be explored.

9.7.1.3 Emphasis on Influence Processes

Investigators have already enumerated specific processes underlying peer influences – for example, distinguishing emulation, differentiation, and example setting in sibling relationships, or exploring modeling and normative regulation in friendships. A fuller understanding of various influence mechanisms is vital to the design of effective prevention/intervention efforts because practitioners need to understand not only *who* fosters positive development but *how* they do so. We found hardly any evidence of specific processes within romantic relationships. Modulation of these influence patterns across age and across different stages of relationships also requires attention.

9.7.1.4 Consensus on Defining Prosocial Behavior

Finally, and more fundamentally, it would be helpful to achieve some consensus on the definition and operationalization of "prosocial behavior." Measurement of this term varies from cataloging specific behaviors (cooperation, sharing) to identifying the absence of problematic behaviors (percentage of one's friends who do not use drugs). These very different metrics make it difficult to compare findings across studies.

9.7.2 Implications for Intervention

Attempts to co-opt the peer system for the purposes of prevention/intervention or even enhancement of youth development are fraught with danger because the system is designed, especially in adolescence, to resist subjugation to adult control. There are numerous examples of iatrogenic effects in response to peer based interventions designed by adults (e.g., Dishion et al. 1999; Mahoney et al. 2001). Particularly in view of the limited research to date on positive peer effects, our three recommendations should be considered tentative.

9.7.2.1 Appreciate the Positive Potential of the Peer System

Although the evidence we cite is limited, it indicates remarkable potential for peers to foster positive youth development in numerous ways. Mindful of this, adults should approach the peer system from a positive perspective, seeking to harness the system to support prosocial norms and behaviors rather than attempting to impede the system's inclination to encourage antisocial behavior. The infamous "just say no" campaign is an example of how a fundamental misunderstanding of the peer system can lead to a fatally flawed approach to prevention. On the other hand, efforts to foster prosocial group norms and supportive relationships at the dyadic level appear to be especially useful.

9.7.2.2 Recognize Developmental Dynamics

Just as children and youth grow and change, so do the structure and operation of their peer system. Interventions must be carefully calibrated to the developmental features of dyadic and group relationships. Close friendships take on stronger support functions in adolescence than they manifest in childhood; with age, friendship groups grow more stable. These developmental changes affect the capacities of various facets of the peer system to foster positive development and to respond to adult guidance in this mission.

9.7.2.3 Leave Well Enough Alone

For most young people, the peer system works effectively to promote positive development. It does not require much in the way of adult tampering. This system fosters a variety of positive outcomes, including nurturing youths' desires to assume more responsibility for and autonomy over their affairs. In many cases, the best thing that adults can do is to simply let it be.

9.8   A Closing Caveat

Our mission has been to illustrate the potential of the child and adolescent peer system to foster positive development and to encourage more research from this perspective. Yet, the capacity of peers to be a destructive, health-compromising force in young people's lives cannot be denied. The best approach to research and intervention is the most challenging: to recognize and respect peers' capacity to enhance as well as undermine individual development. Keeping a balanced view should help adults to guide young people to more effective, rewarding relationships with their peers so that these relationships, in turn, can serve the best interests of positive youth development.

References

Adler, P. A., & Adler, P. (1998). *Peer power: Preadolescent culture and identity*. Piscataway: Rutgers University Press.

Aikins, J. W., Bierman, K. L., & Parker, J. G. (2005). Navigating the transition to junior high school: The influence of pre-transition friendship and self-system characteristics. *Social Development, 14*, 42–60.

Alfaro, E. C., & Umaña-Taylor, A. J. (2010). Latino adolescents' academic motivation: The role of siblings. *Hispanic Journal of Behavioral Sciences, 32*(4), 549–570.

Altermatt, E. R., & Pomerantz, E. M. (2003). The development of competence-related and motivational beliefs: An investigation of similarity and influence. *Journal of Educational Psychology, 95*, 111–123.

Barry, C. M., & Wentzel, K. R. (2006). Friend influence on prosocial behavior: The role of motivational factors and friendship characteristics. *Developmental Psychology, 42*, 153–163.

Benner, A. D. (2011). Latino adolescents' loneliness, academic performance, and the buffering nature of friendships. *Journal of Youth and Adolescence, 40*(5), 556–567.

Berndt, T. J., & Hoyle, S. G. (1985). Stability and change in childhood and adolescent friendships. *Developmental Psychology, 21*, 1007–1015.

Bissell-Havran, J. M., & Loken, E. (2009). The role of friends in early adolescents' academic self-competence and intrinsic value for math and English. *Journal of Youth and Adolescence, 38*(1), 41–50.

Blomfield, C., & Barber, B. (2010). Australian adolescents' extracurricular activity participation and positive development: Is the relationship mediated by peer attributes? *Australian Journal of Educational and Developmental Psychology, 10*, 114–128.

Bouchey, H. A., Shoulberg, E. K., Jodl, K. M., & Eccles, J. S. (2010). Longitudinal links between older sibling features and younger siblings' academic adjustment during early adolescence. *Journal of Educational Psychology, 102*(1), 197–211.

Brody, G. H., Kim, S., Murry, V. M., & Brown, A. C. (2003). Longitudinal direct and indirect pathways linking older sibling competence to the development of younger sibling competence. *Developmental Psychology, 39*(3), 618–628.

Brown, B. B., & Larson, J. (2009). Peer relationships in adolescence. In R. M. Lerner & L. Steinberg (Eds.), *Handbook of adolescent psychology* (3rd ed., pp. 74–103). New York: Wiley.

Cairns, R. B., Leung, M.-C., Buchanan, L., & Cairns, B. D. (1995). Friendships and social networks in childhood and adolescence: Fluidity, reliability, and interrelations. *Child Development, 66*, 1330–1345.

Clasen, D. R., & Brown, B. B. (1985). The multidimensionality of peer pressure in adolescence. *Journal of Youth and Adolescence, 14*, 451–468.

Connolly, J. A., & Johnson, A. M. (1996). Adolescents' romantic relationships and the structure and quality of their close interpersonal ties. *Personal Relationships, 3*, 185–195.

Cook, T. D., Deng, Y., & Morgano, E. (2007). Friendship influences during early adolescence: The special role of friends' grade point average. *Journal of Research on Adolescence, 17*, 325–356.

Crosnoe, R., Cavanagh, S., & Elder, G. H., Jr. (2003). Adolescent friendships as academic resources: The intersection of friendship, race and school disadvantage. *Sociological Perspectives, 6*, 331–352.

de la Haye, K., Robins, G., Mohr, P., & Wilson, C. (2011). How physical activity shapes, and is shaped by, adolescent friendships. *Social Science & Medicine, 73*, 719–728.

Dishion, T. J., McCord, J., & Poulin, F. (1999). When interventions harm: Peer groups and problem behavior. *American Psychologist, 54*, 755–764.

Duncan, S. C., Duncan, T. E., & Strycker, L. A. (2005). Sources and types of social support in youth physical activity. *Health Psychology, 24*, 3–10.

Dunphy, D. C. (1963). The social structure of urban adolescent peer groups. *Sociometry, 26*, 230–246.

Eccles, J. S., & Templeton, J. (2002). Extracurricular and other after-school activities for youth. *Review of Research in Education, 26*, 113–180.

Elliott, D. S., & Menard, S. (1996). Delinquent friends and delinquent behavior: Temporal and developmental patterns. In J. D. Hawkins (Ed.), *Delinquency and crime: Current theories* (pp. 28–67). New York: Cambridge University Press.

Ellis, W. E., & Zarbatany, L. (2007). Peer group status as a moderator of group influence on children's deviant, aggressive, and prosocial behavior. *Child Development, 78*, 1240–1254.

Erath, S. A., Flanagan, K. S., Bierman, K. L., & Tu, K. M. (2010). Friendships moderate psychosocial maladjustment in socially anxious early adolescents. *Journal of Applied Developmental Psychology, 31*, 15–26.

Fox, C. L., & Boulton, M. J. (2006). Friendship as a moderator of the relationship between social skills problems and peer victimization. *Aggressive Behavior, 32*, 110–121.

Guo, J., Hill, K. G., Hawkins, J. D., Catalano, R. F., & Abbott, R. D. (2002). A developmental analysis of sociodemographic, family, and peer effects on adolescent illicit drug initiation. *Journal of the American Academy of Child and Adolescent Psychiatry, 41*, 838–845.

Haselager, G. J. T., Hartup, W. W., van Lieshout, C. F. M., & Riksen-Walraven, J. M. A. (1998). Similarities between friends and nonfriends in middle childhood. *Child Development, 69*, 1198–1208.

Hendrickx, K. P., & Hilde Avonts, D. (2008). Correlates of safe sex behaviour among low-educated adolescents of different ethnic origin in Antwerp, Belgium. *The European Journal of Contraception & Reproductive Health Care, 13*, 164–172.

Henry, D. B., Schoeny, M. E., Deptula, D. P., & Slavick, J. T. (2007). Peer selection and socialization effects on adolescent intercourse without a condom and attitudes about the costs of sex. *Child Development, 78*, 825–838.

Hodges, E. V. E., Malone, M. J., & Perry, D. G. (1997). Individual risk and social risk as interacting determinants of victimization in the peer group. *Developmental Psychology, 33*, 1032–1039.

Hodges, E. V. E., Boivin, M., Vitaro, F., & Bukowski, W. M. (1999). The power of friendship: Protection against an escalating cycle of peer victimization. *Developmental Psychology, 35*, 94–101.

Kapadia, F., Frye, V., Bonner, S., Emmanuel, P. J., Samples, C. L., & Latka, M. H. (2012). Perceived peer safer sex norms and sexual risk behaviors among substance-using Latino adolescents. *AIDS Education and Prevention, 24*, 27–40.

Kindermann, T. A. (1993). Natural peer groups as contexts for individual development: The case of children's motivation in school. *Developmental Psychology, 29*, 970–977.

Kowal, A. K., & Blinn-Pike, L. (2004). Sibling influences on adolescents' attitudes toward safe sex practices. *Family Relations, 53*(4), 377–384.

Li, Y., Lynch, A. D., Kalvin, C., Liu, J., & Lerner, R. M. (2011). Peer relationships as a context for the development of school engagement during early adolescence. *International Journal of Behavioral Development, 35*, 329–342.

MacDonald, D. J., Côté, J., Eys, M., & Deakin, J. (2011). The role of enjoyment and motivational climate in relation to the personal development of team sport athletes. *Sport Psychologist, 25*, 32–46.

Mahoney, J. L., Stattin, H., & Magnusson, D. (2001). Youth recreation centre participation and criminal offending: A 20-year longitudinal study of Swedish boys. *International Journal of Behavioral Development, 25*, 509–520.

Maxwell, K. A. (2002). Friends: The role of peer influence across adolescent risk behaviors. *Journal of Youth and Adolescence, 31*, 267–277.

Mays, D., DaPilla, L., Thompson, N. J., Kushner, H. I., & Windle, M. (2010). Sports participation and problem alcohol use: A multi-wave national sample of adolescents. *American Journal of Preventive Medicine, 38*, 491–498.

McHale, S. M., Kim, J.-Y., & Whiteman, S. D. (2006). Sibling relationships in childhood and adolescence. In P. Noller & J. A. Feeney (Eds.), *Close relationships: Functions, forms and processes* (pp. 127–149). Hove: Psychology Press/Taylor & Francis.

Padilla-Walker, L. M., & Bean, R. A. (2009). Negative and positive peer influence: Relations to positive and negative behaviors for African American, European American, and Hispanic adolescents. *Journal of Adolescence, 32*, 323–337.

Padilla-Walker, L. M., Harper, J. M., & Jensen, A. C. (2010). Self-regulation as a mediator between sibling relationship quality and early adolescents' positive and negative outcomes. *Journal of Family Psychology, 24*, 419–428.

Patrick, K., Norman, G. J., Calfas, K. J., Sallis, J. F., Zabinski, M. F., Rupp, J., et al. (2004). Diet, physical activity, and sedentary behaviors as risk factors for overweight in adolescence. *Archives of Pediatrics & Adolescent Medicine, 158*, 385–390.

Patrick, M. E., Morgan, N., Maggs, J. L., & Lefkowitz, E. S. (2011). "I got your back": Friends' understandings regarding college student spring break behavior. *Journal of Youth and Adolescence, 40*, 108–120.

Prinstein, M. J., Boergers, J., & Spirito, A. (2001). Adolescents' and their friends' health-risk behavior: Factors that alter or add to peer influence. *Journal of Pediatric Psychology, 26*, 287–298.

Raudsepp, L., & Viira, R. (2008). Changes in physical activity in adolescent girls: A latent growth modelling approach. *Acta Paediatrica, 97*, 647–652.

Richmond, M. K., Stocker, C. M., & Rienks, S. L. (2005). Longitudinal associations between sibling relationship quality, parental differential treatment, and children's adjustment. *Journal of Family Psychology, 19*, 550–559.

Rothon, C., Head, J., Klineberg, E., & Stansfeld, S. (2011). Can social support protect bullied adolescents from adverse outcomes? A prospective study on the effects of bullying on the educational achievement and mental health of adolescents at secondary schools in east London. *Journal of Adolescence, 34*, 579–588.

Ryan, A. M. (2001). The peer group as a context for the development of young adolescent motivation and achievement. *Child Development, 72*, 1135–1150.

Schwartz, D., Dodge, K. A., Pettit, G. S., & Bates, J. E. (2000). Friendship as a moderating factor in the pathway between early harsh home environment and later victimization by the peer group. The Conduct Problems Prevention Research Group. *Developmental Psychology, 36*, 646–662.

Smart, R. G., & Stoduto, G. (1997). Interventions by students in friends' alcohol, tobacco, and drug use. *Journal of Drug Education, 27*, 213–222.

Vance, J. E., et al. (2002). Risk and protective factors as predictors of outcome in adolescents with psychiatric disorder and aggression. *Journal of the American Academy of Child and Adolescent Psychiatry, 41*, 36–43.

Vaquera, E. (2009). Friendship, educational engagement, and school belonging: Comparing Hispanic and White adolescents. *Hispanic Journal of Behavioral Sciences, 31*, 492–514.

Wentzel, K. R. (1998). Social relationships and motivation in middle school: The role of parents, teachers, and peers. *Journal of Educational Psychology, 90*, 202–209.

Wentzel, K. R., & Caldwell, K. A. (1997). Friendships, peer acceptance, and group membership: Relations to academic achievement in middle school. *Child Development, 68*, 1198–1209.

Whiteman, S. D., & Christiansen, A. (2008). Processes of sibling influence in adolescence: Individual and family correlates. *Family Relations, 57*, 24–34.

Whiteman, S. D., McHale, S. M., & Crouter, A. C. (2007). Explaining sibling similarities: Perceptions of sibling influences. *Journal of Youth and Adolescence, 36*, 963–972.

Wilson, D. M., Gottfredson, D. C., Cross, A. B., Rorie, M., & Connell, N. (2010). Youth development in after-school leisure activities. *Journal of Early Adolescence, 30*, 668–690.

Witkow, M. R., Bellmore, A. D., Nishina, A., Juvonen, J., & Graham, S. (2005). Mutual antipathies during early adolescence: More than just rejection. *International Journal of Behavioral Development, 29*, 209–218.

Chapter 10
The Emotional Warmth Approach to Professional Childcare: Positive Psychology and Highly Vulnerable Children in Our Society

Colin Maginn and R.J. Seán Cameron

Treatment is not just fixing what is broken, it is nurturing what is best. (Seligman and Csikszentmihalyi 2000, p. 7)

10.1 Introduction

In an ideal world, all children would enjoy loving attached relationships with the adults responsible for their care and would lead happy and fulfilling lives exploring, discovering, and learning about the world that they live in and the people they live with. Sadly, not all children are happy: too many do not receive the care and upbringing they need for a fulfilling life, some live in situations which are frightening, painful, and emotionally damaging, and a number have to grow up in environments where they suffer all of these undeserved and life-limiting conditions.

Penelope Leach in her introduction to *The Pledge for Children* touches on society's complacency about this dark side of life for some children:

> … of course we can see our treatment of children as humane and respectful if we compare it with the treatment of children swept around Eastern Europe in an orgy of "ethnic cleansing" or shot as vermin in the streets of Brazil. (Leach 2011)

The ugly truth is that in every town and city in the world, there are children and young people who have been abandoned, rejected, neglected, abused, and exploited: these children do not live in a world of well-being and opportunity, for them, life is a struggle for survival.

In the United Kingdom, we have extensive laws and regulations supported by a small army of lawyers, social workers, foster parents, and residential childcare workers

C. Maginn (✉) • R.J.S. Cameron
Business & Innovation Centre, The Pillars of Parenting,
Wearfield, Sunderland SR5 2TA, UK
e-mail: colinmaginn@pillarsofparenting.co.uk; r.cameron@ucl.ac.uk

C. Proctor and P.A. Linley (eds.), *Research, Applications, and Interventions for Children and Adolescents: A Positive Psychology Perspective*, DOI 10.1007/978-94-007-6398-2_10, © Springer Science+Business Media Dordrecht 2013

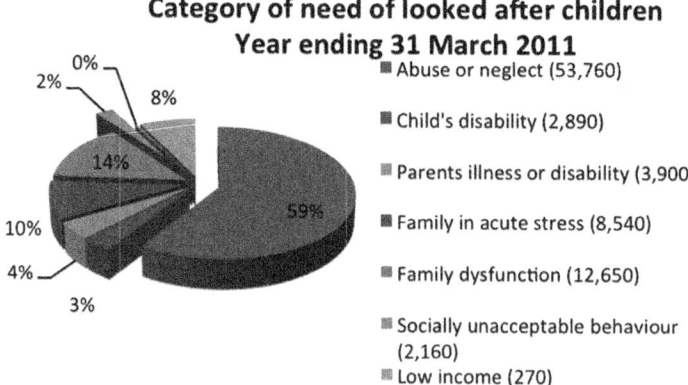

Category of need of looked after children Year ending 31 March 2011

- Abuse or neglect (53,760)
- Child's disability (2,890)
- Parents illness or disability (3,900)
- Family in acute stress (8,540)
- Family dysfunction (12,650)
- Socially unacceptable behaviour (2,160)
- Low income (270)

Fig. 10.1 Department for Education information on the reasons for children and young people being received into public care (Department for Education 2011a. Statistical First Release data. This information can be accessed at: http://www.education.gov.uk/rsgateway/DB/SFR/s001026/index.shtml)

who are employed to safeguard and protect children from harm by ensuring that they have a safe and nurturing place to grow and thrive. In most cases, a child or young person needing public care would be placed with foster parents. In 2011, out of a total of 65,520 children in care, 74 % were in foster homes and just over 10 % were living in children's homes, secure children's homes, and other residential settings (the remainder were living under supervision with parents and close relatives).[1]

While many children and young people have successfully settled into their new homes, there are also some children, whose emotional pain-based behavior has resulted in moves to a succession of foster homes or children's homes. As a result, the psychological trauma resulting from their pre-care neglect or abuse is likely to be compounded by further failed emotional attachments and perceived rejection. Such experiences can be either debilitating for the child or act as triggers for a variety of reactions which range from slow-burning anger to violent and destructive behavior, thereby making it even more difficult to find a permanent home for "the problem child".

This view of the child as "the problem" is endemic within the care system, which has both historical and philosophical roots in a pathogenic paradigm. Historically, the provision of care for needy children in England was left to the church and charities. Charitable giving to the "deserving poor" was formalized by The Poor Law of 1601, an Act of Parliament which placed a duty on parishes to provide for orphans and children in poverty, who were too young to work. Previously, many abandoned, neglected, and abused children had been left to fend for themselves, viewed as responsible for their own situation and therefore "undeserving".

This perception of "feral youth blighting society" still occasionally emerges in the media, yet recent government statistics (Fig. 10.1) show that only 2 % of the children received into care were there primarily because of *their* socially unacceptable behavior, a figure that implies most are there through the faults of others.

---

[1] Department for Education (2011a). Statistical First Release. This information can be accessed at: http://www.education.gov.uk/rsgateway/DB/SFR/s001026/index.shtml.

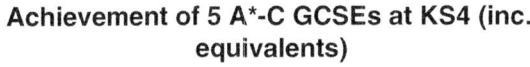

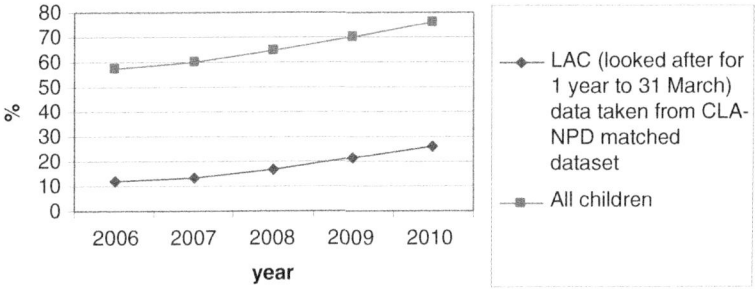

Fig. 10.2 Educational outcomes for children looked after by local authorities in England and Wales matched with data contained within the National Pupil Database (Department for Education 2010; Department for Children, Schools and Families 2008)

10.2   One Big Initiative for Change

For over a decade in the U.K., considerable sums of public money have been directed towards improving outcomes for children in public care, much of this being targeted on what seems like the worthy objective of improving their educational attainments (and hopefully, their life outcomes). While the result has been a modest improvement in the number of young people in public care achieving five A* to C grades at GCSEs (General Certificate of Secondary Education) Key Stage 4, the comparable gains for *all children* have also improved (Fig. 10.2), so not only have the positive outcomes for looked-after children fallen short of what was hoped for, but it could be argued that many of the small improvements which took place in this group might have happened without such a large financial input. Indeed, the number of care leavers who were not in education, employment, or training increased from 32 % in 2010 to 33 % in 2011.

However, low academic attainment is only the tip of the life problem iceberg for children in public care: other life-limiting outcomes in early adulthood can be inferred by the information that some 80 % of *The Big Issue* sellers had been in care; more than a third of young people leaving care were unemployed; half of all prostitutes had been looked after; and up to 50 % of the prison population under 25 had been through the care system. In short, too many care leavers end up homeless, jobless, friendless, and incarcerated.

In their survey of children in care, Blower et al. (2004) concluded that chronic and disabling mental health problems were suffered by a majority of children in their sample and this was despite early recognition of their difficulties, attempts at solutions, and supportive care settings. In a large sample comparison study between looked after children and children living in private households, Ford et al. (2007) found that "children who are looked after by the local authority have a higher prevalence of both psychosocial adversity and psychiatric disorder than the most socio-economically disadvantaged children living in private households..." (p. 323) and concluded that "residential social workers are dealing with many children with serious psychiatric disorders, and yet many have little training or support for the identification and management of these difficulties" (p. 325).

Particularly disturbing was the information gleaned in a survey published in the journal *Community Care* (to which only one third of English councils responded), which revealed that over 2000 children in the care of these authorities had gone missing in 2010 and although most were found within a week, 75 had been missing for more than 3 months, and a further 45 had still not been found (Pemberton 2011). With dismal outcomes like the ones listed above, the population of looked-after children and young people must qualify as one of the most vulnerable in our society today.

Major changes in the public care system are urgently needed but, given the historical context of childcare and some residual and entrenched attitudes to childcare, changing the system is not going to be an easy task, nor is it likely to be achieved quickly. However, there are some reasons for optimism, a report by a cross-party group of members of Parliament reporting in 2009, stated:

> We believe that the greatest gains in reforming our care system are to be made in identifying and removing whatever barriers are obstructing the development of good personal relationships, and putting in place all possible means of supporting such relationships where they occur. (House of Commons 2009, p. 27)

Similarly, the *Children Act 1989 Guidance and Regulations Volume 4: Fostering Services* set out a clear expectation that foster parents would build "long term bonds and attachments" (Department for Education 2011b, p. 16) while the Key Principles and Values section of the *Children Act 1989 Guidance and Regulations Volume 5: Children's Homes* states that "the best outcomes are achieved when the children and young people are cared for by well trained, supportive and actively engaged adults, with whom they can develop appropriate attachments and make positive relationships" (Department for Education 2011c, p. 6).

Advocating the use of positive psychology in residential childcare, Houston (2006) noted that much of the previous work in this area had "fallen prey to a deficit-oriented approach to treatment and therapeutic help" (p. 184). They concluded with the challenging statement: "At the heart of residential care, some might argue, lies a negative mindset..." (p. 198) and that "managers cannot expect their staff to act positively to the young people under their charge if they manage through a negative psychology, one that is critical, risk-aversive, bureaucratically informed, and obsessed with complaints" (p. 198).

Clearly, the childcare profession requires a "mindshift" away from such perspectives as the *problem child* and *keeping a professional distance* stance to one which encourages emotional warmth, accesses professional expertise from psychology, and taps into the healthy strengths, and interests of young people. Childcare needs to reproduce the shift of emphasis, which Seligman and Csikszentmihalyi (2000) achieved from an exclusively problem-focused psychology to positive psychology. Such a mindshift already exists within a minority of highly committed foster parents and residential care staff, who go against the prevailing "risk aversion" and "touch taboo" expectations in social care and who show affection, thoughtfulness, warmth, and kindness to the children in their care: their positive and powerful impact on the children's lives will ripple through future generations and it is from empowering them and modeling their approach that we find the greatest cause for optimism for children in public care. Indeed, the authors are frequently humbled by their selfless dedication to their children and believe that these individuals should be at the forefront of change since they know and intuitively provide what is needed. The task of applied psychologists is to ensure that front line carers and foster parents are supported with the knowledge and skills to see beyond the often-challenging behavior, to increase the likelihood of achieving trusting attachments and the positive life outcomes for young people in their care.

10.3 Achieving the Mindshift: The Emotional Warmth Model of Professional Child Care

In a number of publications over the past 5 years, the authors of this chapter have provided details of a childcare model, designed to empower foster parents and residential child care staff with the psychological knowledge and skills which underpin best practice (see Cameron and Maginn, 2008, 2009, 2011 for the rationale, the processes, and procedures involved in this approach).

The Pillars of Parenting Social Enterprise was set up to inform, train, and support residential and foster carers in their everyday work, which can be both challenging and rewarding. The starting questions were: (a) what are the psychological needs of these children? (b) how can residential and foster carers be enabled to meet these subtle, complex, and often challenging needs? and (c) how can we shift the emphasis in childcare from an overconcentration on young people's problems to an additional focus on their potential?

The *Emotional Warmth* approach, provided by the Pillars of Parenting, offers a systematic approach to professional childcare, that has its roots firmly planted in psychological theory, research, and practice and which enables carers to bring about positive changes in the lives of these vulnerable young people. In brief, there are five important components of the Emotional Warmth approach and these are as follows:

- Empowering carers to support young people in their journey towards *Adaptive Emotional Development* using the three phases of the Cairns (2002) explanation of posttraumatic stress and the carer activities, which support these children and young people through these common post-trauma phases.
- Providing carers with a simple but effective set of strategies which enables them to understand and manage the pain based and frequently-disruptive, self-defeating, and sometimes-violent behavior which children in care often exhibit (see Cameron and Maginn 2009).

- Helping residential carers and foster parents to meet the parenting needs of these children and young people through the eight *Pillars of Parenting* and the accompanying staff support activities, which underpin and support each pillar (see Cameron and Maginn 2009).
- Ensuring that the child can grow and develop emotionally, socially, and academically by teaching carers how to identify a child or young person's *signature (or character) strengths* and helping the child to utilize these effectively in his or her everyday life (cf. Seligman 2002; Linley 2008; Linley et al. 2010; Hooper 2012).
- Providing ongoing advice, support, and training for residential/foster carers in their everyday work by regular consultation sessions led by an experienced applied psychologist (cf. Kennedy et al. 2009).

10.4 Tackling Problems Through the Emotional Warmth Approach

No one working in childcare could ignore the very real problems, which are commonly observed in the looked-after population. The Department for Education and Skills (2001) defined a "mentally healthy individual" as one who can: develop emotionally, creatively, intellectually, and spiritually; initiate, develop, and sustain mutually satisfying personal relationships; face problems, resolve them, and learn from them; be confident and assertive; be aware of others and empathize with them; use and enjoy solitude; play and have fun, and laugh, both at themselves and at the world. Clearly, after missing out on the positive developmental experiences that children require and being subjected to rejection, neglect, and abuse, few looked-after children could claim to have met many (or sometimes, any) of these mental health criteria. Therefore, the first two of the Emotional Warmth components – *support for post-trauma stress* and *the management of self-defeating behavior* – fall squarely into the deficit-orientated approach, the two short sections which follow outline the specific processes involved in the Emotional Warmth approach to these two major problem areas in professional childcare.

10.4.1 Support for Post-trauma Stress

A simplified description of a child's emotional journey through developmental trauma stress has been provided by Cairns (2002) and her work has been extended in the Emotional Warmth model to include the type of support and management required by traumatized children during the period when they are attempting to make sense of the traumatic event(s), which have occurred in their lives (see Table 10.1 for an overview of the three phases of the Cairns (2002) model and a few examples from the menu of carer activities, which can support children and young people through each of these phases).

Table 10.1 The model of trauma and loss, together with some good practice suggestions by carers

Stabilization	Integration	Adaptation
Providing a safe and predictable physical and psychological environment	Aiding a child or young person in the processing of the trauma, i.e., putting the past in its place	Enabling the reestablishment of social connectedness, personal efficacy, and the rediscovering of the joy of living
Some examples of good practice suggested by carers		
Protecting the child from teasing bullying and intimidation	Stressing the normality of feelings associated with previous traumatic events	Helping the child to recognize and accept the changes, which have occurred
Establishing a clear and predictable pattern of daily events for the child	Helping the child to manage post-trauma feelings of shame, guilt and anger	Supporting the child's own efforts to adapt to the changed circumstances
...and others, based on each child's needs	...and others, based on each child's needs	...and others, based on each child's needs

Adapted from Cairns (2002)

The Cairns (2002) overview of post-trauma stress is particularly useful, since it can help residential and foster carers to view a child's often-disruptive behavior within a bigger picture. The model highlights the need to establish a safe and stable environment where the child is able to talk about and learn more about the circumstances surrounding his or her trauma (*stabilization*), to deal with the often-conflicting feelings which accompany such information, to process, control, and manage any resulting psychological or physiological reactions (*integration*), and finally, to receive the type of support which reestablishes social connectedness, develops personal efficacy, achieves a satisfactory level of emotional adjustment to the negative events which have been experienced, and to develop a more optimistic view of the future (*adaptation*).

For each of the three stages of the Cairns (2002) model, there is a menu of post-trauma stress activities, from which the applied psychologist consultant and the carers can discuss, choose or add to and agree, and two or three activities which will provide the most appropriate support for the child through the particular emotional phase, at that point in time. In a children's home, all the carers would agree to carry out these selected support activities when appropriate opportunities present themselves, while foster carer(s) will be able to involve partners, relations and their birth children in these support activities.

10.4.2   Managing Pain Based and Self–Defeating Behavior

In designing their parent-friendly model of behavior management, Westmacott and Cameron (1981) drew upon the considerable body of research in behavioral psychology which showed that disruptive and disturbing behaviors were often initiated and maintained by environmental controlling factors. This way of examining behavior, both functional and dysfunctional, has enabled parents and carers to consider the most likely factors associated with their child's problem behavior and to generate strategies which change some of these controlling conditions, so as to reduce disruptive behavior and to promote positive alternatives. The factors of the ABC (antecedents, background, consequences) approach to behavior management, which can be found in three key areas, are:

A. *Antecedents* (events which precede problem behavior). Such information can lead to strategies for the proactive, preventative management of potentially disruptive behavior.
B. *Background events* (relevant features of the setting or context). Data resulting from an examination of this dimension can be used to create an environment a learning environment which minimizes disruption and encourages positive and adaptive behavior.
C. *Consequences* (those proximal and distal events which follow a problem behavior). A consideration of consequent events can generate more effective and positive adult management of a child's problem behavior, after it has occurred.

The advantage of the ABC model is that it permits an examination of the complex relationship between behaviors (both positive and problematic) and their controlling conditions. This is accomplished by asking parents or carers to keep a record of the antecedents, the background, and the consequences surrounding a particular problem behavior for discussion during a group consultation session. At this meeting, the psychologist consultant can introduce a further element – the *communication function* of the behavior. The key question here is: "what particular need or desire is the child attempting to communicate/convey by his or her disruptive behavior?"

The inclusion of such a cognitive dimension, first advocated by Dreikurs and Soldz as early as 1964, is an important element in the behavior management equation, especially when it comes to understanding and managing persistent, well established, or complex behavior problems which children exhibit (Dreikurs and Soldz 1964). These two theorists had argued that there were at least five commonly occurring messages being communicated through the disruptive behavior of children (and also of adults) namely:

- Obtaining particular objects, situations, or events
- *Seeking attention* (initiating social contact)
- *Attempting to obtain power or/control* (e.g., returning to particular and preferred situations)
- *Wishing to withdraw/escape from a particular situation* (increasing stimulation by escaping from boredom)
- *Seeking revenge* (getting back at someone who has thwarted, refused, or hurt in some way)

Since it represents an extension of the ABC approach, the additional "communication" dimension means that the combined cognitive-behavioral method can be referred to as the *ABCC + model of behavior*. It is this extra *C + factor* which permits a detailed investigation of a child's behavior, which not only illuminates some of the more subtle or difficult to spot antecedents, background events, and consequences surrounding the problem behavior, but can also generate better informed, more sophisticated individual child focused management strategies for reducing the unwanted behavior and/or indicating an alternative or competing response which would reduce the duration and/or frequency of the unwanted behavior.

10.5   The Positive Psychology-Emotional Warmth Connection

Peterson (2006) has argued that positive psychology has three big components: "(a) *positive subjective experience* (happiness, pleasure, gratification, fulfillment), (b) *positive individual traits* (strengths of character, talents, interests, values), and (c) *positive institutions* (families, schools, businesses, communities, societies)" (italics added, p. 20). This framework provides a useful series of links between our Emotional Warmth Model of Professional Child Care and its theoretical antecedents in positive psychology and these will now be discussed.

10.5.1   Positive Subjective Experience and the Pillars of Parenting

The greatest happiness in life, is "to love and be loved" a quotation attributed to George Sands, a nineteenth century author. The word *love* may not be one which is often used in professional childcare – psychologists may refer to "healthy attachments" and the carers may use the term "close relationships" but regardless of the words we use, at the core of human development is the need for a close and warm relationship with a least one other person.

In his hierarchy of needs, Maslow (1971) viewed "belonging" and "love" as being placed after our biological, physiological, and safety needs, however, given recent evidence from the neurobiological sciences, we may need to include love and attachment as one of the basic human needs. Studies from neurological brain scans point to the conclusion that being "securely attached" to a protective adult is not just "nice" but that such attachments are essential for a child's emotional survival. It appears that our brains are "hard wired" to maintain these emotional attachments and that separation and rejection by loved ones on whom we depend, will cause the same reactions in the brain as physical pain. Lieberman and Eisenberger (2009) reported this phenomenon in *Science* magazine, explaining that "for both caregiver and infant to feel pain upon separation ensures social connection and thus offspring survival" (p. 891).

Viewed from this cognitive-neuropsychology perspective, it would be true to say that just as vital as food and shelter, an important task of professional care is to ensure that each child has the subjective experience of feeling wanted, valued, listened to…and of course, loved. The joint NICE/SCIE (National Institute for Health and Clinical Excellence/Social Care Institute for Excellence 2010) guidelines on promoting the quality of life of looked-after children, highlights this perspective of good childcare by stating: "The child's need to be loved and nurtured is fundamental to achieving long-term physical, mental and emotional wellbeing." (p. 9). The challenge for the care profession is how to turn this laudable aspiration into everyday practice, and the Emotional Warmth Model of Professional Child Care sets out to meet this challenge (see Cameron and Maginn 2011).

10.5.2   The Pillars of Parenting

To achieve such a mindshift we need long-term thinking and action, and a rejection of the coldness of those childcare practices which result from currently-employed, professional concepts, such as "looked after" and "caring" for a much-needed emphasis on "parenting". Professional parenting involves a long-term commitment and a task which cannot be left to trial and error: the skills and knowledge required need to be unpacked, analyzed, understood, and implemented, often in difficult circumstances.

The eight Pillars of Parenting, which are illustrated in Table 10.2 are closely linked with underpinning research from the psychology knowledge base and also represent a thoughtful answer to the question, "What would a good parent do?" When planning a program designed to meet a child's parenting needs, the psychologist consultant and the group of foster parents or residential carers would select the pillar which is most likely to meet the child or young person's priority parenting need at that particular point in time. For each of the eight pillars, there is a menu of parenting activities, from which carers can use their detailed knowledge of a young person to choose the two or three activities: these will then be implemented by everyone concerned to provide the most appropriate support the child in the particular pillar (see Table 10.2).

10.5.3   Positive Individual Traits

Seligman (2002) believes that each person possesses several *signature strengths*, which are those strengths of character that a person self-consciously owns, celebrates and (if he or she can) incorporates into everyday activities like maintaining relationships, work, and leisure. The full list of signature strengths (which includes obvious contenders like a love of learning, a sense of fairness, the ability to use humor in everyday life, and enthusiasm) can be found in Seligman's (2002) book, but some of the less obvious ones, which may apply particularly to children in public care have been set out in Table 10.3.

We have consistently found that the awareness and insights gained from the *Realise 2* workshop are transferred and applied by foster parents and residential carers

Table 10.3 A sample of the many possible signature/character strengths of young people

Oodles of Energy	*Creativity*
I like to be up and doing	I can often think outside the box
I can work hard on tasks I like doing	I can usually come up with a good idea
Total Commitment	*Empathy*
If I say I will do something, I will	I usually understand how people feel
I like to see a task through until it's done	I feel deeply for the problems of others
Passion	*Flexibility*
I feel very strongly about certain issues	I can adapt to most situations
I want to change things that I feel are wrong	I enjoy trying out new things
Anticipation	*Friendship*
I look forward to good things in my life	I can make friends easily
I can also solve problems	I can keep friends
Trust	*Loyalty*
I can trust all my friends and family	I stick by friends and family
People trust me	My friends/family stick by me: I stick by them

Collated by Dr. Sean Cameron from suggestions made by the Doctorate in Educational and Child Psychology course members at the University of East London and University College London (December 2009) ©Pillars of Parenting Social Enterprise

to uncover the often-hidden character strengths in the children and young people in their care. When this happens, children feel valued because their strengths skills and talents are noticed, using their strengths is energizing, life becomes more fun, pleasure is gained from spending time doing the things which they enjoy and when an element of difficulty or challenge is added to the activity, successful mastering of the game, task or activity can lead to spontaneous feeling of joy and the experience of optimal experience/flow as described by Csikszentmihalyi (1990).

Having identified the character strengths of individual children and young people in their care, the psychologist consultant and the group of residential carers or foster carer(s) can discuss how to provide opportunities (or to be on the lookout for appropriate windows of opportunity) which allow the child or young person to employ their signature strengths and to enjoy the experience of just how powerful their character strengths can be.

As part of the Pillars of Parenting on-going professional development program, residential and foster carers complete the on-line, *Realise2* strengths assessment, designed by the Centre of Applied Positive Psychology in Coventry (http://www.cappeu.com). The report generated by the assessment, details an individual's: "Realised Strengths"; their "Learned Behaviours" (those skills which do not come naturally but have had to be acquired through considerable practice); their "Weaknesses"; and their "Unrealised Strengths". This assessment gives carers and foster parents the personal and professional information on what they are good at and helps them to appreciate what gives them energy and joy in life. Such information can encourage insights on how to maximize and utilize their individual unrealized strengths and those of the work or support teams.

10.6 Positive Children's Homes and Families

Central government has high expectations about everyone who works with children and young people: they should be ambitious for the child, excellent in their practice, committed to partnership and integrated working, and respected and valued as individuals (Department for Children, Schools and Families 2008). The contribution of those carers, who are working directly with children, is central to the smooth implementation of the Emotional Warmth model described in this chapter, so training, monitoring, and supporting the work of the carers all become organizational priorities. To tackle the twin challenges of providing emotional warmth in their encounters with traumatized children and also enabling a child to move through the bereavement and loss process, residential and foster carers require a combination of personal skills and informed professional expertise. They also need to be resilient and have strong beliefs about the importance of their work; it is not for nothing that Cairns (2002) cautions people not to get involved with children in public care, unless they are prepared to be committed.

While the carers of looked-after children possess detailed knowledge about the child, they also require the most recent information from the knowledge base in psychology to provide them with insight into the complex problems faced by their children, together with the sophisticated strategies required to them to manage these problems. The Emotional Warmth approach provides these key components of professional childcare through a two-pronged program of carer support.

In the first place, carers have immediate access to the knowledge base of psychology through regular child-focused consultations with an experienced consultant psychologist. The protocol for such consultation sessions, which leads to a written and shared individual plan designed to meet the child's personal, social, learning, and development needs can be found in Table 10.4.

Secondly, the on-the-spot learning which occurs in these consultation sessions is consolidated through a continuing professional development program which illuminates their everyday work with the theory, research, and practice underpinning the Emotional Warmth model.

10.6.1 Broaden and Build Inquiry

Identifying, supporting, and ensuring that "positive institutions" flourish, is integral to maintaining the "emotional warmth practice model". The Broaden and Build Appreciative Inquiry approach is used to provide a valuing, informative, and objective report which focuses on: (a) what is going well within the organization and will support the introduction and maintenance of the Emotional Warmth approach; and (b) any areas which could benefit from thoughtful consideration and future development or improvement.

Table 10.4 Protocol for consultation session with an applied psychologist and residential of foster carers' team

Tasks for the psychologist consultant during a group consultation session
1. *Discussion of big and modest successes achieved by staff since the last consultation session*
2. *Update on previous child or young person discussed*
3. *Discussion of management problems of today's child*
Pen portrait of the child or young person
Thumbnail outline of the child's problem(s) and discussion of the ABC and + C factors involved
Changing key ABC factors and teaching new + C skills
Agreed action strategies for management and support
Plan for implementation, monitoring, and evaluation
Summary of agreed action
4. *Discussion and identification of the child's current parenting needs* (using the Pillars of Parenting list and selecting from the staff support activities menu)
5. *Discussion and identification of the child's post-trauma emotional needs* (using the Adaptive Emotional Development model and the menu of staff support activities menu)
6. *Discussion of child's strengths and talents and consideration of the learning opportunities that can arise from these*
7. *Meta-analysis of the session* (reflecting on the process of the consultation process)

The Broaden and Build Appreciative Inquiry approach concentrates mainly on the psychological needs of the child or young person in care, the assumption being that other prerequisites, such as care and protection, are already in place. The report is designed to highlight the key organizational features of a successful residential home (cf. Anglin 2002) and is divided into three main areas:

1. Creating a family living environment *while removing the emotional intensity and negativity of the original family.*
2. Responding to the trauma-based behavior.
3. Developing a sense of normality, security, and belonging *in the new home.*

Since effective leadership in children's homes has been specifically linked with improved outcomes of the young people (see Clough et al. 2006; Hicks et al. 2007), quality of leadership is also considered. As a best practice model of "collaborative team functioning" we have adapted the findings from the large-scale LaFasto and Larson (2001) study to identify the most important tasks that effective team leaders perform. These six behaviors are listed below:

1. Keeps the team focused on the goal
2. Maintains a collaborative climate
3. Builds confidence among members
4. Demonstrates technical competence
5. Sets priorities
6. Manages staff performance

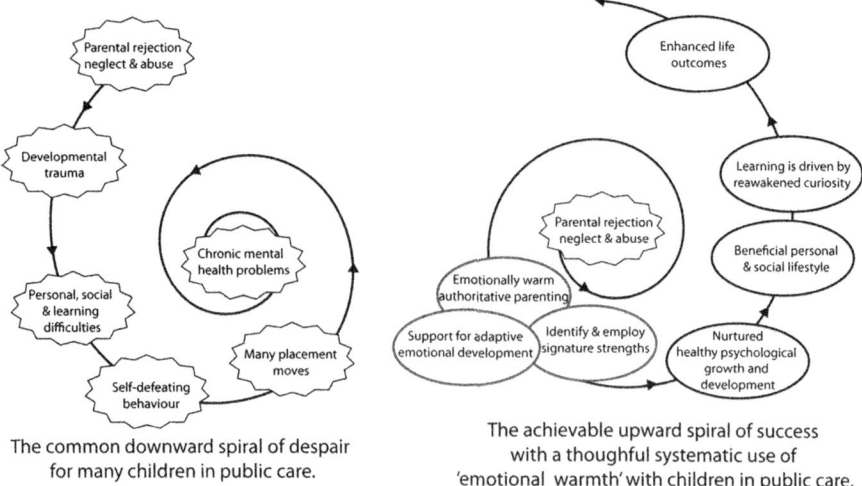

The common downward spiral of despair
for many children in public care.

The achievable upward spiral of success
with a thoughful systematic use of
'emotional warmth' with children in public care.

Fig. 10.3 A comparison of the downward spiral of despair for many children in public care with an achievable, upward spiral of success

Both fostering support groups and children's homes have found the resulting reports useful and practical, since they not only remind them of the worthwhile assets of their organization, but also indicate areas for future discussion and possible improvements. The elements to maintain a "positive organization" create an ongoing dialogue between The Pillars of Parenting and the childcare organization to ensure a functional childcare environment in which the Emotional Warmth approach can grow and flourish.

10.7 The Achievable Upward Spiral

The chapter opened by outlining the downward spiral for many young people in public care which often leads to chronic mental health problems. However, an alternative upward spiral is also possible: this involves emotionally warm parenting' and the systematic use of professional support and evidence-based research to achieve enhanced life outcomes for children in public care (see Fig. 10.3).

We believe that children in public care did not deserve the damaging childhoods that they have had to endure. They do deserve an opportunity to experience kind thoughtful professional support, to enable emotional growth from such adversity.

The Emotional Warmth approach does not shy away from tackling the problems experienced and presented by children and young people in care. However, we do believe that a mindshift from one which mainly focuses on their problems, to one which values and celebrates the healthy side of each child, can be achieved through a combination of skillful parenting, sensitive support for post-trauma stress, building upon the child's signature strengths, and using a psychologist consultant to bring applied psychology into professional child care. Having such a systematic and transparent approach creates an environment, which is safer, and more secure and predictable, within which there are fewer uncertainties and over which children can exert more control.

Such a context is one where children and young people can begin to move from post-traumatic stress to post-trauma growth (cf. Linley and Joseph 2002; Joseph 2012). Their search for meaning and emotional adaptation may be a tough one, but it is also likely to be a worthwhile journey. Our goal for children in public care is that they end up as young adults who are personally stronger and socially more altruistic people who possess a deeper appreciation of some of the things that make living worthwhile.

References

Anglin, J. (2002). *Pain, normality and the struggle for congruence: Reinterpreting residential care for children and youth*. New York: The Haworth Press, Inc.

Blower, A., Addo, A., Hodgson, J., Lamington, L., & Towlson, K. (2004). Mental health of children looked after by local authorities: A needs assessment. *Clinical Child Psychology and Psychiatry, 9*, 117–129.

Cairns, K. (2002). *Attachment, trauma and resilience: Therapeutic caring for children*. London: British Association for Adoption and Fostering.

Cameron, R. J., & Maginn, C. (2008). Professional childcare: The authentic warmth dimension. *British Journal of Social Work, 38*, 1151–1172.

Cameron, R. J., & Maginn, C. (2009). *Achieving positive outcomes for children and young people in public care*. London: Sage.

Cameron, R. J., & Maginn, C. (2011). Living psychology: The emotional warmth dimension of professional childcare. *Educational and Child Psychology, 28*(3), 44–62.

Clough, R., Bullock, R., & Ward, A. (2006). *What works in residential childcare: A review of the research evidence and practical considerations*. London: National Children's Bureau.

Csikszentmihalyi, M. (1990). *Flow: The psychology of optimal experience*. New York: Harper Perennial.

Department for Children, Schools and Families. (2008). *2020 children and young people's workforce strategy*. Nottingham: DfCSF Publication. https://www.education.gov.uk/publicaions/standard/_arc_SOP/Page10/DCSF-01052-2008

Department for Education. (2010). *Outcomes for children looked after by local authorities in England as at 31 March 2010* (SFR 38-2010). London: DfE.

Department for Education. (2011a). *Outcomes for children looked after by local authorities in England as at 31 March 2011*. London: DfE Publication. https://www.education.gov.uk/rsgateway/DB/SFR/s001026/index.shtml

Department for Education. (2011b). Children Act 1989 guidance and regulations: Vol. 4. Fostering services. London: DfE Publication. https://www.education.gov.uk/publications/standard/publicationDetail/Page1/DFE-00023-2011

Department for Education. (2011c). Children Act 1989 guidance and regulations: Vol. 5. Children's homes. London: DfE Publication. https://www.education.gov.uk/publications/standard/publicationDetail/Page1/DFE-00024-2011

Department for Education and Skills. (2001). *Guidance on promotion of mental health within early years and school settings*. Nottingham: DfES Publication. https://www.education.gov.uk/publications/standard/publicationDetail/Page1/DFES-0619-2001

Dreikurs, R., & Soldz, V. (1964). *Children: The challenge*. New York: Hawthorn.

Ford, T., Vostanis, P., Meltzer, H., & Goodman, R. (2007). Psychiatric disorder among British children looked after by local authorities: Comparison with children living in private households. *The British Journal of Psychiatry, 190*, 319–325.

Hicks, L., Gibbs, I., Weatherly, H., & Byeford, S. (2007). *Managing children's homes: Developing effective leadership in small organizations.* London: Jessica Kingsley.

Hooper, J. (2012). *What children need to be happy, confident and successful: Step by step positive psychology to help children to flourish.* London: Jessica Kingsley.

House of Commons. (2009). *Children, schools and family committee, 3rd report: Looked after children.* London: DCSF Publications.

Houston, S. (2006). Making use of positive psychology in residential childcare. In D. Iwaniec (Ed.), *The child's journey through care placement stability, care planning and achieving permanency* (pp. 183–200). Chichester: Wiley.

Joseph, S. (2012). *What doesn't kill us: The new psychology of post-trauma growth.* London: Piatkus.

Kennedy, E. K., Cameron, R. J., & Monsen, J. (2009). Effective consultation in educational and child psychology practice: professional training for both competence and capability. *Educational and Child Psychology, 30*(6), 626–643.

LaFasto, F. M. J., & Larson, C. (2001). *When teams work best: 6000 team members and leaders tell us what it takes to succeed.* London: Sage.

Leach, P. (2011). *The mindful policy group: The pledge for children.* http://www.mindfulpolicy-group.com/the-mpg-pledge-for-children/. Accessed 30 Apr 2012.

Lieberman, M. D., & Eisenberger, N. I. (2009). Pains and pleasures of social life. *Science, 323*, 890–891.

Linley, P. A. (2008). *From average to A+: Realising strengths in yourself and others.* Coventry: CAPP Press.

Linley, P. A., & Joseph, S. (2002). Post-traumatic growth. *Counselling and Psychology, 13*(1), 14–17.

Linley, P. A., Willars, J., & Biswas-Diener, R. (2010). *The strengths book: Be confident, be successful, and enjoy better relationships by realising the best of you.* Coventry: CAPP Press.

Maslow, A. H. (1971). *The farther reaches of human nature.* New York: Viking.

National Institute for Health and Clinical Excellence/Social Care Institute for Excellence (2010). *Promoting the quality of life of looked-after children and young people.* Public Health Guidance PH28. London: NICE.

Pemberton, C. (2011, November 17). Local authorities fail to keep proper records of children missing from care. *Community Care*, 9.

Peterson, C. (2006). *A primer in positive psychology.* New York: Oxford University Press Inc.

Seligman, M. E. P. (2002). *Authentic happiness: Using the new positive psychology to realise your potential for deep fulfilment.* London: Nicholas Brealey.

Seligman, M. E. P., & Csikszentmihalyi, M. (2000). Positive psychology: An introduction. *American Psychologist, 55*(1), 5–14.

Westmacott, E. V. S., & Cameron, R. J. (1981). *Behaviour can change.* Basingstoke: Macmillan.

Part IV
Positive Education

Chapter 11
A Place for Well-Being in the Classroom?

Ian Morris

11.1 Introduction

> Here is Edward Bear, coming downstairs now, bump, bump, bump, on the back of his head, behind Christopher Robin. It is, as far as he knows, the only way of coming downstairs, but sometimes he feels that there really is another way, if only he could stop bumping for a moment and think of it. And then he feels that perhaps there isn't. (Milne 1989, p. 3)

In two crucial areas of life, economics and education, we are in a similarly perplexing position to Winnie-the-Pooh, as these quotes from Martha Nussbaum (2011) and John White (2011) illustrate, respectively:

> For a long time, economists, policy-makers, and bureaucrats who work on the problems of the world's poorer nations told people a story that distorted human experience. Their dominant models asserted that the quality of life in a nation was improving when, and only when, Gross Domestic Product (GDP) per capita was increasing. This crude measure gave high marks to countries that contained alarming inequalities, countries in which a large proportion of people were not enjoying the fruits of a nation's overall economic improvement. Because countries respond to public rankings that affect their international reputation, the crude approach encouraged them to work for economic growth alone, without attending to the living standard of their poorer inhabitants, and without addressing issues such as health and education, which typically do not improve with economic growth. (Nussbaum 2011, p. ix)

> We should have left this sad piece of nonsense [that schooling is centrally about exam success] behind us with the twentieth century. Its schools were caught up in a regime of getting on, doing ever better, getting more and more efficient – but within a system that had lost sight of what it was about…schools should be mainly about equipping people to lead a fulfilling life. (White 2011, p. 1)

Both economics and education have been afflicted by a similar malaise – a measure of success which seems to have ended up harming the very systems it was

I. Morris (✉)
Wellington College, Crowthorne, Berkshire RG45 7PU, UK
e-mail: IRM@wellingtoncollege.org.uk

C. Proctor and P.A. Linley (eds.), *Research, Applications, and Interventions for Children and Adolescents: A Positive Psychology Perspective*, DOI 10.1007/978-94-007-6398-2_11, © Springer Science+Business Media Dordrecht 2013

intended to help. In economics, the arguments are well-rehearsed; that the unrelenting focus on GDP as the only measure of a nation's success has caused governments to lessen their investment in the true ingredients of well-being (such as personal relationships, health, education) preferring to encourage their citizens to become conspicuous consumers in order to feed economic growth, quantifiable in terms of GDP, at a cost both to humans and their environment.

A similar dynamic has taken hold in education. With the laudable aim of raising standards in schools, successive U.K. governments have turned to the narrow and blunt instrument of using examination results as the measure of success. One corresponding effect is a lack of clarity about the aims of education and the perverse situation where, for many, the measure (exam success) has become the aim. This simply will not do. Our aims for education should be coterminous with our deepest wishes for young people and the lives they will lead; to limit this to a clutch of certificates is to sell education short. It must be about something more.

This chapter will argue for just this. In Sect. 11.2, it will argue not just that well-being should play a central role in education, but that well-being should be *the central* aim of education. In Sect. 11.3, it will sketch some ideas of what education needs to do to bring about well-being for all those involved in it. Section 11.4 will glance briefly at what curriculum reform might be needed to better serve the aims of well-being.

11.2   Well-Being as the Aim of Education

Prima facie, it is hard to see why well-being should not serve as the fundamental purpose of our education system, as argued by White (2011):

> Just how *central* an aim should universal well-being be? It is, after all, not the only candidate. Supporting the economy is another. So is preparation for citizenship…It is hard to think of *any* aim, actual or ideal, without *some* link to personal well-being. Economic goals are not ends in themselves; their point is to help people lead more flourishing lives. (p. 121)

But we must be clear what we mean by "well-being". To guide our discussion of well-being in education, I will rely upon a recent and robust definition of the term. In 2008, the U.K. Government Office for Science published the *Foresight Mental Capital and Well-being Project* report, which defined mental capital and mental well-being as follows:

> [Mental capital]…includes [a person's] cognitive ability, how flexible and efficient they are at learning, and their "emotional intelligence", such as their social skills and resilience in the face of stress… [Mental well-being is] a dynamic state in which the individual is able to develop their potential, work productively and creatively, build strong and positive relationships with others, and contribute to their community. It is enhanced when an individual is able to fulfil their personal and social goals and achieve a sense of purpose in their society. (Cooper et al. 2008, p. 10)

So, what needs to be done to realize this aim? One could argue with Claxton (2008), that if we are to make schools centers of genuine, autonomous, and meaningful learning, that well-being, or something like it, would be the end product arising from doing something genuinely challenging and worthwhile. Learning, and a love thereof, is one of many routes to well-being[1] and the job of schools, in conjunction with parents and communities, is to make as many of these different routes to well-being available to children and teachers as possible.

However, at present, well-being only receives adequate focus in schools through the determined efforts of school leaders, teachers, and children despite a system that demands quite different and much narrower things.[2] Claxton's (2008) vision of learning as an instrument of well-being, rather than an instrument of accountability is far from being realized in many schools. White (2007, 2011) argues that the English education system has suffered from a curriculum focused on subjects and content, without overarching aims, restrained by a standards agenda which measures the delivery of this content through holding schools accountable to their exam results. The consequences of this have been a serious undermining of the presence of the ingredients of well-being in schools, as Cigman (2009) observes:

> A standards agenda involves identifying and possibly shaming children and schools that fail. The social consequences of educational failure include disaffection, delinquency, violence and so on: the very problems the standards agenda set out to address. Such an agenda may help some children, but for others, arguably, it makes matters worse by drawing attention to their failures and making them feel unworthy and excluded. (p. 173)

There are other consequences. White (2011) argues that learning is transformed into work, much of which is exam-focused and heteronomous (i.e., externally devised and imposed), which removes the inherent joy of discovery in learning. Genuine learning not only depends upon many of the ingredients of mental well-being in the definition cited above, it also leads to them, creating a virtuous cycle. A related concern is over the confusion of individual aims and institutional ones. When a school sets itself a target to achieve a certain percentage of A grades, it is all too easy for individual children to become lost as means to this end, as expendable statistical contributors to be coerced and manipulated to achieve aims not chosen by them. By reducing learning to a heteronomous process of work, focusing on the accrual of knowledge which results in the acquisition of extrinsic rewards and the potential promise of economic productivity, schools make it much harder for learning and well-being to go together.

---

[1] See for example the New Economics Foundation's "Five Ways to Well-being", which directly references learning http://neweconomics.org/projects/five-ways-well-being, or Seligman's PERMA model (Positive emotions, Engagement (or flow), Relationship/social connections, Meaning (and purpose), Accomplishment; Seligman 2011), which could be argued to subsume learning in engagement and accomplishment.

[2] The explicit requirement to find evidence of the promotion of pupil well-being was removed from the U.K. schools inspection framework in January 2012. The new framework focuses on pupil achievement, quality of teaching, and school leadership and pupils' behavior and safety http://www.publications.parliament.uk/pa/cm201212/cmhansrd/cm120123/text/120123w0001.htm.

White (2011) argues that education should be for well-being; that the life of a school should be built upon this aim. It is here that White's view of education differs significantly from the mainstream. He argues that the mistake we have made in the past is to begin with a list of subjects and graft our aims on to them. White believes that the way to truly bring about well-being in education is to start with well-being as the aim, supported by the development of *dispositions* (i.e., personal qualities), followed by *understanding* (perhaps through the subjects children currently study), with the two (dispositions and understanding) becoming mutually enriching and leading to well-being. As he puts it: "The starting point is that she should have the positive qualities needed for a flourishing life. We would not want her to become brilliant at algebra and Latin, but cripplingly anxious, or cynical, or a sadist. First things first." (White 2011, p. 131)

That an "education for well-being" approach may be considered "radical" by some is a tragedy. Education has been dominated by the insistence solely upon the mastery of a body of knowledge for too long. Of course children need to know about the world they live in, but unless this knowledge is guided by dispositions, which can be encouraged and taught (see discussion below), we leave too much to chance. Qualities such as resilience, persistence, compromise, patience, empathy, and kindness are foundational to everything that children do in schools. That they have been considered "peripheral",[3] or even "ghastly"[4] belies an almost Skinnerian[5] reduction of the role of person and character in learning and a reduction of learning to a caricature of its central role in well-being. It also sets up a false and pernicious dichotomy between "rigorous academic learning" and what are considered by some to be "softer" interpersonal skills. The idea that these two components of learning are in some way separable could only come from a place of very little sympathy for a child trying to master the world in which they live.

White (2011) is, however, guarded about the idea of separate curriculum provision for *well-being* because in his view, if education is truly about well-being through the development of dispositions, the need for a discrete subject to teach it would become obsolete and the stranglehold of the subjects would be loosened. I disagree with him. Elsewhere (see Morris 2012), I have argued that education should serve two functions: *education as happiness* and *education for happiness*. What I mean by this is that every process undertaken in schools should be one that has happiness, or well-being, as its aim and that in every interaction be it in the classroom or the corridor, on the stage or the sports field, is one that can meaningfully contribute to the well-being of the members of the school community. This is not at odds with White's (2011) arguments. Where we part company is on the need

---

[3] In proposed changes to the schools inspection framework in 2010, the Secretary of State for education, Michael Gove announced that schools would no longer be rated on what he termed "peripheral issues", widely thought to be pupil well-being and community cohesion (Harrison 2010).

[4] Nick Gibb, U.K. schools minister, quoted in *Schools strive for pupils' happiness* (Northen 2012), http://www.guardian.co.uk/education/2012/jan/16/children-wellbeing-schools-ofsted?INTCMP=SRCH.

[5] For a discussion of Skinnerian behaviorism, see Kohn (1999), pp. 6–11.

for education for happiness. There is so much research into human well-being and flourishing that time should be made available to run explicit sessions on what well-being and flourishing comprise and how we can apply learning from this research to the activities that children engage in on a daily basis. Children are as entitled to discover what makes for a flourishing life as they are any other knowledge. Furthermore, skills like emotional management, conflict resolution, and finding meaning and purpose are too often expected to emerge through some kind of mysterious osmosis as children encounter the traditional subjects or meet skillful teachers. To assume that learning for well-being would happen across the curriculum, even one with well-being as its aim, when training in well-being is almost completely absent from the education that teachers themselves receive, would be to continue to leave the process to chance.

11.3   Well-Being Education

Just like Winnie-the-Pooh (i.e., Edward Bear; Milne 1989), we have come to the conclusion that there must be another way of coming down the stairs. Our task now is to find out exactly what that might look like. This section will explore examples of the dispositions schools might wish to encourage in order to help children and teachers develop their own well-being and that of others. That I have included teachers here is important. When I trained as a teacher, we were told that all teachers are teachers of literacy and numeracy. Quite so. We are all teachers of well-being too. Young people look to their teachers to role model being human and teachers have a duty, not only to help young people to learn, but also to show them by example the sorts of dispositions that will help them learn and flourish.

   The sketch in this section is based upon the 6-stranded model of well-being that we use at Wellington College,[6] which was informed by the U.K. Government Office for Science's definitions of mental capital and metal well-being presented above (see Cooper et al. 2008). Each strand contains examples of dispositions that can be both explicitly taught in a well-being lesson and ought also to be reflected across the school community by all who belong to it. The brevity of this chapter restricts the scope of the examples discussed. Thus, these should not be seen as exhaustive or prescriptive, but more suggestive of the direction in which to head.

11.3.1   Physical Health

One of the foundations of well-being is an understanding of the functions of our body, what behaviors best serve those functions and a sense (in so far as is possible) of autonomy and choice about our health. These (and others like them) are the

---

[6]The full curriculum can be accessed for free at: http://intranet.wellingtoncollege.org.uk/well-being.

dispositions that will help children to have a positive approach to their health and more importantly, dispositions that can help them to remove the irritating hurdles to flourishing that children often feel imprisoned by. Executive function is just one example of this. Children should find out about the exciting research that has been done into the areas of the brain that affect their executive function and apply this to the kinds of daily temptations that require the ability to delay gratification, such as the choice between computer gaming and playing outside, or answering one more text message and getting to sleep. This can easily be brought to life by reenacting Walter Mischel's classic[7] experiment on delayed gratification using marshmallows and any one of a number of practical strategies for developing executive function (e.g., see Morris 2009). When given the challenge of resisting temptation for homework, our students almost always choose to deal with issues, such as the intrusion of smartphones into studying or conversation, and quickly notice the benefits of being able to manage that intrusion.

A related way of developing this is the use of physical exercise. As Ratey (2001, 2008) has shown, exercise not only depends upon delayed gratification, by putting off more pleasurable things to do it, but it develops it too. Unfortunately, schools have tended to have a history of an excessively competitive approach to physical exercise, with all of the attendant sense of shame and humiliation that can accompany competition (see Kohn 1992). But as Ratey (2008) explains, innovative work has been done to introduce noncompetitive exercise into schools, not just as a way to improve cardiovascular fitness and combat obesity, but to increase children's ability to learn. There is a demonstrable correlation between frequent exercise and improved learning as well as impulse control and once children experience this it can have a profoundly positive impact on their relationship to their physical health. I recently visited a remarkable school in Australia called Timbertop, the mountain campus of Geelong Grammar School. At Timbertop all students *and staff* participate in the running program, which gets steadily more arduous throughout the year, culminating in an 18.5-mile marathon. When I spoke to students about this they spoke not just of stamina or lung capacity, or of cognitive benefits for learning, but also the *dispositional* advantages long distance running brings, such as persistence, a sense of perspective, encouragement of others, and connection with the natural world.

Other components of this strand could include: nutrition and its links to mood and learning; the role of sleep in well-being and how to build good sleep habits; what happens in the brain when we learn and how this awareness can maximize learning; and understanding how to manage excessive stress and capitalize upon the benefits of stress inoculation (see Ratey 2008).

---

[7]For fuller explanation, see Goleman (2004), p. 80.

11.3.2   Positive Relationships

The centrality of our human relationships to our sense of well-being is beyond question, nowhere more so than in schools. McLaughlin and Clarke (2010) in a review of 133 research papers on the impact of the school experience on mental health argue that:

> It is not new to argue that relationships matter but the body of evidence is now quite large and powerful. We can conclude that the connections between people in schools are a driving force in shaping engagement with school. This sense of belonging influences wellbeing, academic outcomes and social development, short and long term…We can also conclude that relationships with teachers and pupils in schools are potentially powerful for all pupils, and particularly so for the more emotionally vulnerable. So engaging with the promotion of positive mental health for young people entails building communities in schools in which young people can have sustaining and meaningful relationships, which they perceive as supportive. These perceptions emerge as important in influencing wellbeing. (p. 20)

Schools have to take seriously their role in helping young people explore how to build positive relationships and they must directly address it. Even if one retains the traditional view of education as being about academic outcomes, the role of the relationships in raising achievement is primary; this is even more the case in an education system that prizes well-being above all.

It is impossible here to detail all of the possible work that could be done in schools to enhance an understanding of relationships and there is already an enormous amount of good work being done. However, there is one contribution to relationships education I would like to highlight.

In recent years, a number of schools have been experimenting with a technique for conflict resolution called "restorative justice" (RJ). Learning to negotiate conflict skillfully draws upon and develops deep understanding of components of relationships, such as empathy, trust, emotional management, the role of shame and pride, compromise, body language, forgiveness, and love. When an offence is committed, a law, rule or norm gets broken and a relationship is harmed in some way. The traditional "criminal justice" approach looks to find which law was broken, who broke it, and how they should be punished, or what they deserve. It tends to remove victim and offender from the process and justice is done to them. The restorative approach explores who has been hurt by the offending, what their needs are, and who has an obligation to meet those needs. It is different because victim and offender collaborate in repairing the harm that offending does to the relationship (Zehr 2002). Instead of imposing punishment on an offender and potentially prolonging the corrosive effects of shame that entails (Nathanson 1992), it seeks to find ways of repairing the harm done to the relationship through the offending, by bringing the victim and the offender together in a carefully conducted meeting that is focused on resolution (cf. Tutu 1999; McCullough 2008).

In schools, where most "offending" is low level, but has a dramatic impact on the quality of relationships, RJ is a powerful tool for dealing with offending *and* repairing the relationships in a more meaningful and lasting way than saying sorry and shaking hands, followed by a detention. Teachers and pupils who use this technique repeatedly find that the RJ process enables both victim and offender to see each other as real people again, rather than the caricatures they can become through a criminal justice approach and in many cases, it can break patterns of antisocial behavior and prevent reoffending.[8]

To be able to resolve conflict constructively could be one of the most important products of school and one of the most significant contributions to well-being both at and beyond it.

11.3.3 Perspective

This aspect of well-being concerns developing what Gilbert (2007) terms a "psychological immune system", or the cognitive ability to respond well to change, challenge, and adversity. This is not concerned with building a psychological suit of armor to deflect the slings and arrows of life, but with the development of a set of resources to help think flexibly and accurately about what happens to us. That we make perceptual errors about what takes place in and around us is not news, but what is news is the idea that schoolteachers can teach a set of skills to children to minimize the emotional and behavioral damage done by unhelpful interpretations of what happens to them.

One of the most renowned examples of this is the Penn Resilience Program (PRP). Originally conceived as a means of responding to childhood depression (Reivich and Shatté 2003) researchers at the University of Pennsylvania devised the PRP to help adolescents become aware of and manage their explanatory style: our thinking response to events in our lives. Beginning with awareness of the effect of thinking on our emotions and behavior (the "ABC" [Adversity, Consequences, Beliefs]) the program runs through a set of skills to deal with the "thinking traps" that can turn past events and future possibilities into problems, develop assertiveness and compromise, and remain calm and focused in stressful situations. There is a rich seam to be mined here for education. Learning is as much about finding ways of getting unstuck as it is about finding things out – schools often focus on the former at the expense of the latter and developing resilience happens accidentally. Worthwhile learning should be challenging as well as enjoyable and children need, deliberately and with guidance, to develop the resources to respond flexibly to adversity. Resilience training does just that.

Another resource that children should develop is the "growth mindset" arising from the research of Carol Dweck. Dweck (2000, 2008) distinguishes between two mindsets, "fixed" and "growth", arising from theories of intelligence. She argues that some people conceive of intelligence as fixed and entity-like, what she calls the "fixed mindset" and others conceive of intelligence as malleable and incremental, what she calls the "growth mindset". Emerging research into the development

---

[8]Further information see: http://www.restorativejustice.org.uk/restorative_justice_works.

of talent (Gladwell 2008; Syed 2010), and neuroplasticity (Doidge 2008) back up the view held by Dweck (2000, 2008) that our mastery of any given discipline is more dependent upon effort and effective practice than it is upon any genetic or trait-like predisposition. In other words, getting good requires working hard and bar a few faculties like eyesight and language, the brain is always capable of learning new things.

What is fascinating about Dweck's research is her evidence that individuals seem to be guided towards either a fixed or a growth mindset by the type of praise they receive (cf. Holt 1982). In a series of remarkable experiments, Dweck (2000) showed that praising children for being clever, or being a "natural" is actually handicapping to their progress because being praised in that way increases the likelihood that children will become more concerned with appearing to be good at a discipline than they will with mastering it. In other words, if a child is told they are clever, they will feel the need to live up to that epithet. The cost of this is significant. Feeling the need to be seen as clever makes students less likely to take risks as learners, more anxious about success and, interestingly, more likely to lie about failure.

It is of fundamental importance that children go through school with an accurate view of how mastery is developed; children who give up at the first try of a new endeavor because they don't perfect it immediately, don't have to suffer in this way. Both resilience and mindset depend upon regular and effective interventions from teachers and this has significant implications for the way that we train for the profession. The teaching of resilience and mindset are not widespread and they need to be if we are to take the well-being of teachers and students seriously.

11.3.4   Engagement

This strand of well-being teaching addresses what might be termed "getting stuck in and staying stuck in", in short what motivates us and how we stay engaged in the activities we choose for ourselves. The Wellington program covers areas such as flow states (Csikszentmihalyi 2002), the significance of positive emotions in broadening our horizons and building our psychological capital (Fredrickson 2009) and the importance of managing feedback in staying engaged. Much of what is done in schools requires high levels of intellectual and emotional engagement and given that "engagement" appears in many inventories of well-being (e.g., Huppert and So 2011) it does not appear to be too much of a stretch to suggest that schools devote time to getting this one right.

One of the most provocative discussions of how we go about getting children motivated to engage comes from Kohn (1999). In a review of studies into human motivation, Kohn (1999) comes to the conclusion that what he calls "pop-behaviorism", that is, the widespread belief (notably in education) that to get anyone to do anything you either have to threaten them with punishment, or promise them a reward, is not only unsuccessful, but harmful.

...students who are motivated by grades or other rewards, typically don't learn as well, think as deeply, care as much about what they're doing, or choose to challenge themselves to the same extent as students who are not grade oriented. But the damage doesn't stop there. Grades dilute the pleasure that a student experiences on successfully completing a task. They encourage cheating and strain the relationship between the teacher and the student. They reduce a student's sense of control over his own fate and can induce a blind conformity to others' wishes – sometimes to the point that students are alienated from their own preferences and don't even know who they are. Again, notice it is not only those who are punished by F's but also those rewarded by A's who bear the cost of grades. (Kohn 1999, p. 204)

Grading increases the likelihood of children becoming "product oriented", rather than "process oriented" in other words, they become more concerned about the end result (the grade) than focusing on the process (learning, practice, and mastery) that will get them there. As mentioned above, this is the perverse situation where the measure becomes the aim.

As Kohn (1999) also points out, the litmus test of the effectiveness of rewards is how well they continue working after they are removed. In experiment after experiment the conclusion repeatedly comes back that as soon as you remove the reward, the desired behavior will cease (Kohn 1999). In schools, this has particular significance for so called "effort-grading" and its implications for lifelong learning. If the investing of effort into learning is made contingent upon the application of rewards and punishment, what happens to our fledgling learners once they leave the reward regime and have to start finding their own motivation to invest effort in the workplace or the university?

In short, if we want young people to engage meaningfully in the processes of learning to be learners and mastering important skills and disciplines, we could do a lot worse than remove grading, of both attainment and effort. A suggestion for what might take its place is made in the next section.

11.3.5   The World

Our children are born into a world that is a product of the GDP focus that Nussbaum's (2011) sketch describes. Just a few minutes spent watching a commercial children's television channel is clear evidence that there are immense forces at work encouraging our young people to consume and consume conspicuously. The harmful consequences of competitive consumption are already well-known (Klein 2000; James 2007; Cooper et al. 2008), and need no rehearsal here, and the assertion that young people need help deciphering the many messages they are flooded with has already led to interesting programs in schools.[9]

In terms of dispositions, Schwartz (2004) provides us with a list of 11 antidotes to dealing with the paralyzing effect of choice available to consumers, being aware

---

[9] One such example is Adbusters' "Media Empowerment Kit", see: http://www.adbusters.org/cultureshop/mediakit.

of adaptation, comparing ourselves less with others, and learning how to "satisfice" more (knowing when something is good enough and not hankering after perfection). Another resource for learning to manage living in a technology-rich, consumer society can be found at: http://www.lifesquared.org.uk, a website providing free publications designed to provoke the reader to stop, think, and question the consuming habits that our economy can encourage us to develop. So much of this work can be described as "the art of living" found in the philosophy of Aristotle and the Stoics:

> In [the Stoic] view, philosophy did not consist in teaching an abstract theory – much less in the exegesis of texts – but rather in the art of living…It is a conversion which turns our entire life upside down, changing the life of the person who goes through it. It raises the individual from an inauthentic condition of life, darkened by unconsciousness and harassed by worry, to an authentic state of life, in which he attains self-consciousness, an exact vision of the world, inner peace, and freedom. (Hadot 1995, p. 83)

It should be noted that encouraging children to think critically about how to carve out a sustainable life in the face of pressure to consume and use technology is not a moral crusade. It is not motivated by a value judgment that books and nature are preferable to TV and shopping malls – everything has its place – it is rather motivated by genuine concerns for the physical and mental health of young people. The simple fact is, that if a child spends their life watching TV or gaming or loitering in shopping centers, their chances of being healthy and happy are greatly reduced, and part of the job of a well-being education is to show children that a balance may be struck and that true fulfillment may lie elsewhere.

11.3.6 Meaning and Purpose

Both Seligman's (2011) PERMA model and Huppert and So's (2011) well-being measure contain explicit reference to the impact of perceiving that one's life has meaning and purpose on our well-being. Frankl (2004) believed its importance so fundamental that he conceived an entire form of therapy around it. That children should leave school with a sense of the direction and value of their own existence seems to be beyond question, but education needs to tread warily here. It would be all too easy for this kind of work to be hijacked by a more prescriptive, sinister, or narcissistic agenda. One only need recall Maggie Smith's 1969 portrayal of Muriel Spark's (1961) tragic Jean Brodie, to remember the risks inherent in trying to exert undue influence over what children believe their lives to be for.

The development of a personal sense of meaning requires many of the other dispositions hinted at throughout this chapter, but this does not mean it should be a discussion shunted to the end; in an education that values well-being, discussions of meaning and purpose should be a regular feature. Providing the outcomes are not controlled and students are provided with a rich and diverse array of material to reflect upon, the moment of school leaving should be one filled with genuine optimism about the range of possible trajectories available, rather than feeling like Winnie-the-Pooh when he reached the bottom of the stairs.

11.4   Well-Being and the Curriculum

Our aim and our dispositions are in place, but what of *understanding*, the space traditionally occupied by the academic subjects? White (2011) argues that schools should have more freedom to promote dispositions by finding ways to work outside the traditional framework of subjects. He also argues that improvements need to be made to teaching and teacher training to encourage teachers to develop *wholehearted* engagement in learning and also to enable children to have more autonomy over what they learn and when. *Wholeheartedness* and *autonomy* could be promoted, he suggests, through more collaborative forms of learning (as opposed to individuals plowing through work to prepare them for exams) and by more cross-curricular learning, where students are given projects to work on which draw upon different disciplines. Furthermore, White (2011) suggests that our traditional approach to assessing learning (i.e., through the use of terminal exams) be replaced by a process of continuous assessment of dispositions and understanding by the people who know the child best: the teachers who teach them (as opposed to the anonymous examiner) and, interestingly, the parents.

In the UK, the freedom to take innovative approaches to teaching and learning already exists, because the curriculum does not specify how to teach. However, very few schools seem to experiment with the kinds of approaches suggested by White (2011) and it may be that until a systematic method of innovating with the curriculum is demonstrated, that many schools simply stick to the safety of what has always been done.

There is an interesting assessment framework that might make innovation more likely. The Middle Years Programme (MYP), developed by the International Baccalaureate,[10] offers tremendous autonomy to schools in developing their own programs of study, keeps assessment of learning in house, and is structured to encourage not only interdisciplinary investigation, but also explicitly requires students to engage with questions of how they go about and improve their own learning.

The real beauty of the program, however, is the absence of terminal exams. Over the course of the program students produce work that is returned with formative comments from teachers, which advise on how to improve and are awarded a numerical grade at the end. In an ideal, Kohn-like world, even this grade would be absent, being replaced instead by a statement of achievement, recording the development of dispositions and understanding, written by the people who know the student best. But the MYP is an excellent start. The continual assessment and process orientated feedback supports the development of both a resilience and growth mindset, and the relative absence of "rewards" enables students to develop an intrinsic motivation to learn. In this way, the MYP is structured to encourage the development of the dispositions that underpin not only mastery of learning, but well-being too.

---

[10] See further http://www.ibo.org/myp/.

11.5   Conclusion

Questions about the place of well-being in education, particularly in the light of recent work done to define well-being, are in fact more fundamental questions about the very purpose of our schools. In responding to these questions we have a duty to be bold and do our best to avoid the narrow vision of schooling sketched at the start of this chapter, and also to avoid the predicament of poor Winnie-the-Pooh. An education system which has well-being as its aim and which prioritizes dispositions over understanding is not so very different from what we have now, because this is often what informs the vocation of most teachers. However, the system, comprising teacher training, the silos of the subjects, and measuring outcomes constrain this. These things need to be changed to provide the education our children deserve. Primarily, teacher training must focus much more on recruiting and preparing educators first and subject specialists second; it must also train teachers to help children develop the kinds of dispositions that can lead to flourishing. Secondly, the curriculum needs reform. As mentioned above, there is a possible model in the International Baccalaureate MYP that could, with tweaking, support the aim of well-being much more fully. Finally, governments need to find much more inventive and much less reductionist approaches to measuring the effectiveness of our schools.

Well-being is now, through the years of work into human flourishing, a robust concept and one that is fit to guide our education system. It is neither ghastly nor peripheral, but utterly central to our deepest wishes for what education can achieve for children.

References

Cigman, R. (2009). Enhancing children? In R. Cigman & A. Davies (Eds.), *New philosophies of learning* (pp. 205–220). Chichester: Wiley.

Claxton, G. (2008). *What's the point of school? Rediscovering the heart of education*. Oxford: OneWorld.

Cooper, C. et al. (2008). *Foresight mental capital and well-being project*. London: The Government Office for Science.

Csikszentmihalyi, M. (2002). *Flow*. London: Random House.

Doidge, N. (2008). *The brain that changes itself: Stories of personal triumph from the frontiers of brain science*. London: Penguin.

Dweck, C. S. (2000). *Self-theories*. Philadelphia: Taylor & Francis.

Dweck, C. S. (2008). *Mindset*. New York: Ballantine.

Frankl, V. (2004). *Man's search for meaning*. London: Rider.

Fredrickson, B. L. (2009). *Positivity: Groundbreaking research reveals how to embrace the hidden strength of positive emotions, overcome negativity, and thrive*. New York: Crown Publishers.

Gilbert, D. (2007). *Stumbling on happiness*. London: Harper Perennial.

Gladwell, M. (2008). *Outliers: The story of success*. London: Penguin.

Goleman, D. (2004). *Emotional intelligence*. London: Bloomsbury.

Hadot, P. (1995). *Philosophy as a way of life*. Oxford: Blackwell.

Harrison, A. (2010). Schools inspections slimmed down. *BBC News, Education & Family*. http://www.bbc.co.uk/news/education-11400774. Accessed February 14, 2012.

Holt, J. (1982). *How children fail*. New York: Merloyd Lawrence.

Huppert, F. A., & So, T. T. C. (2013). Flourishing across Europe: Application of a new conceptual framework for defining well-being. *Social Indicators Research, 110*(3), 837–861. doi:10.1007/s11205-011-9966-7.

James, O. (2007). *Affluenza*. London: Random House.

Klein, N. (2000). *No logo*. London: Flamingo.

Kohn, A. (1992). *No contest: The case against competition*. New York: Houghton Mifflin.

Kohn, A. (1999). *Punished by rewards*. New York: Houghton Mifflin.

McCullough, M. E. (2008). *Beyond revenge: The evolution of the forgiveness instinct*. San Francisco: Jossey-Bass.

McLaughlin, C., & Clarke, B. (2010). Relational matters: A review of the impact of school experience on mental health in early adolescence. *Educational and Child Psychology, 27*(1), 95–107.

Milne, A. A. (1989). *Winnie-the-pooh and some bees*. London: Methuen.

Morris, I. (2009). *Learning to ride elephants: Teaching happiness and well-being in schools*. London: Continuum.

Morris, I. (2012). Going beyond the accidental: Happiness, education and the Wellington College experience. In I. Boniwell, A. Conley-Ayes, & S. David (Eds.), *The Oxford handbook of happiness*. Oxford: Oxford University Press.

Nathanson, D. (1992). *Shame and pride: Affect, sex, and the birth of the self*. New York: W. W. Norton and Company.

Northen, S. (2012, January 12). Schools strive for pupils' happiness. *The Guardian, Education*. http://www.guardian.co.uk/education/2012/jan/16/children-wellbeing-schools-ofsted?INTCMP=SRCH. Accessed June 4, 2012.

Nussbaum, M. (2011). *Creating capabilities: The human development approach*. Cambridge: Belknap.

Ratey, J. (2001). *A user's guide to the brain*. New York: Random House.

Ratey, J. (2008). *Spark*. New York: Little, Brown and Company.

Reivich, K., & Shatté, A. (2003). *The resilience factor*. New York: Broadway Books.

Schwartz, B. (2004). *The paradox of choice*. New York: HarperCollins.

Seligman, M. E. P. (2011). *Flourish*. London: Nicholas Brealey.

Spark, M. (1961). *The prime of Miss Jean Brodie*. New York: HarperCollins.

Syed, M. (2010). *Bounce*. London: Fourth Estate.

Tutu, D. M. (1999). *No future without forgiveness*. New York: Doubleday.

White, J. (2007). *What schools are for and why*. Philosophy of Education Society of Great Britain.

White, J. (2011). *Exploring well-being in schools*. Abingdon: Routledge.

Zehr, H. (2002). *The little book of restorative justice*. Intercourse: Good Books.

Chapter 12
Positive Education, or Just Education

Hans Henrik Knoop

12.1   One and a Half Educational Paradigm

The quality, sustainability, and future perspective of any modern society depend on the quality of its educational system. The globalization of information, trade and travel, along with the increased level of competition following it, has put an immense focus on education everywhere. Cultures and societies stand and fall with their ability to foster citizens able to carry the torch further onward; and willing to, as they find it worthwhile. However, many of the initiatives taken to improve education over the last decades have failed to impress, and have often come at a high price, with many pupils and teachers suffering demotivation, stress, and even depression. Currently, the overwhelmingly dominating paradigm around the world is one of centralized control over content combined with decentralized economy, predominantly top-down-management, monitored through standardized testing, comparative statistics in form of rankings, often sadly tempered by a culture of low trust and a sense of diminishing professional autonomy. This paradigm is very much in line with the so-called New Public Management paradigm taken from organizational leadership studies, which in many ways function similarly to what is squarely known as privatization of public institutions dating back to the Reagan-Thatcher era in the 1980s. It is by and large an extension and elaboration of the industrial type of mass education that has been dominating for more than two centuries, but it has been continuously "refined" by use of still more detailed curricular demands and sophisticated evaluation technologies for centralized monitoring. The paradigm does hold some merit in that it is able to bring a population together in a shared "form", and teach specified content as to ensure common language, knowledge, values, and practices.

H.H. Knoop (✉)
Department of Education, University of Aarhus, Niels Juels Gade 84, building 2110,
room 139, 8200 Aarhus N, Denmark
e-mail: knoop@dpu.dk

C. Proctor and P.A. Linley (eds.), *Research, Applications, and Interventions for Children and Adolescents: A Positive Psychology Perspective*, DOI 10.1007/978-94-007-6398-2_12,
© Springer Science+Business Media Dordrecht 2013

This was initially important in order to transform a more analogue farmer culture into a more digital factory worker culture, and it is important today as the increasing cultural complexity poses a constant threat of cultural dissolution. In some cases, the strict monitoring of school performances also seems to prevent educational "catastrophes" yet, in most countries it seems to rather foster mediocrity than excellence, despite many attempts at the latter through targeted talent development, prizes for excellent performances, and sometimes combinations of the two in the form of television shows like "Britain's Got Talent", and so forth (e.g., OECD PISA [Organisation for Economic Co-operation and Development Programme for International Student Assessment 2000, 2003, 2006, 2009]).[1] However, there are a number of far more controversial consequences of this paradigm also. The most important of these may be that it tends to stratify its population into layers, classes, tiers, and lifestyles based on differences in economic wealth. As such, what is reproduced by this model is the status quo rather than social reform, even if it does seem to have helped large population groups in many countries towards economic growth in the early phases of their industrialization, rising above recent extreme poverty and continues to do so to this day with Singapore and South Korea as two well-known examples. Even more relevant in this context though is that much of the psychology indirectly "applied" by this system flies in the face of what we know about effective learning and human flourishing. For example, the extensive use of extrinsic rewards almost certainly tends to undermine learners' interest in learning – a grave fact eerily in line with evidence from the business world showing how actions taken to *improve the efficiency of various outcomes by a third party's use of extrinsic rewards* have failed, and indeed been counterproductive in all markets studied to date (Winston 2006). It is on the shoulders of this paradigm that positive education comes into the world.

12.2   Positive Education as a Tentative Alternative in the Making

It is understandable if the term "positive education" sounds like the marriage of an insult to an oxymoron to many. How can such a term not insinuate that the rest of education is more or less negative, obviously offending some? Others may, based on their first-hand experience, seriously ask how something as dull as education can possibly be positive. Yet, it is precisely connotations to education implied in such sentiments that make the specific approaches of positive education so important today. For education worth its name needs to be everything but a negative and boring experience to pupils and teachers. Learning marked by negativity is almost by definition counterproductive in that it tends to shy people away from learning, and boring learning is at best highly ineffective. Education needs first and foremost to

---

[1] OECD PISA (2000, 2003, 2006, 2009) results can be found at: http://www.pisa.oecd.org.

be a positive and inspiring experience if it is to serve the citizens depending on it, which is pretty much everyone. So what is positive education?

Positive education has been defined in a variety of ways but generally people seem to agree that it is about the application of psychological knowledge regarding individual strengths, well-being, social relations, and leadership in ways that go beyond what has been done so far, based on state-of-the-art psychological evidence. Obviously, it transcends the limits of this chapter to review all relevant evidence in detail, so in what follows, rather than presenting scattered studies from many subareas and with mixed results, I chose to outline some of the most robust positive psychological theories on which education, along with many other fields of practice, can confidently expect to benefit significantly, if only application is done properly. For the sake of overview I have roughly grouped these theories in those before the formal inception of the positive psychology movement around year 2000, and those that have emerged later, acknowledging the great overlap between the two. And as I hope to make clear, the psychological evidence presented is both strong, convincing, and peculiarly absent in much public debate about "what works" in education, one-sidedly focused on hard evidence regarding non-psychological features such as grades, rankings, drop-out-rates, and money.

12.3 Early Psychological Findings of Particular Educational Importance

Some of the first direct strides towards what eventually became positive psychology were made through the acknowledgement that people are not born as blank slates, that they are living organisms, with needs of their own – to be satisfied in order to live a full life. Abraham Maslow (1954), maybe stronger than anyone else, paved the way for this understanding by arguing for a third type of psychology, a humanistic psychology. Indeed, he even coined the term "positive psychology" as something close to being a synonym to humanistic psychology, focusing on human strengths rather than their deficits, as it was predominantly the case within the up until then highly influential behavioristic and psychoanalytic paradigms of psychology. To this day, many of Maslow's basic observations remain valid and much of what is known as "progressive" and "creative" in education has been strongly informed and inspired by humanistic thought of this kind, as has much of the so-called "human relation/resource management" in work-life. The growth-directed psychotherapeutical approach of Carl Rogers (1961, 1969) remains of premiere influence among therapists also and is but another example of how humanistic psychology continues to flourish. Indeed, Rogers expressed a humanistic approach to education as forcefully as anyone: "If we value independence, if we are disturbed by the growing conformity of knowledge, of values, of attitudes, which our present system induces, then we may wish to set up conditions of learning which make for uniqueness, for self-direction, and for self-initiated learning" (Rogers 1961, p. 24), echoing progressive ideas of John Dewey (1916/2009) half a century earlier.

On the shoulders of Maslow and peers, an almost equally important theoretical contribution has come from Ed Deci and Richard Ryan's (2000) work on self-determination.[2] Over more than 40 years they have developed a robust theory of human motivation elaborating and corroborating humanistic psychology, especially by convincingly showing how human beings are well understood as biological organisms that depend on an organismic understanding of themselves, strongly in line with Maslow, but also acknowledging that these organisms are very sophisticated mammals capable of, indeed fundamentally requiring, communication, social relatedness, learning, creativity and autonomous action at a level unparalleled in any other species on the planet.

Self-determination theory obviously has strong implications for education as, in the words of C. P. Niemiec and Ryan (2009) it

> …assumes that inherent in human nature is the propensity to be curious about one's environment and interested in learning and developing one's knowledge. All too often, however, educators introduce external controls into learning climates, which can undermine the sense of relatedness between teachers and students, and stifle the natural, volitional processes involved in high-quality learning … A large corpus of empirical evidence based on SDT suggests that both intrinsic motivation and autonomous types of extrinsic motivation are conducive to engagement and optimal learning in educational contexts. In addition, evidence suggests that teachers' support of students' basic psychological needs for autonomy, competence, and relatedness facilitates students' autonomous self-regulation for learning, academic performance, and well-being. (p. 133)

Of particular educational importance here are numerous findings showing how individual and social flourishing in all age groups depends directly on the personal experience of autonomous motivation. In other words, self-determination theory argues forcefully for giving priority to intrinsic motivation in almost any kind of learning environment, if the particular type of learning is to be effective and joyful enough to be self-reinforcing (Deci and Ryan 2000). Many other findings from biology, evolutionary psychology, and systems science are in line with this research, and have produced insights compatible, or indirectly corroborating self-determination theory (e.g., Camazine et al. 2001; Csikszentmihalyi 1993, 1996; Kauffman 2000; Pinker 2002).

Almost "synergistically" with self-determination theory stands Albert Bandura's (1994) equally robust theory of self-efficacy. Self-efficacy is "the belief in one's capabilities to organize and execute the courses of action required to manage prospective situations" (Bandura 1995, p. 2). In other words, self-efficacy is a belief in one's own ability to meet coming and important challenges successfully. Self-efficacy has been proven highly predictive of individuals' performances in many different settings, ironically in line with the famous quote by Henry Ford: "Whether you think you can, or you think you can't – you're usually right", and potentially directly related to placebo effects. Pupil's self-efficacy thus being the learner's expectation regarding own performance can meaningfully be understood as complementary to the teachers' expectation towards the learners yielding the so-called

---

[2] See: http://www.selfdeterminationtheory.org.

Pygmalion-effect, originally studied by Robert Rosenthal (Rosenthal and Jacobson 1992). Also Bandura's (e.g., 1977, 1994) work has fundamental implications for education, where most pupils have first-hand experience of insurmountable failure as they found themselves stalling, gradually being sorted into classes, categories, levels of status, as they saw their more competent peers proceed and advance themselves. The predictive value of self-efficacy, and its precise and rather easily manageable measures, compared to related but more vague concepts such as self-confidence, have made it popular not only in psychology but also in many bordering areas of study such as stress-research and preventive medicine (e.g., Zachariae 2011). Maybe the most important educational implication of the research on self-efficacy is that it provides an irrefutable argument for ensuring that all students experience school learning as an overall successful venture because self-efficacy grows from own experience of success, that is: for a learner, success requires previous success. This is another reason why rigidly standardized teaching, learning, and testing is bound to discourage a large percentage of pupils as they come to see learning as a no-win-game. In support of this point, Robert Rosenthal offers his only conclusion of prescriptive nature from his decades of research: "Superb teachers can teach the "unteachable"; we know that. So, what I think this research shows is that there's a moral obligation for a teacher: if the teacher *knows* that certain students can't *learn*, that teacher should get out of that classroom" (Rhem 1999, p. 4).

Contrasting, yet almost complementing, both self-determination theory and self-efficacy theory is the theory of learned helplessness (Seligman and Maier 1967; Overmier and Seligman 1967). This theory explains how it is possible to brutalize animal, and humans, into complete passivity and apathy by removing their sense of control over their own situation. Also this theory, though obviously running counter to any educational endeavor, has important explanatory power in the cases of young people burning out in school due to continuous failure to succeed meaningfully.

Of maybe unparalleled theoretical importance in expanding humanistic psychology towards the positive psychology movement, are the contributions of Mihaly Csikszentmihalyi (1990, 1993, 1996). Csikszentmihalyi's work is best known though the concept of "flow", which is a construct developed to frame the optimal experience in which an engaged person is completely immersed in activity to a degree that the activity becomes autotelic, a goal in itself, ultimately completely intrinsically motivating, worth doing for its own sake (Csikszentmihalyi 1990). A glimpse of how deep this theory goes, not the least in the context of education, may be given by a simple reflection on time and life quality. Thus, if one is asked what one finds really worth doing in life it quickly becomes clear that almost nothing done in a state of haste qualifies. By and large, hurrying things through it is simply not worthwhile – at least not for those who do it (others may cynically benefit from it, of course). Obviously, this is not the place for a detailed investigation of the philosophy of time, but the implications of this as regards an educational system being run by digital time-frames for over two centuries should be fairly clear even so. Moreover, flow-theory is embedded in a much deeper appreciation of complexity elaborated in the masterpiece *The evolving self: A psychology for the third millennium* (Csikszentmihalyi 1993). The groundbreaking understanding of flow and complexity has had profound influence in many fields, but arguably most directly in education as the concept of flow serves as an almost perfect description of play in academic terms, with play being the preferred state of consciousness for children during their early years: as indeed it remains to be throughout life if the concept of flow is elaborated a bit to encompass also the play-like state people find themselves in when studying really exciting material, through curious exploration. There is massive evidence of the effectiveness of play and flow on learning, with the research of Csikszentmihalyi and colleagues specifically demonstrating that the more intrinsically motivated learners are: the more they enjoy learning, the more they will learn, the more inclined they will be to learn more, and the more inclined they will be to contribute to the greater good (e.g., Anderson et al. 1976; Csikszentmihalyi and Rathunde 1993; Csikszentmihalyi et al. 2005; Deci and Ryan 2000; Fredrickson 2009; Harter 1978; Knoop 2011; Ryan 1995; Shernoff and Hoogstra 2001).

Again, many other lines of psychological study contribute to the foundation of today's positive psychology, but those mentioned above have proven so robust that it will be unsurprising if they each prove themselves universal, and thus of universal importance to educators also. They provide a firm and congruent basis of understanding that does not reduce or discard important contributions from other domains of psychological inquiry, and most importantly, cannot be neglected if education is to function optimally. On a further note, the scholars mentioned seem to share an ambition of going beyond the "ism-game", gradually leaving the battle of psychological paradigms behind, aiming to synthesize psychological science at a higher level. To be sure, this has not prevented positive psychology from being perceived as a new paradigm by many, but it seems to be a widely shared ambition in the field to stay firmly within established scientific boundaries.

12.4   Recent Findings in Positive Psychology of Particular Educational Importance

More recent psychological evidence, of course still standing on the shoulders of what went before, include the authoritative mapping the negativity-bias – a tendency to experience bad (negative) aspects of life stronger than good ones, relating to almost every aspect of live (Baumeister et al. 2001; Rozin and Royzman 2001). This finding is so important that Linley et al. (2010) have described it as no less than the main challenge for positive psychology, almost the raison d'etre of positive psychology as it pervades every aspect of human life and interaction, and more than any other single factor explains why it is necessary to give special attention to, and foster, the brighter sides of life. The understanding of the negativity-bias has tremendous implications for education, in that an optimal educational experience requires positivity quantitatively overwhelming negativity in individuals, groups, and cultures, which seems downright impossible without an informed strategy for this.

Directly related to the pivotal challenge of keeping negativity within limits, are two ground-breaking findings by Barbara Fredrickson and colleagues regarding positivity. First, the discovery of the link between positive emotions and learning though the Broaden-and-Build theory (Fredrickson 2009) stands out. The theory shows how humans react to positive emotions in ways that broaden their capacity to learn and consequently tend to learn more (build). Secondly, the mathematical exposure of the positivity ratio, stating that a person needs at least three times as many positive emotions as negative ones in order to flourish, is important (Fredrickson and Losada 2005). It is hard to find a better argument than these two theories for ensuring the individual experience of positive emotions as an essential part of any educational experience.

A third major contribution to positive psychology in recent years regards the mapping and advanced use of individual strengths. To be sure, within general psychology individual strengths have long been studied as traits, intelligences, styles, interest and values, but data from thousands of users of online surveys such as the Clifton Strengths Finder, the Values-in-Action – Inventory of Strengths (VIA-IS) measuring character strengths, and the Realise2[3] are opening inspiring both new theoretical developments and applications of strengths in daily life. In education these positive strength-approaches are running across the traditional divisions of disciplines lighting up a host of human qualities (strengths) that have hitherto been difficult to see because the sciences, arts, and crafts often do not readily reveal them. Thus, for instance the strength of perseverance may obviously be of great use in any domain but typically not a strength that is given particular attention, let alone that is graded in education (though it certainly can contribute to performances that are).

The VIA Classification (Peterson and Seligman 2004) and VIA-IS are used by researchers and practitioners around the world (Niemiec 2012), making it one of the most substantial initiatives to emerge from the burgeoning science of positive psychology to date. Research on the VIA Classification (Peterson and Seligman 2004) is flourishing and like other practitioners educators are working to find ways to apply the research to their practices while maintaining prudence with the findings, as this research defines fairly new territory. Research on character strengths across "educational" disciplines is seen in positive psychotherapy (Seligman et al. 2006); in various forms of coaching, ranging from executive to life, health, and parent coaching; use with children, adolescents, teachers, and school systems (Fox Eades 2008; Proctor and Fox Eades 2011; Park and Peterson 2009); in positive education (e.g., Geelong Grammar School and St Peters College in Australia; a significant number of schools in Denmark; the Penn Resiliency Program[4]); positive institutions, business, and Appreciative Inquiry (Cooperrider 2009; Cooperrider and Whitney 2005); and faculty development and teaching (McGovern and Miller 2008).

When zooming in on the educational applications of strengths broadly, Lopez and Louis (2009) find that there are generally five recommendable principles of strengths-based education: measurement, individualization, networking, deliberate

---

[3] See: http://www.strengthsfinder.com, http://www.viacharacter.org, http://www.cappeu.com.

[4] See: http://www.ggs.vic.edu.au, http://www.stpeters.sa.edu.au, http:www.ppc.sas.upenn.edu/prp-sum.htm.

application, and intentional development. Lopez and Louis (2009) argue that through a parallel process, educators practice the principles of strengths-based education when advising and teaching while students learn to put their strengths to work in learning and social situations. It should be clear how these recommendations are in line with the central elements of self-determination theory, that show how individuals function at optimal levels and are most authentically motivated when three psychological needs are met: competence, autonomy, and relatedness (Deci and Ryan 2000). Lopez and Louis (2009) highlight how helping students understand the connection between their strengths and their personal goals, and offering guidance in the application of their strengths in the most effective ways, may elicit feelings of competence. Further, providing students with choices and opportunities for self-direction can support their need for autonomy: "When educators establish a learning culture where students view themselves and others through "strengths-colored glasses" (Clifton et al. 2006, p. 73), they help to foster appreciation for differences, highlight the value of collaboration and teamwork, and establish a powerful sense of relatedness." (Lopez and Louis 2009).

To sum up, all the elements of well-being presented so far, including positive emotion, engagement, meaning and positive social relations, positive expectations, and the individually energizing strengths found through surveys like the Clifton Strength Finder, the VIA-IS, and the Realise2 survey provide a basis for educational practice that obviously should no longer be neglected if education is to function optimally. The most important causal relations implied in the presented theories are illustrated in Fig. 12.1 in order to serve both as a kind of visual summary, and as a launch pad for the final part of this chapter sharing experiences and findings from application of positive psychology in Danish schools and a few more general ideas and concerns regarding the future of positive psychology in the broader societal context.

12.5   An Education to Its Fullest

Since 2005 systematic measures of pupils' positive emotions, engagement, meaning, social relations, and possibilities of individualized learning has been conducted as integrated elements in research-based school development projects (Knoop 2010). An estimated total of 20,000 pupils in elementary and lower secondary school have participated along with approximately 2,500 teachers and leaders at around 50 schools. This is not the place for a detailed description of these projects, but the common ambition as regards applied positive psychology in all these projects has been for high-trust collaborations between dedicated practitioners and researchers in order to optimize the well-being and thereby academic performance of the pupils and the teachers, as well as to allow the researchers anonymous access to substantial amounts of data. In other words, all these projects have had a double ambition of stimulating pedagogy while producing reliable data for scientific purposes. The results have been mostly positive, yet somewhat mixed, being highly dependent on the specific interest and sense of ownership of the teachers involved.

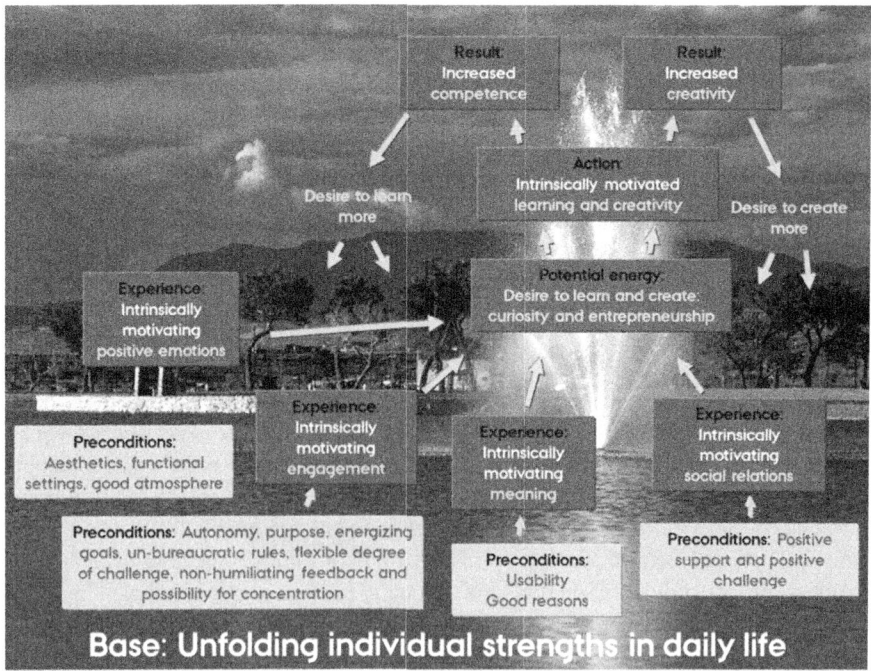

Fig. 12.1 How well-being, learning, creativity, and performance is energizingly related in a person (*blue boxes*) – and how elementary organizational preconditions (*yellow boxes*) and the unfolding of individual strengths enables such human flourishing (Knoop 2009, 2011) (Color figure online)

The categories surveyed over 6 years are by and large those represented in Fig. 12.1, though revisions have continuously advanced the degree of detail and precision in line with scientific progress and practical feasibility. Currently, a whole new and very promising instrument is being developed under the name Live'n'Learn. dk[5] that allows for health, well-being and learning to be survey coherently (Knoop et al. in press). The academic rationale is to apply the most fundamental categories of well-being to schools by educating teachers in understanding and applying them, by facilitating teachers and pupils in administrating the web based survey, and by offering ideas and other feedback based on the survey-results – both immediately and in the longer term. Finally, it is no minor detail that we are doing this work in a cultural setting that may be hypothesized as being as supportive of well-being and strengths-based approaches as anywhere in the world. In brief, the basis for this assumption is that Denmark are among the highest ranking countries in the world regarding economic equality, personal autonomy, social trust, avoidance of corruption, satisfaction with life/happiness, flourishing, creativity, private homes online at broadband-level, and material wealth. Taken together this means that we have

---

[5]See: http://www.Live&Learn.dk.

the chance of developing and/or using sophisticated measures of well-being and strengths in a context that to a very high degree seems to support many of the most important sources for well-being and strengths-based activity. To be sure, this rather fortunate basis may make it harder to improve on some measures but Danish education suffers more than enough even so and there continues to be all good reasons for infusing new energy, more intrinsic motivation, and more self-reinforcing quality in education.

12.6 Epilogue

So far, education has had three functions. Qualifying young people for life's challenges, socializing young people into cultural traditions, and selection of young people for different working positions available in society. It is strongly debatable how well education has succeeded in overcoming, or better: living up to these tasks, and one can (un-)comfortably argue, that only the last function is fulfilled if ever so unjust. That only the selective function has worked insofar people have been divided horizontally into domains and field and vertically into unequally privileged layers of society. To be sure, it is difficult to imagine a modern society where some kind of horizontal and vertical division of labor is not in place, but importantly in this context is to note how positive psychology harbors an ideal flying in the face of all graver forms of inequality as it aims at securing everyone sufficient social appreciation, everyone sufficient positive experiences, and everyone future perspectives making their lives worthwhile.

Positive psychology is clearly much more about optimizing specific types of processes to be applied generally rather than about specific aims and specific content. As such positive psychology is both apolitical and neutral as regards academic and professional disciplines. Yet, the findings coming from the research within positive psychology indirectly favor high levels of economic equality, and high levels of equality when comparing the social status of the many positions in the labor market. Because, simply, the evidence shows that high levels of equality in democratic (equal-vote-based, at least in principle) countries predict high levels of well-being, that high levels of equality among co-workers strongly furthers co-working, and that high levels of equality promotes social responsibility because it is broadly considered fair and therefore worth reciprocating. Other findings, like those pointing to the diminishing benefit of material good, may indirectly be seen as political messages as well. Yet, in this chapter I shall not discuss these important aspects further but limit myself to underscoring how positive psychology may be at odds with all of the three main functions of education as they have been managed so far: as already indicated the brute selection into very unequal positions in society does not sit well with the aims of helping everybody into worthwhile living; the socialization in factory-like settings that are of very little use in the future seems equally outdated; and the qualification process known by rote learning of academic content to be forgotten even faster than it is learned obviously can not be defended from any evidence-based finding coming from positive psychology either. As such, and quite ironical, the sweet and smooth and harmless and mellow air of positive psychology perceived by so many at first blush turns out to have a strong critical edge, providing serious leverage to social and cultural reforms for those taking it seriously on board.

References

Anderson, R., Manoogian, S. T., & Reznick, J. S. (1976). The undermining and enhancing of intrinsic motivation in preschool children. *Journal of Personality and Social Psychology, 34*, 915–922.

Bandura, A. (1977). Self-efficacy: Toward a unifying theory of behavioral change. *Psychological Review, 84*, 191–215.

Bandura, A. (1994). Self-efficacy. In V. S. Ramachaudran (Ed.), *Encyclopedia of human behavior* (Vol. 4, pp. 71–81). New York: Academic.

Bandura, A. (1995). *Self-efficacy in changing societies*. Cambridge/New York: Cambridge University Press, Cambridge.

Baumeister, R. F., Bratslavsky, E., Finkenauer, C., & Vohs, K. D. (2001). Bad is stronger than good. *Review of General Psychology, 5*, 323–370.

Camazine, S., Deneubourg, J. L., Franks, N. R., Sneyd, J., Theraulaz, G., & Bonabeau, E. (2001). *Self-organization in biological systems*. Princeton: Princeton University Press.

Clifton, D. O., Anderson, C. E., & Schreiner, L. A. (2006). *StrengthsQuest: Discover and develop your strengths in academics, career, and beyond* (2nd ed.). New York: Gallup Press.

Cooperrider, D. L. (2009, June). *The discovery and design of positive institutions: Definitions and a framework for research*. Paper presented at the International Positive Psychology Association conference, Philadelphia, PA.

Cooperrider, D. L., & Whitney, D. (2005). *Appreciative inquiry: A positive revolution in change*. San Francisco: Berrett-Koehler.

Csikszentmihalyi, M. (1990). *Flow: The psychology of optimal experience*. New York: Harper & Row Publishers.

Csikszentmihalyi, M. (1993). *The evolving self: A psychology for the third millennium*. New York: HarperCollins.

Csikszentmihalyi, M. (1996). *Creativity: Flow and the psychology of discovery and invention*. New York: HarperCollins.

Csikszentmihalyi, M., & Rathunde, K. (1993). The measurement of flow in everyday life: Towards a theory of emergent motivation. In J. E. Jacobs (Ed.), *Developmental perspectives on motivation 1992: Nebraska symposium on motivation* (Vol. 40, pp. 57–97). Lincoln: University of Nebraska Press.

Csikszentmihalyi, M., Abuhamdeh, S., & Nakamura, J. (2005). Flow. In A. J. Elliot & C. S. Dweck (Eds.), *Handbook of competence and motivation* (pp. 589–608). New York: The Guilford Press.

Deci, E. L., & Ryan, R. M. (2000). The 'what' and 'why' of goal pursuits: Human needs and the self-determination of behavior. *Psychological Inquiry, 11*, 227–268.

Fox Eades, J. M. (2008). *Celebrating strengths: Building strengths-based schools*. Coventry: CAPP Press. Danish translation published 2011.

Fredrickson, B. L. (2009). *Positivity: Groundbreaking research reveals how to embrace the hidden strength of positive emotions, overcome negativity, and thrive*. New York: Crown.

Fredrickson, B. L., & Losada, M. (2005). Positive affect and the complex dynamics of human flourishing. *American Psychologist, 60*, 678–686.

Harter, S. (1978). Effectance motivation reconsidered: Toward a developmental model. *Human Development, 1*, 661–669.

Kauffman, S. A. (2000). *Investigations*. New York: Oxford University Press.

Knoop, H. H. (2009). En fremtid mellem kontrol og uforudsigelighed. *Copenhagen: Kognition & Pædagogik, 19*(74), 66–71.

Knoop, H. H. (2010). Positiv psykologi i Danmark i 2010: Om ordentlig uorden. *Copenhagen: Kognition & Pædagogik, 20*(75), 2–13.

Knoop, H. H. (2011). Education in 2025: How positive psychology can revitalize education. In I. Stewart, S. I. Donaldson, M. Csikszentmihalyi, & J. Nakamura (Eds.), *Applied positive psychology: Improving everyday life, health, schools, work, and society* (pp. 97–116). New York: Routledge Academic, Copemhagen.

Knoop, H. H., Okholm, M., & Poulsen, K. (in press). *Live'n'Learn: Measuring what really counts.* Aarhus University & Rambøll.

McGovern, T. V., & Miller, S. L. (2008). Integrating teacher behaviors with character strengths and virtues for faculty development. *Teaching of Psychology, 35*(4), 278–285.

Niemiec, R. (2012). VIA character strengths – Research and practice: The first 10 years. In H. H. Knoop & A. Delle Fave (Eds.), *Well-being and cultures: Perspectives from positive psychology (cross-cultural advancements in positive psychology).* Dordrecht: Springer.

Niemiec, C. P., & Ryan, R. M. (2009). Autonomy, competence, and relatedness in the classroom: Applying self-determination theory to educational practice. *Theory and Research in Education, 7*, 133–144.

Linley, A., Willars, J., & Biswas-Diener, R. (2010). *The strength book.* Cambridge: CAPP Press, Coventry.

Lopez, S. J., & Louis, M. C. (2009). The principles of strengths-based education. *Journal of College and Character, 10*(4), 1–8.

Maslow, A. (1954). *Motivation and personality.* New York: Harper.

Overmier, J. B., & Seligman, M. E. P. (1967). Effects of inescapable shock upon subsequent escape and avoidance responding. *Journal of Comparative and Physiological Psychology, 63*, 28–33.

Park, N., & Peterson, C. (2009). Strengths of character in schools. In R. Gilman, E. S. Huebner, & M. J. Furlong (Eds.), *Handbook of positive psychology in schools* (pp. 65–76). New York: Routledge.

Peterson, C., & Seligman, M. E. P. (2004). *Character strengths and virtues – A handbook and classification.* New York: Oxford University Press.

Pinker, S. (2002). *The blank slate – The modern denial of human nature.* London: BCA.

Proctor, C., & Fox Eades, J. (2011). *Strengths gym: Build and exercise your strengths!* St Peter Port: PPRC.

Rhem, J. (1999). Pygmalion in the classroom. *The National Teaching & Learning Forum, 8*(2), 1–2. http://www.ntlf.com/issues/v8n2/v8n2.pdf

Rogers, C. (1961). *On becoming a person: A therapist's view of psychotherapy.* London: Constable.

Rogers, C. (1969). *Freedom to learn: A view of what education might become* (1st ed.). Columbus: Charles Merill.

Rosenthal, R., & Jacobson, L. (1992). *Pygmalion in the classroom (expanded ed.).* New York: Irvington.

Rozin, P., & Royzman, E. B. (2001). Negativity bias, negativity dominance, and contagion. *Personality and Social Psychology Review, 5*(4), 296–320.

Ryan, R. M. (1995). Psychological needs and the facilitation of integrative processes. *Journal of Personality, 63*, 397–427.

Seligman, M. E. P., & Maier, S. F. (1967). Failure to escape traumatic shock. *Journal of Experimental Psychology, 74*, 1–9.

Seligman, M. E. P., Rashid, T., & Parks, A. (2006). Positive psychotherapy. *American Psychologist, 61*, 774–778.

Shernoff, D. J., & Hoogstra, L. (2001). Continuing motivation beyond the high school classroom. *New Directions for Child and Adolescent Development, 93*, 73–87.

Winston, C. (2006). *Government failure versus market failure.* Washington, DC: Brookings Institution Press.

Zachariae, R. (2011, December 8). *Positive psychology, health and stress.* Psychology Lecture, Aarhus University.

Chapter 13
Enhancing Well-Being in Adolescents: Positive Psychology and Coaching Psychology Interventions in Schools

Lisa Suzanne Green and Jacolyn Maree Norrish

13.1 Well-Being in Schools: Then and Now

There is increasing consensus that well-being is an important aspect of school life. Gill (2009) argues "human flourishing should be the core aim of education, and that education ought to be directed at the child as a whole, nurturing their diverse qualities and virtues as well as their inner integrity and harmony" (p. 6). Huitt (2010) also acknowledges the change of paradigm occurring in education whereby schools are now being seen as institutions whose role extends beyond academic competence to preparing the "whole child".

This greater focus on the development of the whole child and the enhancement of well-being in schools is supported by a growing body of scientific research suggesting that well-being is related to social, emotional, and academic capability and prosocial behavior (Durlak et al. 2011). Additionally, research supports scientifically grounded well-being initiatives in playing a crucial preventative role in reducing depression, anxiety and stress within the school environment (Neil and Christensen 2007; Greenberg et al. 2003).

Green et al. (2011) suggest that historically schools have aimed for academic excellence as primary evidence for their success, however they note that there are growing numbers of schools who are now acknowledging the need to develop students in a more holistic way, with a stronger focus on well-being. For example, Geelong Grammar School and Knox Grammar School in Australia and Wellington College in the United Kingdom have made whole-school commitments to positive

L.S. Green (✉)
Coaching Psychology Unit, University of Sydney, 2000, Sydney, NSW, Australia
e-mail: suzy@thepositivityinstitute.com.au

J.M. Norrish
Mind Set Go Psychology, 5 Glusshouse Road, Collingwood, Victoria, Australia
e-mail: jaccinorish@gmail.com

C. Proctor and P.A. Linley (eds.), *Research, Applications, and Interventions for Children and Adolescents: A Positive Psychology Perspective*, DOI 10.1007/978-94-007-6398-2_13, © Springer Science+Business Media Dordrecht 2013

education programs that aim to help students to flourish psychologically, socially, and academically. Green et al. (2011) conclude that this recognition is also in response to the increasing statistics on psychological distress and mental illness in children and adolescents, and the need to take a more proactive rather than reactive approach to mental health.

Whilst well-being is not a new item on the school agenda, an historical review would suggest that the approach to well-being has primarily been deficit-focused. Akin-Little et al. (2003) note this particularly in regard to educational psychology services whereby they suggest these services are mostly available only after students demonstrate difficulties with learning or behavior. Damon (2004) argues that this problem-based focus in education and educational services has directed a huge share of the available resources to attempting to remediate the incapacities of young people with labels like Attention-Deficit/Hyperactivity Disorder and "learning disorder". Morrison et al. (2006) suggest that this is hardly surprising given that educational systems and external agencies usually provide extra support services and personnel on the basis of documentation of a pupil's assessed problems, deficits, and difficulties.

However, McGrath (2009) notes a shift in focus on well-being initiatives over time, beginning with the focus on self-esteem in the 1970s, which moved to social skills programs in the early 1990s, and then to resilience programs in early 2000. McGrath (2009) suggests from then on there has been a strong focus on anti-bullying initiatives, values programs, and student well-being initiatives including social and emotional learning programs. Noble and McGrath (2008) suggest that "… there are many examples of educational psychology practice slowly moving away from a model of deficit-focused service delivery toward more positive and preventative models that focus on the strengths of pupils, schools and families" (p. 121; Chafouleas and Bray 2004; Fagan and Wise 2000; Reschly 2000; Wilson and Reschly 1996).

This movement towards more positive and preventative models has been more recently supported by the emergence of *positive education* (Seligman et al. 2009). Initiatives that fall under the umbrella of positive education or "positive psychology in education" are aimed at increasing well-being and resilience. Such approaches do not ignore or discount the needs of students' with specific difficulties or challenges but acknowledge the value of promoting holistic well-being in conjunction with supporting students' specific needs. Moreover, it is proposed that helping students to develop their strengths and capacities has a beneficial and preventative effect on a wide range of challenges and difficulties that student's experience (Jenson et al. 2004).

13.2 Positive Education

Professor Martin Seligman formally identified the field of positive education in 2009. Seligman et al. (2009) defined positive education as "education for both traditional skills and for happiness" (p. 293). Seligman's interest in education began with rigorous research aimed at solving the question "Can well-being be taught in Schools?" (Seligman et al. 2009, p. 297). Seligman identifies both the Penn Resilience Program (PRP; Brunwasser et al. 2009) and Strath Haven Positive Psychology Curriculum (Seligman et al. 2009) as two evidence-based approaches that give support to a positive response to this question. The PRP is designed to prevent depression and hence falls under the prevention banner. Seligman et al. (2009) notes that PRP is "one of the most widely researched programs designed to prevent depression in young people" (p. 297), quoting over 17 studies conducted over 20 years providing evidence for its use in reducing depression. The Strath Haven program has a stronger focus on the promotion of well-being. Seligman et al. (2009) suggests the major goals of this program are: (1) to help students identify their signature character strengths; and (2) to increase students' use of these strengths in their day-to-day life. This program has also been scientifically evaluated and was shown to increase student's enjoyment and engagement in school and improve their social skills.

Seligman et al. (2009) concludes that there are three primary reasons why well-being should be taught in schools: (1) as an antidote to depression; (2) as vehicle for increasing life satisfaction; and (3) as an aid to better learning and more creative thinking.

More recently, it has been suggested that a broader and more useful definition of positive education is "applied positive psychology in education" (Green et al. 2011). Positive psychology itself has been defined as an umbrella term encompassing theory and research in relation to what makes life worth living (Noble and McGrath 2008). Whilst the study of happiness falls under this umbrella, so do other psychological constructs such as meaning, wisdom, creativity and many more, all which may be seen as relevant to the school setting to assist in the understanding and development of high levels of psychological well-being in students, staff, and school. Beyond the well-being programs identified previously (i.e., PRP/Strath Haven), there are an increasing number of schools-based positive psychology interventions (PPIs) being created and utilized in schools in an attempt to teach and enhance the well-being of students.

13.3 School-Based Positive Psychology Interventions

The implementation of positive psychology in school settings is garnering substantial attention. As identified previously, schools are a central developmental context in adolescents' lives and, along with their families and communities, play a critical role in the development of crucial life and social skills.

School-based PPIs are defined as initiatives that explicitly aim to enhance well-being or build competence within the school context. Whilst there has been substantial research into school-based programs that aim to prevent or treat mental distress, pathology, or risk behaviors (see Neil and Christensen 2007; Spence and Shortt 2007), studies into school-based programs that promote well-being are less common. While the field is young, PPIs focused on building capabilities and strengths, versus approaches that aim to alleviate problems or fix deficits, are inherently attractive to educational professionals due to their constructive and holistic focus.

Positive psychology can be implemented in school settings explicitly, such as through structured programs or PPIs, or implicitly through practices that support positive psychology principles across various areas of school life. Thus far, the majority of research in school-based positive psychology has focused on explicit PPIs and programs. These programs can be divided into single component PPIs that focus on one key construct, such as hope (Marques et al. 2011) or gratitude (Froh et al. 2008), or multi-component PPIs that integrate several key positive psychology concepts into a comprehensive approach.

13.3.1 Examples of Single-Component PPIs

Gratitude involves positive feelings, such as thankfulness or appreciation, which are related to perceived good fortune or the prosocial behaviors of others (Froh et al. 2010; Wood et al. 2010). In adolescent samples, gratitude has been related to beneficial psychological outcomes, such as high subjective well-being and optimism, as well as social benefits, such as pro-social behaviors and social support (Froh et al. 2009b). In a study of 700 adolescents (aged 10–14), Froh et al. (2010) found that adolescents with high gratitude at one time point reported higher life satisfaction and more social integration 6-months later than those with initial low gratitude, supporting the benefits of gratitude over time.

There are two published studies of interventions that focus on cultivating gratitude in students. Froh et al. (2008) conducted a study of a counting blessings intervention where students were required to deliberately pay attention to up to five positive events daily for a 2-week period. Eleven classes of students were randomly allocated to the gratitude condition, a comparison condition that required students to pay attention to daily hassles, or a non-intervention control condition. Students allocated to the gratitude condition reported more satisfaction with school experience than students allocated to the other two conditions; and enhanced well-being relative to students in the hassles condition. In a second gratitude PPI study, Froh et al. (2009a) matched students ($N=89$; age range 8–19) by school grade and then randomly allocated them to a gratitude visit condition or a comparison condition that involved writing about daily events. Students allocated to the gratitude visit condition were invited to write a gratitude letter to someone who was important in their lives and deliver it in person. While overall there were no significant differences between the groups, a key finding was that positive affect moderated the relationship between the study condition and student well-being over the 2-month follow-up time period. This suggests that students with low initial levels of positive affect may benefit the most from gratitude PPIs.

Snyder (2002) proposed that hope is a cognitive-motivational process based on three interconnected components: (1) goals; (2) pathways or strategies to achieve the goals; and (3) agency or motivation to implement the pathways. Valle et al.

(2006) investigated hope and life satisfaction in 860 students and found that high hope at the commencement of the study predicted high life satisfaction 1 year later after controlling for initial levels of life satisfaction. Hope was also associated with fewer internalizing behaviors over time. Marques et al. (2011) conducted a study where 31 adolescents took part in a 5-week hope program and a matched sample of 31 adolescents formed a comparison control. Students in the hope condition reported increased self-worth, life satisfaction, and hope relative to controls post-intervention and at an 18-month follow-up time point.

13.3.2 Examples of Multi-component PPIs

Multi-component PPIs focus on helping students to develop positive psychology skills in several key domains. An example is the Strath Haven Positive Psychology Program identified earlier, which integrates learning related to the 24 character strengths in the Values in Action framework (Peterson and Seligman 2004). The program runs over 20–25 weeks and integrates efforts to build character strengths, with efforts to cultivate positive emotions, explore sources of meaning in life, and develop resilience (Seligman et al. 2009). In an evaluation of the program, 347 year 9 students were randomly allocated to the Strath Haven curriculum or the school's usual language arts condition (Seligman et al. 2009). Over the 2-year follow-up time frame, students who completed the Strath Haven curriculum demonstrated increased engagement with school, as measured by self and teacher reports, and improved social skills, as measured by mother and teacher reports; however, there were no significant improvements for symptoms of depression or anxiety. It may be that PPIs that aim to build strengths and capacities are most effective at promoting holistic well-being when used in conjunction with efforts to prevent or treat mental ill-health.

Strengths Gym is a similar example of a multi-component positive psychology program (Proctor et al. 2011). Strengths Gym provides a flexible curriculum for developing the 24 VIA character strengths through various strengths exercises and challenges, in-class activities, philosophical discussions, stories, and real-world homework activities (see Proctor, Chap. 2, this volume). Proctor et al. (2011) examined the effectiveness of Strengths Gym in a study of 319 adolescents (mean age = 12.98; SD = .50). Classes of students in two schools were allocated to the Strengths Gym condition or a comparison control condition. Teachers administered the Strengths Gym curriculum over a 6-month period. Post-intervention, students allocated to Strengths Gym reported significantly higher life satisfaction (r = .51) than students allocated to the comparison condition after controlling for age, gender, school, year, and baseline life satisfaction scores. In addition, while findings were non-significant, trends suggested benefits for the Strengths Gym condition in terms of positive affect, negative affect, and self-esteem. Taken together, these results provide promising evidence of the effectiveness of strengths programs in enhancing student well-being.

13.4   Evidence-Based Coaching as a PPI

The term "evidence-based coaching" was coined by Grant (2003) to distinguish between professional coaching that is explicitly grounded in broader empirical and theoretical knowledge base and coaching that was developed from the "pop psychology" personal development genre. Evidence-based coaching is underpinned by the field of coaching psychology. Coaching psychology, is a complementary field to positive psychology, and similar to positive psychology, is also concerned with optimal functioning and well-being enhancement. Its focus however is on understanding and applying relevant psychological theories and techniques to a collaborative relationship to enhance goal attainment and increase self-regulation for the "normal, non-clinical population" (Grant 2005). Coaching psychology has been defined as an "applied positive psychology" (Australian Psychological Coaching Psychology Interest Group 2012), whereby "coaching" (including the methodology and relationship) provides the opportunity for the application of positive psychology research, such as strengths identification and use (Linley et al. 2010). The role of positive psychology in coaching has also been discussed previously in the literature, however further research in regard to its specific applications is needed (see Linley and Harrington 2005; Kaufmann 2006; Biswas-Diener and Dean 2007).

13.5   Evidence Based Coaching in Schools

At this point in time, there is increasing interest on utilizing coaching in schools, both for students and staff. For example, the University of East London's Coaching Psychology Unit, offer students a dedicated module on Coaching and Mentoring in Education and held an International Conference on Coaching and Positive Psychology in Education in 2010.

However, there is currently limited research on applications of coaching psychology and evidence-based coaching in the education sector. Despite this there is interest growing in this field with over 2,590 citations in the database ERIC (in October 2010 using the keywords *coaching* and *education*) and over 537 citations in the database PsycINFO. It should however be noted that the majority of this literature is focused on *academic coaching* for students to enhance learning, or overcome literacy or learning difficulties (e.g., Merriman and Codding 2008; Plumer and Stoner 2005).

A study by Green et al. (2007) has given preliminary support for the use of evidence-based coaching in educational settings for students. Green et al. (2007) conducted a randomized wait-list control group study of evidence-based life-coaching with an adolescent population. Participants were randomly assigned to receive either a 10-week cognitive-behavioral solution-focused life coaching program or a wait-list control. They found that the 28 female senior high school students in the coaching program experienced a significant increase in levels of cognitive hardiness, hope, and a significant decrease in levels of depression, compared to the wait-list control group.

Furthermore, a recent pilot study was conducted by Madden et al. (2011) utilizing strengths-based coaching for primary school boys in a within-subject design study. Thirty-eight year five male students (mean age = 10.7 years) participated in a strengths-based coaching program as part of their Personal Development/Health program at an independent, private primary school in Sydney, Australia. Participants were randomly allocated to groups of four or five with each group receiving eight coaching sessions over two school terms. The Values in Action-Youth (Park and Peterson 2006) survey was used to highlight participant's character strengths, and the participants were coached in identifying personally meaningful goals, and in being persistent in their goal-striving, as well as finding novel ways to use their signature strengths. They also completed a "letter from the future" that involved writing about themselves at their best. The strengths-based coaching pilot program was associated with significant increases in the students' self-reported levels of engagement and hope. The authors concluded that strengths-based coaching programs may be considered as a potential mental health prevention and promotion intervention in a primary school setting to increase students' well-being and may also form an important part of an overall positive education program.

Whilst these studies provide promising support for the ongoing use of evidence-based coaching in educational settings, further research is required.

13.6 Strategic Integration of Positive Psychology and Coaching Psychology

Green et al. (2011) have argued for the integration of coaching psychology and positive psychology in the school setting to facilitate student, staff, and whole school optimal functioning and well-being. Whilst both positive psychology and coaching psychology can be utilized to enhance well-being and optimal functioning, they suggest that both approaches have primarily been applied independently of each other and require further integration. For example, schools who may be utilizing single or multi-component PPIs may not have even considered coaching or be mindful of what it has to offer a school, believing it to be primarily utilized in organizational settings. Similarly, a school implementing coaching for academic performance or for the broader purposes of enhancing well-being, such as the Madden et al. (2011) study may not have considered also offering class or group based PPIs.

Whilst research supports that both positive psychology and coaching psychology approaches lead to increased well-being, it may not be necessary to utilize both approaches simultaneously. However, Green et al. (2012) suggest that whilst a school may choose to select either approach as a means to create enhanced well-being and optimal functioning for both students and staff, school leadership should consider a strategic integration of both approaches. They argue that any training in positive psychology principles could be enhanced through the use of evidence-based coaching to support the transfer of training and sustain application in daily life. For example, if a student was learning about "strengths", they could set a personal goal to leverage a particular character strength. The student then takes ownership of the goal with the learning becoming more personalized. If coaching was offered on a continuing basis to the student (either individually or in a group) there is opportunity to offer ongoing support and track progress of that goal.

Green et al. (2012) suggest that goals may be set in regard to the application of any positive psychology concept including gratitude, kindness, forgiveness. In this manner, they argue, positive psychology is "brought to life" whereby the concepts are applied meaningfully and practically to a student's academic or personal life, drawing on the goal-setting and goal-striving methodologies of evidence-based coaching.

As such, we would suggest schools consider carefully how applications of both positive psychology and coaching psychology, either separately or as an integrated approach, could help create, enable and sustain well-being for students and staff.

13.7 Future Research and Implications

Future research is required on both school-based PPIs and evidence-based coaching in schools. In addition to supporting the use of both PPIs and evidence-based coaching in schools, further research will yield a more sophisticated understanding of the benefits of the two approaches for students with different needs and characteristics potentially enabling the targeting of interventions for maximum effect. In an attempt to resolve some of these questions, the authors are currently undertaking comparative research on these two fields involving a randomized controlled trial with senior high schools students in Sydney, Australia (Harvard University, Institute of Coaching Grant 2011).

We would also suggest that even more importantly, research is required on how these two complementary fields may be more closely integrated to enhance outcomes for students, staff, and schools. Larger scale positive education initiatives, such as the one currently being conducted at Knox Grammar School, in Sydney Australia, are utilizing and combining both approaches in an attempt to increase student, staff, and whole school well-being (Green et al. 2011). Independent scientific evaluation will provide further support for these types of programs.

In addition further research is required in regard to the mental health of those undergoing positive education interventions. PPIs and evidence-based coaching interventions are often promoted as "mental health prevention/promotion" and are usually aimed at a normal population rather than a clinical population with broad-sweeping assumptions on the mental health of those undergoing such interventions. This is particularly so in regard to coaching whereby many coaches assume that those wanting to engage a coach fall within the normal population. Fortunately this assumption has been questioned by three scientific studies showing that 25–52 % of people attending for coaching interventions present with significantly high levels of psychological distress (Green et al. 2006; Spence and Grant 2007; Kemp and Green

2010). We would suggest that these mental health or "screening" issues have not yet been raised or discussed adequately within the positive psychology literature or in terms of screening for PPIs. Given there is scant literature supporting the use of PPIs or coaching with clinical populations, there are real concerns that such interventions may lead to a negative outcome, rather than the intended positive one. Green et al. (2012) also highlight this issue and provide the example of a school student who may undertake a "strengths-based coaching intervention", fail to apply their strengths sufficiently or achieve their goals, due to an underlying clinical disorder such as depression, potentially worsening the clinical disorder, rather than improving the child's well-being.

Overall, the understanding of the impact of PPIs on adolescents who are not mentally well is limited. A priority for both research and the application of positive education is a greater understanding of the experience of students with symptoms of mental illness, and how such students can be supported to obtain the help and support they need without excluding them from school wide well-being practices. It is argued that positive education initiatives will work best when efforts to promote well-being and efforts to treat mental illness are applied in an complementary, integrated, and sustained way (Norrish and Vella-Brodrick 2009).

As previously mentioned, positive education includes both explicit structured education and implicit practices that support key learning in more informal ways. For example, students may explore their character strengths as part of a positive education program – this learning may then be supported and developed implicitly via school-wide practices such as exploring strengths at assemblies, educating parents on the importance of strengths, or creating a school-culture where the strengths language is used frequently (Fox Eades 2008). Similarly, the goal setting strategies that students learn as part of a coaching program may be developed by opportunities for students to set and work towards their goals in various classes and extracurricular activities. It is proposed that student learning is greatest when key messages are reinforced across numerous levels of the school environment and when core ideas are communicated between school staff, families, and the wider community (Weare 2000). However, while the whole school approach is potentially the most powerful in terms of promoting student well-being, it is also inherently more challenging to measure via rigorous research techniques, (such as randomized controlled trials), as it requires the manipulation of naturally occurring factors and the pervasiveness of the approach precludes the creation of control groups. Balancing the importance of rigorous research techniques with ecological factors such as the importance of the school-wide practices that support and deepen learning is one of the greatest challenges of positive education moving forward.

13.8   Conclusion

In conclusion, we argue that both positive psychology and coaching psychology have much to offer adolescents in schools in not only enhancing well-being, but also improving their overall optimal functioning including their learning and achievement.

We have suggested that the strategic use of both positive psychology and coaching psychology by a school should be a key consideration by leaders, particularly in terms of these interventions underpinning a larger scale *positive education program.*

Finally, we concur with Clonan et al. (2004) who suggest that "no two school systems would implement positive school psychology in an identical fashion" (p. 105) and the need for schools to create bespoke programs that meet the individualized need of their school's students and staff. Whether schools look to implement smaller scale PPIs or evidence-based coaching or alternatively are wishing to create a larger scale positive education program, there is a pressing need for further research to support such initiatives to support the widespread adoption of such programs in schools globally to increase the overall flourishing of not only our adolescent population, but for all students and staff.

References

Akin-Little, K. A., Little, S. G., & Delligatti, N. (2003). A preventative model of school consultation: Incorporating perspectives from positive psychology. *Psychology in the Schools, 41*(1), 155–162.

Australian Psychological Society, Coaching Psychology Interest Group. (2012). Retrieved from http://www.groups.psychology.org.au/igcp/. Accessed on 16 March 2012.

Biswas-Diener, R., & Dean, B. (2007). *Positive psychology coaching: Putting the science of happiness to work for your clients.* Hoboken: Wiley.

Brunwasser, S. M., Gillham, J. E., & Kim, E. S. (2009). A meta-analytic review of the Penn Resiliency Program's effects on depressive symptoms. *Journal of Consulting and Clinical Psychology, 77*(6), 1042–1054.

Chafouleas, S. M., & Bray, M. A. (2004). Introducing positive psychology: Finding its place within school psychology. *Psychology in the Schools, 41,* 1–6.

Clonan, S. M., Chafouleas, S. M., McDougal, J. L., & Riley-Tillman, T. C. (2004). Positive psychology goes to school: Are we there yet? *Psychology in the Schools, 41*(1), 101–110.

Damon, W. (2004). What is positive youth development? *Annals of the American Academy of Political and Social Science, 591,* 13–23.

Durlak, J. A., Weissberg, R. P., Dymnicki, A. B., Taylor, R. D., & Schellinger, K. B. (2011). The impact of enhancing students' social and emotional learning: A meta-analysis of school-based universal interventions. *Child Development, 82*(1), 405–432.

Fagan, T. K., & Wise, P. S. (2000). *School psychology: Past, present and future.* Bethesda: National Association of School Psychologists.

Fox Eades, J. (2008). *Celebrating strengths: Building strengths-based schools.* Coventry: CAPP Press.

Froh, J. J., Sefick, W. J., & Emmons, R. A. (2008). Counting blessings in early adolescents: An experimental study of gratitude and subjective well-being. *Journal of School Psychology, 46,* 213–233.

Froh, J. J., Kashdan, T. B., Ozimkowski, K. M., & Miller, N. (2009a). Who benefits the most from a gratitude intervention in children and adolescents? Examining positive affect as a moderator. *The Journal of Positive Psychology, 4,* 408–422.

Froh, J. J., Yurkewicz, C., & Kashdan, T. B. (2009b). Gratitude and subjective well-being in early adolescence: Examining gender differences. *Journal of Adolescence, 32,* 633–650.

Froh, J. J., Bono, G., & Emmons, R. (2010). Being grateful is beyond good manners: Gratitude and motivation to contribute to society among early adolescents. *Motivation and Emotion, 34,* 144–157.

Gill, S. (2009, July). *Monitoring and promoting well-being in education principles and possible approaches to child well-being indicators* (Working Paper Education for Well-Being Europe Consortium).

Grant, A. M. (2003). The impact of life coaching on goal attainment, metacognition and mental health. *Social Behavior and Personality: An International Journal, 31*(3), 253–264.

Grant, A. M. (2005). What is evidence-based executive, workplace and life coaching? In M. Cavanagh, A. M. Grant, & T. Kemp (Eds.), *Evidence-based coaching: Vol. 1. Theory, research and practice from the behavioural sciences* (pp. 1–12). Bowen Hills: Australian Academic Press.

Green, L. S., Oades, L. G., & Grant, A. M. (2006). Cognitive-behavioural, solution focused life coaching: Enhancing goal striving, well-being and hope. *The Journal of Positive Psychology, 1*, 142–149.

Green, L. S., Grant, A. M., & Rynsaardt, J. (2007). Evidence-based coaching for senior high school students: Building hardiness and hope. *International Coaching Psychology Review, 2*(1), 24–31.

Green, S., Oades, L., & Robinson, P. (2011, April). Positive education: Creating flourishing students, staff and schools. *InPsych*, pp. 16–18.

Green, L. S., Oades, L. G., & Robinson, P. L. (2012). Positive psychology and coaching psychology in schools. In C. van Nieuwerburgh (Ed.), *Coaching in education: Getting better results for students, teachers and parents*. London: Karnac.

Greenberg, M. T., et al. (2003). Enhancing school-based prevention and youth development through coordinated social, emotional, and academic learning. *American Psychologist, 58*, 466–474.

Harvard University, Institute of Coaching Grant. (2011). *Enhancing well-being and self- regulation in a general adolescent population: Comparing evidence-based coaching and positive psychology interventions*. Total funding US$39,829. Investigators: Green, L. S. Norrish, J. M., Vella-Brodrick, D. A., & Grant, A. M.

Huitt, W. (2010). Analyzing paradigms used in education and schooling. *Educational psychology interactive*. Valdosta: Valdosta State University. Retrieved from http://www.edpsycinteractive. org/topics/intro/paradigm.html

Jenson, W. R., Olympia, D., Farley, M., & Clark, E. (2004). Positive psychology and externalising students in a sea of negativity. *Psychology in the Schools, 41*, 67–79.

Kauffman, C. (2006). Positive psychology: The science at the heart of coaching. In D. R. Stober & A. M. Grant (Eds.), *Evidence based coaching handbook: Putting best practices to work for your clients* (pp. 219–253). Hoboken: Wiley.

Kemp, T., & Green, L. S. (2010). *Executive coaching for the normal "non-clinical" population: Fact or fiction?* Paper presented at the Fourth Australian Conference on Evidence-Based Coaching, University of Sydney.

Linley, P. A., & Harrington, S. (2005). Positive psychology and coaching psychology: Perspectives on integration. *The Coaching Psychologist, 1*(1), 13–14.

Linley, P. A., Nielsen, A. M., Gillett, R., & Biswas-Diener, R. (2010). Using signature strengths in pursuit of goals: Effects on goal progress, need satisfaction, and well-being, and implications for coaching psychologists. *International Coaching Psychology Review, 5*(1), 8–17.

Madden, W., Green, S., & Grant, A. (2011). A pilot study evaluating strengths-based coaching for primary school students: Enhancing engagement and hope. *International Coaching Psychology Review, 61*(1), 71–83.

Marques, S. C., Lopez, S. J., & Pais-Ribeiro, J. L. (2011). "Building hope for the future": A program to foster strengths in middle-school students. *Journal of Happiness Studies, 12*, 139–152.

McGrath, H. (2009). *An evidence-based positive psychology approach to student well-being*. Paper presented at the 1st Australia Positive Psychology in Education Symposium, University of Sydney.

Merriman, D. E., & Codding, R. S. (2008). The effects of coaching on mathematics homework completion and accuracy of high school students with attention-deficit/hyperactivity disorder. *Journal of Behavioral Education, 17*, 339–355.

Morrison, G. M., Brown, M., D'Incau, B., O'Farrell, S. L., & Furlong, M. J. (2006). Understanding resilience in educational trajectories: Implications for protective possibilities. *Psychology in the Schools, 43,* 19–31.

Neil, A. L., & Christensen, H. (2007). Australian school-based prevention and early intervention programs for anxiety and depression: A systematic review. *The Medical Journal of Australia, 186,* 305–308.

Noble, T., & McGrath, H. (2008). The positive educational practices framework: A tool for facilitating the work of educational psychologists in promoting pupil wellbeing. *Educational and Child Psychology, 25,* 119–134.

Norrish, J. M., & Vella-Brodrick, D. A. (2009). Positive psychology and adolescents: Where are we now? Where to from here? *Australian Psychologist, 1,* 1–9.

Park, N., & Peterson, C. (2006). Moral competence and character strengths among adolescents: The development and validation of the values in action inventory of strengths for youth. *Journal of Adolescence, 29*(6), 891–909.

Peterson, C., & Seligman, M. E. P. (2004). *Character strengths and virtues: A handbook and classification.* New York: Oxford University Press.

Plumer, P. J., & Stoner, G. (2005, August). The relative effects of classroom peer tutoring and peer coaching on the positive social behaviours of children with ADHD. *Journal of Attention Disorders, 9*(1), 290–300.

Proctor, C., Tsukayama, E., Wood, A. M., Maltby, J., Fox Eades, J. M., & Linley, P. A. (2011). Strengths gym: The impact of a character strengths-based intervention on the life satisfaction and well-being of adolescents. *The Journal of Positive Psychology, 6*(5), 377–388.

Reschly, D. J. (2000). The present and future status of school psychology in the United States. *School Psychology Review, 29,* 507–522.

Seligman, M. E. P., Ernst, R. M., Gillham, J., Reivich, K., & Linkins, M. (2009). Positive education: Positive psychology and classroom interventions. *Oxford Review of Education, 35,* 293–311.

Snyder, C. R. (2002). Hope theory: Rainbows in the mind. *Psychological Inquiry, 13,* 249–275.

Spence, G. B., & Grant, A. M. (2007). Professional and peer life coaching and the enhancement of goal striving and well-being: An exploratory study. *The Journal of Positive Psychology, 2,* 185–194.

Spence, S. H., & Shortt, A. L. (2007). Research review: Can we justify the widespread dissemination of universal, school-based interventions for the prevention of depression among children and adolescents? *Journal of Child Psychology and Psychiatry, 48,* 526–542.

Valle, M. F., Huebner, E. S., & Suldo, S. M. (2006). An analysis of hope as a psychological strength. *Journal of School Psychology, 44,* 393–406.

Weare, K. (2000). *Promoting mental, emotional and social health. A whole school approach.* London: Routledge.

Wilson, M. S., & Reschly, D. J. (1996). Assessment in school psychology training and practice. *School Psychology Review, 25,* 9–23.

Wood, A. M., Froh, J. J., & Geraghty, A. W. A. (2010). Gratitude and well-being: A review and theoretical integration. *Clinical Psychology Review, 30,* 890–905.

Part V
Positive Youth Development:
Practice, Policy, and Law

Chapter 14
Sociomoral Development for Behaviorally At-Risk Youth: Mac's Group Meeting

John C. Gibbs, Granville Bud Potter, and Ann-Marie DiBiase

14.1 Introduction

In 1993, at a juvenile correctional facility in Columbus, Ohio, a group of eight residents and a staff group leader were having a mutual help meeting. The focus of the meeting was an incident reported by 15-year-old Mac, one of the group members. Mac had resisted and yelled profanities at a staff member who, in accordance with institutional policy, had begun to inspect his carrying bag. The group and Mac agreed that Mac's defiance and profanity represented, in the language of the program, an Authority Problem, but the group wanted to know the *meaning* of that problem, its underlying "thinking error" or cognitive distortion. Angry as he thought about the incident and his subsequent disciplinary write-up, Mac explained that the bag contained something very special and irreplaceable – photos of his grandmother – and that he was not going to let anyone take the photos from him. Mac's peers understood his point of view but saw it as one-sided: Mac thought only of safeguarding his photos. He did not for a moment consider the staff member's perspective or the facility's rules: she was only carrying out institutional policy concerning inspection for possible contraband. Nor did Mac consider that she was not abusive and that he thus had no reason to assume that the photos

J.C. Gibbs (✉)
Department of Psychology, The Ohio State University,
1835 Neil Avenue, Columbus, OH 43210, USA
e-mail: gibbs.1@osu.edu

G.B. Potter
EQUIP consultant, 5015 Charlbury Drive, Columbus, OH 43220, USA
e-mail: budpotter@att.net

A.-M. DiBiase
Department of Graduate and Undergraduate Studies, Faculty of Education, Brock University,
500 Glenridge Ave, St. Catherines, ON, Canada L2S 3A1
e-mail: Ann-Marie.DiBiase@brocku.ca

C. Proctor and P.A. Linley (eds.), *Research, Applications, and Interventions for Children
and Adolescents: A Positive Psychology Perspective*, DOI 10.1007/978-94-007-6398-2_14,
© Springer Science+Business Media Dordrecht 2013

would be confiscated. In the language of the program, Mac had Self-Centered and Assuming the Worst thinking errors; this distorted thinking had generated the surface behavior identified as an "authority problem". Furthermore, Mac's anger at staff for his write-up was identified as an Easily Angered problem and was attributed to a Blaming Others thinking error. After all, Mac had no one but himself to blame for the incident report.

As they helped Mac deal with his one-sided viewpoint and develop his positive potential, the group used certain tools or equipment, acquired elsewhere in the program. This equipment included the reasons for the institution's inspection policy, how Mac could have corrected his thinking errors and used other skills to manage his anger, and how he could have expressed his concern to the staff member in a balanced and constructive fashion.

As the meeting progressed (it lasted more than an hour), Mac's anger dissipated considerably, and he began to regret his verbal assault on the staff member. He started to take into account her perspective. In other words, he began to "see" the other person (and the way the facility she served had to work) in a genuine sense. He could see the unfairness of his behavior toward her, empathize with her, and appropriately attribute blame (i.e., correct his Blaming Others thinking error). Over the course of subsequent sessions, sometimes as he helped others in the group, Mac continued to work on correcting or remedying his cognitive limitations and taking the perspectives of others in various ways. With encouragement, accountability, and practice, social perspective-taking became easier, more spontaneous for Mac. Constructive and responsible behavior was increasingly evident as Mac's Authority and Easily Angered problems attenuated. As Mac made gains toward responsible thought, so he also made gains toward responsible behavior.

14.2   The EQUIP Program

Mac's mutual help meeting illustrated part of EQUIP (Gibbs et al. 1995, 2009), a group-based cognitive-behavioral intervention program for behaviorally at-risk or antisocial youth like Mac. Based on developmental theory (Gibbs 2013), EQUIP posits that the fundamental problem generating much antisocial behavior pertains to self-centered (egocentrically biased, self-serving, or imbalanced) attitudes, thoughts, or perceptions of people and events. Mac's one-sided viewpoint meant that he often did not take into account other persons' legitimate feelings and expectations. Everyone is egocentric to some extent, and Mac's life had not been easy. Yet Mac's pervasively self-centered approach to problems in his life had only made those problems worse. Hence, the fundamental goal of a treatment program for antisocial youth should be to facilitate socio necessary moral development in a broad sense, that is, to provide social perspective-taking opportunities that can remedy self-centered cognitive limitations, facilitate growth beyond the superficial in social and moral life, and induce responsible thought and behavior.

This chapter describes the approaches and applications involved in the EQUIP program. We will describe how EQUIP combines two major treatment approaches and emphasizes cognitive restructuring as well as social perspective-taking. We will conclude with a consideration of how EQUIP might be supplemented with more intense social perspective-taking techniques for severe offenders.

14.2.1 First, the Mutual Help Approach: Transform the Group's "Culture" So That Group Members Are Motivated to Help One Another

Mac's group meeting specifically illustrated the first approach used in the EQUIP program, namely, our cognitive version of *Positive Peer Culture* (Vorrath and Brendtro 1985), or, more generally, what we call the mutual help approach. Such interventions address the challenge of a negative youth culture. In their analysis of the moral atmosphere or moral climate of a Bronx, New York, high school, Kohlberg and Higgins (1987) identified certain *oppositional* or "counter norms" (in our terms, culturally normative cognitive distortions), such as "look at me the wrong way and you're in for a fight" (another example of Assuming the Worst) and "it's your fault if something is stolen – you were tempting me" (p. 110) (another example of Blaming Others). In correctional settings, the negative youth culture is generally "characterized by opposition to institutional rules and goals, norms against inform- ing authorities about rule violations, and the use of physical coercion as a basis of influence among inmates" (Osgood et al. 1985, p. 71).

The aim of Positive Peer Culture is to transform this negative (self-centered, dis- torted, harmful) culture of antisocial youth into a mutual help culture, i.e., a positive group in which members listen to and work with one another's perspectives. Techniques for accomplishing this aim include: selecting for the initial peer group relatively positive (or at least less limited) peers; the cognitive-behavioral technique of relabeling, reframing, or cognitive restructuring (e.g., characterizing helping others as a *strong* rather than weak or sissy thing to do); confronting or reversing responsibility (see below); encouraging the honest sharing of personal histories ("life stories"); iso- lating and redirecting specific negative group members; and providing community service (cf. Hart et al. 2006) as well as faith-building opportunities (see Vorrath and Brendtro 1985). A helping group culture promotes amenability to treatment and moti- vates these youths to become – as was Mac's group – genuine and serious about help- ing one another. Antisocial youths' (such as Mac's) typical problems with authority, anger, stealing, lying, and so forth are identified in terms of a standard problem list, of which a key term is Inconsiderate of Others – implying the need for remediation through taking others' perspectives (precisely what Mac did *not* do).

The "confronting" technique, through which group members (such as Mac) are made aware of the effects of their actions on others, is especially relevant to social perspective-taking. Essentially, the group or group leader respectfully but forthrightly challenges the youth to put himself or herself in others' positions, to consider their legitimate expectations, feelings, and circumstances. Confronting thereby directly challenges Self-Centered and Blaming Others thinking errors (see below). Agee (1979) argued that effectively confronting violent offenders typically requires concrete, personal, and "blunt" techniques if they are to grasp the harm their violence has caused others. For example, if a violent offender has a sister and cares about her, that is an opening. The therapist might frame a female victim as someone's sister and appeal to moral reciprocity: "If it's okay for you to do that to someone else's sister, is it okay for them to do it to your sister?" (pp. 113–114). Yochelson and Samenow (1977) suggested that confrontation should include teaching "the chain of injuries" (p. 223) – extended to absent and indirect victims – resulting from every crime. Hoffman (2000) suggested that "the confrontings should also include the other's life condition beyond the immediate situation ... which the delinquents seem to ignore on their own" (p. 292). Agee's (1979) emphasis on bluntness notwithstanding, Vorrath and Brendtro (1985) stressed that, to be effective, confronting must be conveyed in a constructive and caring fashion.

Outcome evaluation studies of Positive Peer Culture and related interventions have yielded a mixed picture. Although these valuable programs have generally been found to promote youths' self-concept or self-esteem, reductions in recidivism are not typically found (see Gibbs et al. 1996). Worse, some peer group programs have actually had deleterious effects (see Dishion et al. 1999).

In our view, mutual help-only programs have had only mixed success because they do not adequately address the perspective-taking and helping-skill limitations of antisocial youth. Such programs can succeed for a while in inducing erstwhile antisocial youths to become "hooked on helping", perhaps because, as Vorrath and Brendtro (1985) suggested, the helper in the process "creates his own proof of worthiness" (p. 6) and thereby a genuine basis for self-respect. Furthermore, the confronting technique – if done properly – can induce genuine social perspective-taking. In the absence of constructive skills or tools for helping recalcitrant peers, however, antisocial youths often fall back on what they know best: putdowns and threats. To investigate mutual help problems and needs for improvement, Brendtro and Ness (1982) surveyed ten schools and facilities using Positive Peer Culture or related programs. Cited as a problem at nine of the ten centers was "abuse of confrontation" (e.g., "harassment, name-calling, screaming in someone's face, hostile profanity, and physical intimidation", p. 322) – going rather beyond Agee's (1979) call for bluntness! The pervasiveness of such abuse should not be surprising: how can a youth with antisocial behavior problems be helped by fellow group members who are trying but who lack skills and maturity for dealing with such problems – indeed, who have such problems themselves?

14.2.2   Limitations of Antisocial Youth: The Three D's

Mac's mutual help meeting illustrated more than traditional Positive Peer Culture techniques. For example, Mac reported and the group discussed not only Mac's Authority and Easily Angered problems but also the underlying thinking errors generating those problems – an innovation that deepens Positive Peer Culture problem work. That is our cognitive version of Positive Peer Culture, which we call the mutual help approach. Even such deeper problem work, however, does not fully address the perspective-taking limitations of anti-social youths and hence their groups.

Reflecting the one-sided orientation of antisocial youths are three main limitations. After extensive work with antisocial adolescents, Dewey Carducci (1980), a Cleveland, Ohio high school teacher, reached three main conclusions regarding the problematic tendencies of such adolescents. Carducci (1980) wrote that the antisocial or behaviorally at risk juvenile is "frequently at a stage of arrested moral/ethical/social/emotional development in which he is fixated at a level of concern about getting his own throbbing needs [or impulses and desires] met, regardless of effects on others" (p. 157). Second, such juveniles "blame others for their misbehavior" (Carducci 1980, p. 157). Third, they "do not know what specific steps [in a social conflict] … will result in [the conflict's] being solved [constructively]" (Carducci 1980, p. 158).

The research literature concerning conduct disorder, opposition defiance, and other patterns of adolescent antisocial behavior (Kazdin 1995) strikingly corroborates Carducci's (1980) impressions. Gibbs et al. (1996) have termed these three limitations, respectively: (1) pronounced egocentric bias and developmental *delay* in moral judgment; (2) self-serving cognitive *distortions*; and (3) social skill *deficiencies* – the "three Ds", so to speak, common among antisocial youths. Although distinguishable, the limitations, as noted, commonly point to a paucity of social perspective-taking (Barriga et al. 2001b; Leeman et al. 1993). We emphasize that these "limitations" are problem tendencies or risk factors, not strict incapacities. We urge practitioners to see their youths as persons with the potential to make more responsible choices, that is, to develop in sociomoral terms, and hence to hold them accountable and capable of rising to a higher standard. Practitioners must also keep in mind, however, that the youths' limitations or problem tendencies can keep them from fully realizing their potential or rising to meet greater expectations. One must, then, retain faith in the youths' potential for responsible thinking and acting even as one addresses the problem tendencies that are currently making it difficult for them to achieve their sociomoral potential. We will briefly consider each of these limitations as a prelude to describing the EQUIP curriculum components that address them.

14.2.2.1 Moral Judgment Developmental Delay: Pronounced Egocentric Bias and Superficiality

First, as is typical of youth around the world who show antisocial behavior, Mac's morality was immature or superficial (that is, egocentric, pragmatic, and concrete). Inappropriately immature moral judgment is our first D, developmental *delay*. The phenomenon of moral judgment developmental delay can be specified. In my

Table 14.1 Cross-cultural samples of male delinquents and non-delinquents in rank order by mean Sociomoral Reflection Maturity Score (*SRMS*)

Country	Sample	Age range (Mean)	n	Global stage range	M
Bahrain	Non-delinquents	17–18 (17.7)	30	3–3/4	313
USA	Non-delinquents	13–19 (15.7)	86	2/3–3	272
Sweden	Non-delinquents	13–18 (15.6)	29	2/3–3	266
England	Non-delinquents	14–16 (15.5)	149	2–3	264
Germany	Non-delinquents	14–16 (15.6)	309	2/3–3	261
Bahrain	Delinquents	14–19 (16.8)	30	2/3–3	254
China	Non-delinquents	13–15 (NR)	10	NR	251
Netherlands	Non-delinquents	NR (15.1)	81	2–3	249
Germany	Delinquents	14–17 (15.6)	39	2–3	243
USA	Delinquents	13–18 (15.9)	89	2–2/3	243
Netherlands	Delinquents	NR (16.5)	64	2–2/3	241
Sweden	Delinquents	13–18 (15.5)	29	2–2/3	228
England	Delinquents	14–17 (15.9)	147	2–2/3	223
Australia	Delinquents	14–18 (16.5)	38	1/2–2/3	211[a]
China	Delinquents	13–15 (NR)	10	NR	182

Adapted from Gibbs et al. (2007), used with permission of Elsevier Science Direct
Note: NR indicates information not reported. Global stage range is estimated on the basis of plus or minus on standard deviation of SRMS. Non-delinquents are generally male high school students selected (sometimes matched) for a comparison study of delinquents
[a]Mean pretest score in an intervention study

conceptualization (Gibbs 2013; revised from Kohlberg 1984), two immature stages, (1) centrations or fixations upon the salient and (2) exchanges, normally tend to decline during adolescence with the growth of two more advanced or mature stages, (3) mutualities and (4) systems (see Gibbs et al. 2007). These two stages of superficial moral judgment reduce morality to salient surface features of people, things, or actions: either with impressive physical appearances or physical consequences (Stage 1) or with concrete, tit-for-tat exchanges of favors or blows, that is, pragmatic reciprocity (Stage 2).

For every culture studied, conduct-disordered adolescents evidence a delay in moral judgment stage, attributable mainly to a more extensive use of moral judgment (Stage 2), compared with their non-delinquent counterparts (Gibbs et al. 2007; Stams et al. 2006; see Table 14.1 – note the lack of overlap between delinquent and non-delinquent mean moral judgment maturity scores). Studies of moral judgment delay by area of moral value (keeping promises, helping others, respecting life, etc.) have found delay in *every* area (Gregg et al. 1994; Palmer and Hollin 1998). The area of greatest delay concerned the reasons offered for obeying the law. Nondelinquents generally gave Stage 3 and Stage 4 reasons, for example, the selfishness of most law-breaking, such as stealing (Stage 3) and its ramifications in society (Stage 4) of chaos, insecurity, or loss of trust. In contrast, like Joey's reasoning (see below), delinquents' reasoning generally concerns the risk of getting caught and going to jail. The qualities of superficiality and pronounced egocentric bias are evident.

It should be emphasized that the superficiality of delayed moral judgment pertains to the *reasons* or *justifications* for moral decisions or values. I (Gibbs) remember discussing moral values and reasons with another 15-year-old named Joey. The year was 1987, about 5 years before my EQUIP program work with Mac and others at a residential facility. Joey seemed earnest and sincere as he emphatically affirmed the importance of moral values, such as keeping promises, telling the truth, helping others, saving lives, not stealing, and obeying the law. "And why is it so important to obey the law or not steal?" I asked Joey. "Because, [pause], like in a store, you may think no one sees you, but they could have cameras!" he replied. His other explanations were generally similar: keeping promises to others is important because if you don't, they might find out and get even, helping others is important in case you need a favor from them later, and so forth. Could Joey be trusted to live up to his moral values in situations where his fear of observers and surveillance cameras is weaker than his egocentric motives and biases? Despite their evaluation of moral values as important, many antisocial juveniles are developmentally delayed and at risk for antisocial behavior given their pronounced egocentric bias and limited grasp of the deeper reasons or bases for the importance of those values and associated decisions.

14.2.2.2   Self-Serving Cognitive Distortions

The second D refers to cognitive *distortions*. Recall that Mac tended to make exceptions for himself (check others' bags, but not his), to assume the worst about others' intentions (she wants to take away my photos forever), and blame others for his aggression (it was her fault I got angry). Although we have already referred to cognitive distortions or thinking errors (Yochelson and Samenow 1976, 1977, 1986; cf. "faulty beliefs" Ellis 1977; cf. "neutralization techniques" Sykes and Matza 1957), some elaboration concerning this important limitation will be helpful. Cognitive distortions are inaccurate or non-veridical frameworks for perceiving events. Cognitive distortions can be self-debasing (and depressogenic), but our main concern here is with *self-serving* cognitive distortions (Barriga et al. 2000). Reviewed below is our typology of self-serving cognitive distortions that, at elevated levels, facilitate aggression and other antisocial behavior.

The Primary Self-Serving Cognitive Distortion: Self-Centered

The longer that the pronounced egocentric bias of moral developmental delay persists, the more it tends to consolidate into a primary self-serving cognitive distortion that we have called Self-Centered. We (Gibbs et al. 1995) have defined Self-Centered as "according status to one's own views, expectations, needs, rights, immediate feelings, and desires to such an extent that the legitimate views, etc., of others (or even one's own long-term best interest) are scarcely considered or are disregarded altogether" (p. 108). The combination of a radically Self-Centered worldview with even the normal array and intensity of egoistic motives constitutes a risk factor for antisocial behavior.

Clinicians working with antisocial youths typically discern a link between the youths' antisocial behavior and a self-centered attitude toward or perception of other people and events. Samenow (1984) quoted a 14-year-old delinquent: "I was born with the idea that I'd do what I wanted. I always felt that rules and regulations were not for me." (p. 160). Redl and Wineman (1951) noted that a youth "justified" his having stolen a cigarette lighter simply on the grounds that he wanted it (pp. 154–155). In our group work with antisocial youth, one group member seemed to think that he had adequately justified his having stolen a car by explaining: "I needed to get to Cleveland." Other group members, reflecting on their shoplifting and other offenses, have recollected that their thoughts at the time concerned whether they could do what they wanted and get away successfully. The only perspective these juveniles took was their own; spontaneous references to the victims' perspectives were totally absent. Indeed, a recent study (Wainryb et al. 2010) found that only 10 % of violent youths (vs. 89 % of comparison youths) referred to their victims' emotions in narrating a time of having harmed someone. Antisocial youths (especially, children with callous and unemotional traits) who do express concern for a victim may do so for self-serving reasons, for example, to make a good impression on an interviewer or therapist (Kahn 2012).

Secondary Cognitive Distortions

To continue his Self-Centered attitude and antisocial behavior, the offender typically develops protective rationalizations, or what we term *secondary* cognitive distortions. These secondary cognitive distortions protect the offender against certain types of psychological stress, such as guilt or threats to self-concept. A serious offender minimized his crime as having no personal relevance: "Just because I shot a couple of state troopers doesn't mean I'm a bad guy." (Samenow 2004, p. 172). A 17-year-old delinquent, reflecting back upon his burglaries, recalled how he assuaged his conscience with a Blaming Others thinking error: "If I started feeling bad, I'd say to myself, tough rocks for him; he should have had the house locked better and the alarm on." (Samenow 1984, p. 115). In our typology and "How I Think" assessment method (Barriga et al. 2001a, 2007; Gibbs et al. 2001), these self-serving protectors of the Self-Centered attitude are termed *Blaming Others*, *Assuming the Worst*, and *Minimizing/Mislabeling*. The categories are fairly self-explanatory. Together, the primary and secondary self-serving cognitive distortions play an important role in the initiation and maintenance of antisocial behavior.

14.2.2.3   Deficiencies in Social Skills

Finally, recall that Mac neglected to balance his concerns with the legitimate expectations of the staff member. Antisocial youths generally evidence not only moral developmental delays and self-serving cognitive distortions but also social skills deficiencies – the third of the three Ds found in the literature. *Social skills* typically refer to the cognitive ability to regulate or maintain balanced and constructive behavior in difficult interpersonal situations. An example is the behavior of a youth who deals constructively with deviant peer pressure by suggesting a nondeviant alternative. Another example is that of a youth who calmly and sincerely offers clarification or apologizes to an angry accuser. Such behavior is "neither aggressive nor obsequious" (Carducci 1980, p. 161); that is, it achieves a fair balance between one's own perspective and that of another. Similarly, Robert Deluty (1979) conceptualized social skills as appropriately assertive responses intermediate between threats or aggression (such as Mac's), on one hand, and submission or running away, on the other (although calmly leaving the scene can be appropriate or balanced in some circumstances). While asserting or explaining his or her own perspective, the socially skilled individual also communicates awareness of the other person's viewpoint, feelings, and legitimate expectations. Ellen McGinnis and Arnold Goldstein (1997) operationalized social skills in terms of "steps" that include constructive self-talk (e.g., "think ahead").

Research on social skills has generally found deficiencies among antisocial youths relative to comparison groups, corroborating Carducci's (1980) impression that they typically "do not know what specific steps [in a social conflict] … will result in [the conflict's] being solved" (pp. 157–158). Freedman et al. (1978) found evidence of extensive social skill deficits or deficiencies among incarcerated male juvenile offenders (cf. Simonian et al. 1991). Such deficiencies are perhaps not surprising given the typical absence of models of constructive problem solving in the youths' home environments (Kazdin 1995). Given our conceptualization of social skills as enabling balanced and constructive interpersonal behavior in difficult situations, socially unskilled behavior involves unbalanced and destructive behavior in two categories of interpersonal situations: (a) irresponsibly submissive behavior in deviant peer pressure situations (an imbalance that favors others and is tantamount to disrespect for self) and (b) irresponsibly aggressive behavior in anger provocation situations (favoring self and tantamount to disrespect for the other). Simonian et al. (1991) found factor analytic support for these submission and aggression factors of socially unskilled or unbalanced behavior. With respect to aggression and covert antisocial behavior, imbalance in favor of the self is perhaps the basic problem of social skills deficiencies – just as pronounced egocentric bias is basic to moral developmental delay and Self-Centered is basic to self-serving cognitive distortion. Wherever and however it manifests among the limitations of antisocial youth, the self-centered orientation implies the need for its remediation through opportunities and encouragement to take into account the perspectives of others.

Implications for Treatment

These self-centered tendencies and limitations across morality, social perception, and social skills meant that Mac usually did not really see or take into account others' perspectives. Typical of his approach to life, Mac did not treat the staff member as a person but instead merely as an interfering object to be resisted and overcome.

Consequences such as write-ups or other acts of accountability were an outrage. Is it any wonder that Mac had problems with authorities and others, had committed felonies, and was chronically angry?

These observations prompt some questions. How is one to remedy these tendencies and limitations so that behaviorally at-risk or problem behavior youth can reach their sociomoral potential? How does one motivate and help youth to see others' perspectives, to engage in responsible thought and behavior so spontaneously and pervasively that it redefines their whole approach to life? These treatment questions are addressed in EQUIP. To answer them, EQUIP uses a combined approach.

14.2.3   Remedying the Limitations: Equipping the Group and Its Members

In EQUIP's combined approach, the mutual help sessions do not stand alone. If the youths are not to become frustrated, they need to acquire psychoeducational or cognitive-behavioral skills or equipment for helping one another and themselves toward responsible thought and behavior. Psychoeducation refers to teaching the knowledge and skills needed for competent daily living. Cognitive-behavioral psychoeducation refers to the facilitation of more mature and accurate cognitive habits and behavioral skills. EQUIP aims to "restructure" the antisocial cognitive habits of at-risk youth in the direction of responsible thought and social behavior. In technical terms, EQUIP is a group-based, comprehensive cognitive-behavioral approach that includes skills training but emphasizes social perspective-taking and cognitive restructuring.

After a few weeks, EQUIP groups begin equipment meetings so that they become not only motivated but also equipped for helping and changing; those meetings are where they cultivate moral judgment maturity, anger management, and social interaction skills. Mac's group applied moral and social tools they had learned to help him more effectively. One facility conducted its mutual help meetings Monday through Wednesday and its equipment meetings on Thursdays and Fridays.

Whereas a peer culture of caring is cultivated during mutual help meetings, the needed social perspective-taking skills and maturity are taught during the equipment meetings. It was during such equipment meetings that Mac learned relevant insights and tools such as: the need for institutions to have rules against contraband; techniques to correct thinking errors and manage anger; and steps of constructive and balanced social behavior. These resources were crucial as Mac worked on his Authority and Easily Angered problems during the meeting and beyond. Put in general terms, participants in the EQUIP program become equipped with skills and maturity that address the limitations just reviewed. Hence, the curriculum components provide a variety of social perspective-taking opportunities and encompass both the cognitive skills training and the cognitive restructuring techniques that together comprise a complete cognitive-behavioral approach (Glick 2006; Glick and Gibbs 2011). The components are: (1) mature moral judgment (or social decision-making); (2) skills (especially cognitive restructuring skills) for managing anger; and (3) social skills (for constructive and balanced behavior). Again, *the three interrelated curriculum components of EQUIP correspond to the three interrelated limitations of antisocial youths.*

The equipment meetings are introduced to the EQUIP groups with the explanation that what group members learn in those meetings will help them to help one another more effectively. Given its emphasis on group members' helping potential rather than on their targeted limitations, this explanation itself tends to promote antisocial youths' amenability to treatment. Litwack (1976) found that both the juvenile offenders' motivation to learn constructive skills and the learning itself improved when they were told that they would subsequently be using the skills to help other adolescents. In contrast, traditional or direct teaching programs may implicitly stigmatize the learner as dependent and inadequate, thereby eliciting defensiveness and exacerbating resistance and noncompliance problems (Reissman 1990).

14.2.4 Synergy Between Mutual Help and Cognitive-Behavioral Approaches

The motivational benefits of introducing the EQUIP curriculum with the Mutual Help rationale make the point that the mutual help approach can enhance the effectiveness of the cognitive-behavioral approach. Indeed, cognitive-behavioral programs may not accomplish much if young offenders' resistance to treatment and negative group norms are not addressed (i.e., if a receptive group is not first cultivated). Yet as noted, the contributions flow in the reverse direction as well. If their good intentions are to fare well, prospective helpers must know how to help constructively (i.e., with skills and maturity). If it is true that the mutual help approach needs the cognitive-behavioral approach, then the reverse is just as true. This bi-directionality or interdependence bears repeating: the two approaches – one motivating, the other equipping – need each other. Synergy can emerge through the integration of mutual help and cognitive-behavioral approaches, as in EQUIP. The best implementations of the EQUIP program achieve such a synergy as youth in equipment meetings motivated and those same youth in mutual help meetings are equipped. And in the positive spiral, the EQUIP-based institution is all the time becoming safer and more humane.

14.2.5 Cognitive Restructuring, Social Perspective-Taking, and EQUIP's Three Curriculum Components

In the EQUIP program, cognitive restructuring and social perspective-taking characterize not only mutual help but also its cognitive-behavioral curriculum. The three-component EQUIP cognitive-behavioral curriculum as taught in the equipment meetings for a typical 10 week/31-session program. Although the self-serving cognitive distortions are assimilated into one component (anger management) of the curriculum, the thinking error language is crucially important for the entire program, not only for the youth culture but for the staff culture as well. Hence, we now recommend introducing the language in a special preliminary session, preferably through use of the *EQUIPPED for Life* game (Horn et al. 2007) designed expressly for that purpose. A comparable game for children is called *Clear Thinking* (Franklin Learning Systems 2005). This game could be used in conjunction with social perspective-taking exercises for children, such as those provided by Norma Feshbach and colleagues (see Feshbach et al. 1983).

The social perspective-taking opportunities provided in the EQUIP curriculum are emphasized in the following description of the curriculum's three components.

14.2.5.1   Component 1: Equipping with Mature Moral Judgment (Social Decision Making)

Morally delayed youths need an enriched, concentrated "dosage" of social perspective-taking opportunities to stimulate them to catch up to age-appropriate levels of moral judgment. These opportunities are provided in EQUIP during a type of equipment meeting called "social decision-making", which features discussion with the goal of reaching maturely reasoned decisions concerning sociomoral problems. Participants must justify their problem-solving decisions in the face of challenges from more developmentally advanced peers (or, in the case of a highly limited group, initially from the group leader). A Stage 1- or Stage 2-thinking participant – who may usually dominate peers – may lose in a challenge from a more mature peer and may accordingly experience an inner conflict or "disequilibration" that could stimulate a more mature moral understanding. As others' perspectives are considered in their own right (not just as a means to one's own ends), more ideal and mutual moral understanding begins to displace superficial and egocentrically biased judgments.

The potential of problem situations to stimulate perspective-taking is exploited through their associated probe questions. The final question pertaining to curriculum material titled "Juan's Problem Situation", for example, asks, "Who might be affected (in addition to Phil himself) if Phil were to commit suicide?" (Gibbs et al. 1995, pp. 94–95; see also Potter et al. 2001). This question prompts group members to take the perspectives of loved ones, specifically, to empathize with the distress and grief caused by suicide and hence to identify the Self-Centered thinking error in Phil's intentions. Similarly, Angelo's Problem Situation, in which Angelo must decide whether to resist or join in a car theft – "Let's say the car is *your* car." (Fig. 14.1, question 6) – directly stimulates the group participants to take the perspective of the prospective victim in the spirit of Stage 3 moral reciprocity. There is a certain clever irony to how this "you're the victim" technique uses Self-Centered against itself! Other questions stimulate group members to consider possible adverse consequences for Angelo's friend (Fig. 14.1, question 8) and Ramon's family. Still other questions remove impediments to perspective taking in that they "plant" secondary cognitive distortions such as

Week 4A   **Angelo's Problem Situation**

> Angelo is walking along a side street with his friend Ramon. Ramon stops in front of a beautiful new sports car. Ramon looks inside and then says, excitedly, "Look! The keys are still in this thing! Let's see what it can do! Come on, let's go!"

What should Angelo say or do?

1. Should Angelo try to persuade Ramon not to steal the car? *(Check one.)*

    ☐ should persuade   ☐ should let steal   ☐ can't decide

2. What if Ramon says to Angelo that the keys were left in the car, that anyone that careless deserves to get ripped off? Then should Angelo try to persuade Ramon not to steal the car? *(Check one.)*

    ☐ should persuade   ☐ should let steal   ☐ can't decide

3. What if Ramon says to Angelo that the car owner can probably get insurance money to cover most of the loss? Then should Angelo try to persuade Ramon not to steal the car? *(Check one.)*

    ☐ should persuade   ☐ should let steal   ☐ can't decide

4. What if Ramon tells Angelo that stealing a car is no big deal, that plenty of his friends do it all the time? Then what should Angelo do? *(Check one.)*

    ☐ should persuade   ☐ should let steal   ☐ can't decide

5. What if Angelo knows that Ramon helps his parents with their household expenses and that they will suffer if Ramon is caught, loses his job, and goes to jail? Then should Angelo try to persuade Ramon not to steal the car? *(Check one.)*

    ☐ should persuade   ☐ should let steal   ☐ can't decide

6. Let's say the car is your car. Then should Angelo try to persuade Ramon not to steal the car? *(Check one.)*

    ☐ should persuade   ☐ should let steal   ☐ can't decide

7. In general, how important is it for people not to take things that belong to others? *(Check one.)*

    ☐ very important   ☐ important   ☐ not important

8. Let's say that Angelo does try to persuade Ramon not to steal the car, but Ramon goes ahead and takes it anyway. Angelo knows that Ramon is in bad shape from being high—he could have a serious accident, and someone could get killed. Then what should Angelo do? *(Check one.)*

    ☐ contact the police   ☐ not contact the police   ☐ can't decide

Fig. 14.1 Sample problem situation in an equipment (social decision-making) meeting (From DiBiase et al. 2012, p. 152. Copyright 2012 by Research Press)

Blaming Others (Fig. 14.1, question 2) and Minimizing/Mislabeling (Fig. 14.1, question 3 and 4) for participants to identify and correct.

Other problem situations and probe questions encourage group members to take the perspective of someone not immediately present in the situation, as when the group decides that stealing a stereo system is wrong even if from a stranger's car, or – considering that the life of one's drug-dependent sister may be at stake – decides against making a drug delivery to her neighborhood. Like the *you're the victim* technique that uses egocentric bias against itself, encouraging participants to imagine harm to someone close to them "is a way of turning empathy's familiarity and here-and-now biases against themselves and recruiting them in the service of prosocial motive development" (Hoffman 2000, p. 29).

14.2.5.2 Component 2: Equipping with Skills to Manage Anger and Correct Thinking Errors

Although egocentric bias is reduced as mature moral judgment is cultivated during the perspective-taking of the Social Decision-Making component, egocentric bias in its consolidated cognitive distortion form, Self-Centered, is such a major, immediate problem that it requires treatment attention in its own right. Beck (1999) was right to characterize righteous self-centeredness (the key problem of the reactive offender) as "the eye ('I') of the storm" (p. 25) of anger in antisocial behavior. Mac was typical of this type of antisocial youth.

Cognitive restructuring of self-serving thinking errors is crucial in anger management. In one session, for example, the group leader uses the exercise Gary's Thinking Errors (depicting a stabbing; see Fig. 14.2) to bring home the connection between distorted thinking and violence and, accordingly, the importance of correcting thinking errors before it is too late. For example, to correct Self-Centered thinking, one group member at the 1993 meeting suggested that, like the hypothetical Gary, Mac could say to himself, "I'd be mad, too, if I was her. She has a right to expect better from me."

If Gary – or group members in such a situation – are to become more fair and empathic, then, they must also learn to identify and "talk back to" or correct their secondary thinking errors. Group members have suggested that Blaming Others thoughts to the effect that violence against Meagan (see Fig. 14.2) is her fault could be corrected with self-talk such as, "Nobody's forcing me to grab that knife – it's my fault if I do." Assuming the Worst thoughts of hopelessness can be corrected with, "There's hope for us if I start treating her decently." Correcting an intention to "teach her a lesson" (Minimizing/Mislabeling) might be a thought such as, "You don't teach anybody anything by stabbing and maybe killing them."

14.2.5.3 Component 3: Equipping with Social Skills

Anger-managing skills are requisite to the use of social skills: after all, as long as rage grows rather than declines in difficult situations, balanced and constructive behavior is virtually impossible. Following the learning of anger management skills, then, EQUIP group members learn 10 social skills (cf. Goldstein and McGinnis 1997; McGinnis and Goldstein 1997) through four phases: (1) modeling or

Gary's Thinking Errors

Triad Members: _____ Date: _____

Gary is in the kitchen of his apartment. Gary's wife, Meagan, is angry at him for something he did to hurt her. She yells at him. She pushes his shoulder. Thoughts run through Gary's head. Gary does nothing to correct the errors in his thoughts. Gary becomes furious. He screams at Meagan. A sharp kitchen knife is nearby. Gary picks up the knife and stabs Meagan, seriously wounding her.

1. What thoughts ran through Gary's head, do you think, both during the situation and afterward? Suggest some sample thoughts.

_____

_____

2. What are the errors in these thoughts? Meagan was mad at Gary because he did something to hurt her. What do you think that might have been?

_____

_____

3. What might Gary have told himself in this situation? In other words, how might Gary have "talked backed" to his thinking errors? Suggest some things Gary could have said to himself to correct each type of thinking error.

_____

_____

_____

4. If Gary had corrected his thinking errors, would he still have stabbed Meagan?

_____

_____

Fig. 14.2 Sample exercise in an equipment (anger management) meeting (From DiBiase et al. 2012, p. 48. Copyright 2012 by Research Press)

"showing the skill"; (2) role-playing or "trying the skill" (if a group member cannot think of a relevant situation, a list of typical situations is provided); (3) providing feedback on the role-play or "discussing the skill"; and (4) practicing the skill (at the facility or in the community).

Social skills can in many instances be construed as step-by-step, practical training in reducing self-centration or taking the perspectives of others in specific social situations. Perspective-taking is implicitly involved in many of the social skills and is an explicit step in several of them (e.g., "How might the other person feel at the start of the stressful situation? Why?" in Preparing for a Stressful Conversation, or think "What is the other person accusing me of? Is he or she right?" in Dealing Constructively with Someone Accusing You of Something).

14.3   Adaptation and Evaluations of EQUIP: Issues of Implementation

Since its introduction in the early 1990s, the EQUIP Program has been implemented, adapted, and (to some extent) evaluated at various facilities or institutions in North America and Europe. The institutions include juvenile correctional facilities, community-based adult correctional facilities (or halfway houses), and middle schools; the young persons served have ranged in age from preadolescence through adulthood.

Implementations of EQUIP typically involve adaptations and include the program in an array of services. Peter Langdon and colleagues (Langdon et al. 2013) have adapted EQUIP for use with male offenders with intellectual disabilities. Another implementation of EQUIP has been accomplished at the Minnesota Correctional Facility in Red Wing, which provides treatment, education, and transition services for serious and chronic male juvenile offenders. The Red Wing implementation has adapted and focused on use of the Cognitive Distortions (Minimizing is separated from Mislabeling). To promote coherence across programs, the Red Wing staff use their adapted version of the EQUIP problem and thinking error language throughout the facility's diverse programs: Restorative Justice, Reflection Journaling, Substance Abuse Treatment, Sex Offender Treatment, and Relapse Prevention programs. Some implementations are only partial; for example, the Alvis House, a halfway house for adults in Columbus, Ohio, does not include Mutual Help meetings in its adaptation.

Some adaptations have modified or even eliminated the EQUIP name. Although Colorado's Youthful Offender System (YOS) does not identify EQUIP by name, much of the material, in consultation with Potter, has been assimilated into the YOS core program interventions (the Colorado consultation resulted in our *EQUIP Implementation Guide*; Potter et al. 2001). Potter has also adapted EQUIP for use at Ohio's Franklin County Community-Based Correctional Facility, where it is called Responsible Adult Culture (RAC; Potter et al. 2013). DiBiase and colleagues innovated a prevention version of EQUIP for behaviorally at-risk middle and high school youth, a version now called *Teaching Adolescents to Think and Act Responsibly: The EQUIP Approach* (DiBiase et al. 2012).

EQUIP should in theory be at least as effective as other cognitive-behavioral interventions, given that EQUIP also addresses motivational issues. One year recidivism (re-adjudication) at Red Wing declined from 53 to 21 % following implementation of EQUIP in 1998 (a comparison sample was not available; Handy, personal communication, February 21, 2008). Recidivism following the RAC version of EQUIP was also at 21 %, compared to 29 % at a facility that was equivalent except that it did not include cognitive restructuring but was otherwise comparable (see Devlin and Gibbs 2010).

Nonetheless, like that of other programs, EQUIP's effectiveness appears to vary with quality of implementation. Landenberger and Lipsey's (2005) meta-analysis of studies comparing cognitive-behavioral with other programs found an overall effectiveness for the cognitive-behavioral programs, for example, a mean recidivism rate substantially less than that of the non-cognitive-behavioral programs

(37 % vs. 53 %, respectively) (see also Lipsey et al. 2001). Lipsey et al. (2001) and Landenberger and Lipsey (2005) noted that the weakest recidivism results were found at cognitive-behavioral programs "low in strength and fidelity of implementation" (p. 155), for example, inadequate staff training, two or three rather than five weekday meetings, and high turnover among participants. Three outcome evaluation studies of EQUIP conform to Lipsey et al. (2001) pattern: a high-fidelity implementation of EQUIP was found to have substantial institutional conduct and recidivism effectiveness (12 month recidivism at 15.0 % vs. 40.5 % for the mean of the control groups; see Leeman et al. 1993), in contrast to weaker or negligible results for lower-fidelity implementations (Liau et al. 2004; Nas et al. 2005; cf. Helmond et al. 2012). EQUIP can be included among the referents for Lipsey et al. (2001) conclusion that "a great deal of improvement may be possible in the implementation of [cognitive-behavioral] programs" (p. 155).

14.4 Social Perspective-Taking for Severe Offenders

Outcome evaluation studies suggest, then, that given adequate implementation, EQUIP can induce responsible behavior among broad groups of initially antisocial youth. To be effective with groups of more severe offenders, however, EQUIP perspective-taking may require supplementation. EQUIP can be strengthened through integration with programs emphasizing even more intensive and extensive modes of social perspective-taking. Quite compatible with EQUIP, for example, are 12-step and victim awareness programs (see Gibbs 2013). These programs aim to induce perspective-taking and empathy for victims through specific depicted situations, as well as other stimulations of victim awareness through video or film presentations, newspaper or magazine articles, guest speakers (especially recovering victims or family survivors of murder victims), role-plays, personal journals, homework, and reminder posters.

A particular type of powerful or intense role-play that deserves special attention entails the violent youth's reenactments of his crime as both perpetrator and victim. Such re-enactive role-play has been used in the Texas Youth Commission Capital Offender Group program (Alvarez-Sanders and Reyes 1994), an intensive 4 month therapy designed "to break a participant's psychological defenses to force him to see his victim's suffering, to help him discover his conscience and feel remorse" (Woodbury 1993, p. 58). The juveniles role-play many aspects of their own histories, including family relationships and the homicidal events themselves. In a role-played reenactment of a crime, the perpetrator must remain at the scene even though in the actual event he typically had fled. He is urged by the group and the leader to hear the pleas and *see* the blood of the victim (played by a group peer), to experience the victim's suffering (and thereby experience empathic distress and guilt) – ("great care must be taken", however, to insure that the role-play does not instead elicit violent or predatory desires among the group members; Marshall et al. 1999, p. 90). In a second re-enactive role-play, the perpetrator must directly put himself in the victim's place: this time the perpetrator feels what it is like to be the victim by taking the victim's role (cf. reverse role-play activity, Beck 1999).

Outcome evaluations of the Capital and Serious Violent Offenders Treatment Program have indicated substantial reductions in re-arrest and re-incarceration (Texas Youth Commission 2011). Basing the program in EQUIP might make it even more effective.

Agee and McWilliams (1984; cf. Pithers 1999) used vivid crime reenactment role-play to achieve therapeutic breakthroughs with violent juvenile offenders in the context of a mutual help program. Following one such role-play reenactment of a horrific crime, an adolescent sex offender named Larry faced a stunned group and group leader and found himself "stunned by the enormity of what he had done" (Agee and McWilliams 1984, p. 182). At court months later, instead of displaying his previous unrepentant and even cocky demeanor, Larry seemed genuinely contrite. Although Larry continued to need therapy to prevent relapse, a perspective-taking breakthrough was evident.

Role reversal or crime reenactment role-plays, then, illustrate a useful supplementary technique for EQUIP social perspective-taking and may be especially needed in working with the severe offender population.

14.5   Conclusion

Whether their histories are more or less severe, youths who present with antisocial or externalizing problem behavior need mutual help and cognitive-behavioral programs that include skills training but emphasize cognitive restructuring and social perspective-taking. Such opportunities and practice in a group such as Mac's – that is to say, one that is serious about change and equipped with the skills and maturity to accomplish it – can facilitate sociomoral development and hence responsible thought and behavior among its members. Accordingly, the institution becomes safer and more humane, and recidivism declines (Power 2010). With opportunities, encouragement, and practice in EQUIP and like programs, erstwhile youths like Mac can spontaneously see – really see – the other person.

References

Agee, V. L. (1979). *Treatment of the violent incorrigible adolescent*. Lexington: Lexington Books.
Agee, V. L., & McWilliams, B. (1984). The role of group therapy and the therapeutic community in treating the violent juvenile offender. In R. Mathais (Ed.), *Violent juvenile offenders* (pp. 283–296). San Francisco: National Council on Crime and Delinquency.
Alvarez-Sanders, C., & Reyes, L. S. (1994). *Capital offender group program*. Giddings: Giddings State Home and School of the Texas Youth Commission.
Barriga, A. Q., Landau, J. R., Stinson, B. L., Liau, A. K., & Gibbs, J. C. (2000). Cognitive distortion and problem behaviors in adolescents. *Criminal Justice and Behavior, 27*, 333–343.

Barriga, A. Q., Gibbs, J. C., Potter, G. B., & Liau, A. K. (2001a). *How I Think (HIT) questionnaire manual*. Champaign: Research Press.

Barriga, A. Q., Morrison, E. M., Liau, A. K., & Gibbs, J. C. (2001b). Moral cognition: Explaining the gender difference in antisocial behavior. *Merrill-Palmer Quarterly, 47*, 532–562.

Barriga, A. Q., Gibbs, J. C., Potter, G. B., Konopisos, M., & Barriga, K. T. (2007). *The How I Think about drugs and alcohol (HIT-D & A) questionnaire*. Champaign: Research Press.

Beck, A. T. (1999). *Prisoners of hate: The cognitive basis of anger, hostility, and violence*. New York: HarperCollins.

Brendtro, L. K., & Ness, A. E. (1982). Perspectives on peer group treatment: The use and abuse of guided group interaction/positive peer culture. *Children and Youth Services Review, 4*, 307–324.

Carducci, D. J. (1980). Positive peer culture and assertiveness training: Complementary modalities for dealing with disturbed and disturbing adolescents in the classroom. *Behavioral Disorders, 5*, 156–162.

Deluty, R. H. (1979). Children's action tendency scale: A self-report measure of aggressiveness, assertiveness, and submissiveness in children. *Journal of Consulting and Clinical Psychology, 47*, 1061–1071.

Devlin, R., & Gibbs, J. C. (2010). Responsible adult culture (RAC): Cognitive and behavioral changes at a community-based correctional facility. *Journal of Research in Character Education, 8*, 1–20.

DiBiase, A. M., Gibbs, J. C., Potter, G. B., & Blount, M. R. (2012). *Teaching adolescents to think and act responsibly: The EQUIP approach*. Champaign: Research Press.

Dishion, T. J., McCord, J., & Poulin, F. (1999). When interventions harm: Peer groups and problem behavior. *American Psychologist, 54*, 755–764.

Ellis, A. (1977). Rational-emotive therapy: Research data that support the clinical and personality hypothesis of RET and other modes of cognitive-behavior therapy. *The Counseling Psychologist, 7*, 2–42.

Feshbach, N. D., Feshbach, S., Fauvre, M., & Ballard-Campbell, M. (1983). *Learning to care: Classroom activities for social and affective development*. Glenview: Scott, Foresman, & Co.

Franklin Learning Systems. (2005). *Clear thinking [game]*. Westport: Franklin Learning Systems.

Freedman, B. J., Rosenthal, L., Donahoe, C. P., Schlundt, D. G., & McFall, R. M. (1978). A social behavioral analysis of skills deficits in delinquent and nondelinquent adolescent boys. *Journal of Consulting and Clinical Psychology, 46*, 1148–1462.

Gibbs, J. C. (2013). *Moral development and reality: Beyond the theories of Kohlberg, Hoffman, and Haidt* (3rd ed.). New York: Oxford University Press.

Gibbs, J. C., Potter, G. B., & Goldstein, A. P. (1995). *The EQUIP program: Teaching youth to think and act responsibly through a peer-helping approach*. Champaign: Research Press.

Gibbs, J. C., Potter, G. B., Barriga, A. Q., & Liau, A. K. (1996). Developing the helping skills and prosocial motivation of aggressive adolescents in peer group programs. *Aggression and Violent Behavior, 1*, 285–305.

Gibbs, J. C., Potter, G. B., DiBiase, A.-M., & Devlin, R. (2009). The EQUIP program – Social perspective taking for responsible thought and behavior. In B. Glick (Ed.), *Cognitive behavioral interventions for at-risk youth* (vol. 2, pp. 9–2 to 9–27J). Kingston: Civic Research Institute.

Gibbs, J. C., Barriga, A., & Potter, G. (2001). *The How I Think questionnaire*. Champaign: Research Press.

Gibbs, J. C., Basinger, K. S., Grime, R. L., & Snarey, J. R. (2007). Moral judgment development across cultures: Revisiting Kohlberg's universality claims. *Developmental Review, 27*, 443–500.

Glick, B. (2006). History and development of cognitive behavioral interventions. In G. Glick (Ed.), *Cognitive behavioral interventions for at-risk youth* (pp. 1–1–1–16). Kingston: Civic Research Institute.

Glick, B., & Gibbs, J. C. (2011). *Aggression replacement training: A comprehensive intervention for aggressive youth* (3rd ed.). Champaign: Research Press.

Goldstein, A. P., & McGinnis, E. (1997). *Skillstreaming the adolescent: New strategies and perspectives for teaching prosocial skills* (Rev. ed.). Champaign: Research Press.

Gregg, R. V., Gibbs, J. C., & Basinger, K. S. (1994). Patterns of developmental delay in moral judgment by male and female delinquents. *Merrill-Palmer Quarterly, 40*, 538–553.

Hart, D., Atkins, R., & Donnelly, T. M. (2006). Community service and moral development. In M. Killen & J. G. Smetana (Eds.), *Handbook of moral development* (pp. 633–656). Mahwah: Erlbaum.

Helmond, P., Overbeek, G., & Brugman, D. (2012). Program integrity and effectiveness of a cognitive behavioral intervention for incarcerated youth on cognitive distortions, social skills, and moral development. *Children and Youth Services Review, 34*, 1720–1728.

Hoffman, M. L. (2000). *Empathy and moral development: Implications for caring and justice.* Cambridge: Cambridge University Press.

Horn, M., Shively, R., & Gibbs, J. C. (2007). *EQUIPPED for life* (3rd ed.). Westport: Franklin Learning Systems.

Kahn, J. (2012, May 13). Trouble, Age 9. *New York Times Magazine*, pp. 34–37 ff.

Kazdin, A. E. (1995). *Conduct disorders in childhood and adolescence* (2nd ed.). Newbury Park: Sage.

Kohlberg, L. (1984). *The psychology of moral development: Essays on moral development* (Vol. 2). San Francisco: Harper & Row.

Kohlberg, L., & Higgins, A. (1987). School democracy and social interaction. In W. M. Kurtines & J. L. Gewirtz (Eds.), *Moral development through social interaction* (pp. 102–108). New York: Wiley-Interscience.

Landenberger, N. A., & Lipsey, M. W. (2005). The positive effects of cognitive-behavioral programs for offenders: A meta-analysis of factors associated with effective treatment. *Journal of Experimental Criminology, 1*, 451–476.

Langdon, P. E., Murphy, G. H., Clare, I. C. H., Palmer, E. J., & Rees, J. (2013). An evaluation of the EQUIP treatment programme with men who have intellectual and other developmental disabilities. *Journal of Applied Research in Intellectual Disabilities, 26*, 167–180.

Leeman, L. W., Gibbs, J. C., & Fuller, D. (1993). Evaluation of a multi-component group treatment program for juvenile delinquents. *Aggressive Behavior, 19*, 281–292.

Liau, A. K., Shively, R., Horn, M., Landau, J., Barriga, A. Q., & Gibbs, J. C. (2004). Effects of psychoeducation for offenders in a community correctional facility. *Journal of Community Psychology, 32*, 543–553.

Lipsey, M. W., Chapman, G. L., & Landenberger, N. A. (2001). Cognitive-behavioral programs for offenders. *Annals of the American Academy of Political and Social Sciences, 578*, 144–157.

Litwack, S. E. (1976). *The use of the helper therapy principle to increase therapeutic effectiveness and reduce therapeutic resistance: Structured learning therapy with resistant adolescents.* Unpublished doctoral dissertation, Syracuse University, New York.

Marshall, W. L., Anderson, D., & Fernandez, Y. (1999). Empathy. In W. L. Marshall, D. Anderson, & Y. Fernandez (Eds.), *Cognitive behavioral treatment of sex offenders.* West Sussex: Wiley.

McGinnis, E., & Goldstein, A. P. (1997). *Skillstreaming the elementary school child: New strategies and perspectives for teaching prosocial skills* (Rev. ed.). Champaign: Research Press.

Nas, C. N., Brugman, D., & Koops, W. (2005). Effects of the EQUIP programme on the moral judgement, cognitive distortion, and social skills of juvenile delinquents. *Psychology Crime and Law, 11*, 421–434.

Osgood, D. W., Gruber, E., Archer, M. A., & Newcomb, T. M. (1985). Autonomy for inmates: Counterculture or cooptation? *Criminal Justice and Behavior, 12*, 71–89.

Palmer, E. J., & Hollin, C. R. (1998). A comparison of patters of moral development in young offenders and non-offenders. *Legal and Criminological Psychology, 3*, 225–235.

Pithers, W. D. (1999). Empathy: Definition, measurement, enhancement, and relevant to the treatment of sexual abusers. *Journal of Interpersonal Violence, 14*, 257–284.

Potter, G. B., Gibbs, J. C., & Goldstein, A. P. (2001). *EQUIP program implementation guide.* Champaign: Research Press.

Potter, G. B., Gibbs, J. C., Robbins, M., & Langdon, P. (2013). *Responsible Adult Culture: A comprehensive cognitive-behavioral program for adult offenders*. Manuscript in preparation.

Power, C. (2010). The moral education miracle at the Franklin county community-based correctional facility: The influence of moral culture. *Journal of Research in Character Education, 8*, xiii–xxii.

Redl, F., & Wineman, D. (1951). *Children who hate: The disorganization and breakdown of behavior controls*. Glencoe: The Free Press.

Reissman, F. (1990). Restructuring help: A human services paradigm for the 1990s. *American Journal of Community Psychology, 18*, 221–230.

Samenow, S. E. (1984). *Inside the criminal mind*. New York: Random House.

Samenow, S. E. (2004). *Inside the criminal mind: Revised and updated edition*. New York: Random House.

Simonian, S. J., Tarnowski, K. J., & Gibbs, J. C. (1991). Social skills and antisocial conduct of delinquents. *Child Psychiatry and Human Development, 22*, 17–22.

Stams, G. J., Brugman, D., Dekovic, M., van Rosmale, L., van der Laan, P., & Gibbs, J. C. (2006). The moral judgment of juvenile delinquents: A meta-analysis. *Journal of Abnormal Child Psychology, 34*, 697–713.

Sykes, G. M., & Matza, D. (1957). Techniques of neutralization: A theory of delinquency. *American Sociological Review, 22*, 664–670.

Texas Youth Commission. (2011). *Capital and serious violent offender treatment program* in *Annual Review of treatment effectiveness*. Austin: Texas Youth Commission.

Vorrath, H. H., & Brendtro, L. K. (1985). *Positive peer culture* (2nd ed.). New York: Aldine.

Wainryb, C., Komolova, M., & Florsheim, P. (2010). How violent youth offenders and typically developing adolescents construct moral agency in narratives about doing harm. In K. McLean & P. Pasupathi (Eds.), *Narrative development in adolescence: Creating the storied self*. New York: Springer.

Woodbury, R. (1993, October 11). Taming the killers. *Time*, pp. 58–59.

Yochelson, S., & Samenow, S. E. (1976). *The criminal personality: Vol. 1. A profile for change*. New York: Jason Aronson.

Yochelson, S., & Samenow, S. E. (1977). *The criminal personality: Vol. 2. The change process*. New York: Jason Aronson.

Yochelson, S., & Samenow, S. E. (1986). *The criminal personality: Vol. 3. The drug user*. Northvale: Jason Aronson.

Chapter 15
Positive Youth Development in Organized Programs: How Teens Learn to Manage Emotions

Natalie Rusk, Reed W. Larson, Marcela Raffaelli, Kathrin Walker, LaTesha Washington, Vanessa Gutierrez, Hyeyoung Kang, Steve Tran, and Stephen Cole Perry

15.1 Introduction

Adults must be able to manage anger, anxiety, and other emotions in order to lead productive and healthy lives. The ability to manage emotions requires handling "hot" emotional situations as they occur, such as finding ways to express anger without lashing out or to regulate anxiety in order to concentrate on one's work (Gross and Thompson 2007). Managing emotions also involves the ability to make use of the functional properties of different feelings, for example, channeling excitement in order to motivate action or responding to guilt with reflection on one's actions (Izard 2009). Emotional management skills are linked to a variety of positive outcomes, and thus understanding the development of these skills is important for the study of positive youth development.

N. Rusk (✉)
MIT Media Lab, Massachusetts Institute of Technology, E14-464B, 77 Massachusetts Ave.,
Cambridge, MA 02139, USA
e-mail: nrusk@media.mit.edu

R.W. Larson
Department of Human and Community Development, University of Illinois at Urbana-Champaign, 2032 Doris Christopher Hall, 904 West Nevada Street, Urbana, IL 61801, USA
e-mail: larsonR@illinois.edu

M. Raffaelli
Department of Human and Community Development, University of Illinois at Urbana-Champaign, 2003 Doris Christopher Hall, 904 West Nevada Street,
Urbana, IL 61801, USA
e-mail: mraffael@illinois.edu

K. Walker
Extension Center for Youth Development, University of Minnesota, 405 Coffey Hall,
1420 Eckles Avenue, St. Paul, MN 55108, USA
e-mail: kcwalker@umn.edu

C. Proctor and P.A. Linley (eds.), *Research, Applications, and Interventions for Children and Adolescents: A Positive Psychology Perspective*, DOI 10.1007/978-94-007-6398-2_15,
© Springer Science+Business Media Dordrecht 2013

But mature adult emotional functioning is by no means a given – it has to be achieved. As young people move into adolescence, they become able to think about emotions in a more conscious and analytic way (Harris et al. 1981). Although emotional development begins in infancy, much of this early development occurs outside of conscious awareness (Calkins and Leerkes 2010). Adolescents acquire new metacognitive and executive skills that allow them to reason deliberately about their thoughts, feelings, and actions (Kuhn 2009). They become able to consciously reflect on their experiences, draw conclusions, and create strategies for navigating complex situations. These new skills equip adolescents to develop and apply skills for recognizing, regulating, and benefiting from emotions as they arise in the diverse situations and contexts of daily life.

In this chapter we examine emotional learning as a focus for understanding positive youth development and how it can be supported. Research and theory indicate that positive development occurs when youth are *active producers* of their own development and learning, especially as they move into the teenage years (Larson 2011a; Lerner 2002). We examine emotional development in the specific context of organized programs (such as arts, technology, and leadership programs) – contexts that afford youth considerable freedom within an overarching, goal-directed structure.

Emotions often arise in organized programs as youth work towards goals. Encountering obstacles can trigger negative emotions, such as frustration and anger; achieving success can trigger positive emotions, such as pride and happiness. This makes organized youth programs a rich context for emotional learning. Indeed, survey research shows that youth report more experiences related to emotion learning in organized programs than in school classrooms (Larson et al. 2006).

This chapter examines youth's processes of emotional development within these contexts and the role of adult program leaders in facilitating this development. We first review the literature on youth programs as contexts for positive development. We then address the question of how adolescents apply their new metacognitive and executive skills to reflect on the puzzling, not-quite logical dynamics of emotional states. We examine how adolescents learn about managing these dynamics. We then examine the practices of program leaders that support youth's emotional development. This is not a simple question: If youth are active producers of their development, what role, if any, can adults play in facilitating this process? Program leaders have the unique opportunity to be present as youth encounter the frustration, excitement, and boredom that arise in their projects. How do they help youth mobilize their cognitive skills to understand and manage these emotional ups and downs in their work?

L. Washington • V. Gutierrez • S. Tran • S.C. Perry
Department of Human and Community Development, University of Illinois at Urbana-Champaign, 274 Bevier Hall, M/C-180, 905 South Goodwin Avenue, Urbana, IL 61801, USA
e-mail: washington.latesha@gmail.com; gutierrez.vanessa86@gmail.com; tran19@illinois.edu; perry7@illinois.edu

H. Kang
Department of Human Development, Binghamton University, State University of New York, P.O. Box 6000, Binghamton, NY 13902-6000, USA
e-mail: hkang@binghamton.edu

15.2 Youth Programs as Contexts for Positive Development

15.2.1 Features of Effective Programs for Adolescents

High-quality youth programs support youth in developing life and career skills (Hirsch et al. 2011). Effective programs have a number of important features that make them conducive to positive development (Eccles and Gootman 2002; Mahoney et al. 2009). We call attention to three that we think particularly important.

First, effective programs engage youth as active participants in program activities (Durlak et al. 2010). In programs for adolescents, the activities often center on projects, such as creating an artwork or a website, conducting a science activity, or planning an event. Youth are given agency in working towards a project goal – they exercise choice in the direction and have a voice in decision-making (Kirshner et al. 2003). Program leaders emphasize to youth that it is "your project": they want youth to experience ownership over it.

A second important feature is that youth typically experience high intrinsic motivation and cognitive engagement in this work (Larson 2000; Vandell et al. 2006). Many adolescents become highly invested in the goals they are trying to achieve, particularly when they can see a connection to their future (Dawes and Larson 2011). As a result, they report being genuinely engaged with the challenges of their projects (Larson 2011b).

A third important feature of effective programs for adolescents is that projects engage youth in real world (or real-world-like) work (Heath 1998). Work on their projects typically confronts youth with complex, real-world demands and challenges. Programs engage youth in open-ended tasks without guarantees about how they will work out. The problems they must solve to reach their goals are often unstructured. Furthermore, youth often receive authentic feedback – they can see if their project has successfully met their goals. For example, when organizing a community event, they can see how many people attend and how the people respond to their work.

These features of youth programs give rise to a range of emotional episodes that resemble those in adult work environments. Because youth are invested in their goals, when events are going well they can experience positive emotions such as excitement and satisfaction. But they also experience negative emotions when they encounter obstacles or things do not work out as they had hoped. Youth are not just learning about emotions, they are learning about the situations that lead to them, their dynamics over time, and how different responses lead to different outcomes. In an intensive case study of youth rehearsing for a high school theater production, Larson and Brown (2007) documented how youth consciously learned to better understand and manage these emotional episodes. This chapter builds on this work, exploring these processes in greater depth.

15.2.2   The Role of Program Leaders in Supporting Youth's Work

Effective program leaders play important roles in facilitating youth's work and learning. They help cultivate the program environment, helping youth feel physically and psychologically safe. Program leaders model and encourage youth to treat each other respectfully and foster collaboration. They also cultivate trust and a sense of belonging, which provide key foundations for youth participation and positive development (Eccles and Gootman 2002; Lerner et al. 2009). Effective youth program leaders often relate to youth in ways that bridge the role of friend, adult mentor, teacher, or parent (Walker 2011). This can provide an opening for youth to seek emotional support and guidance, sharing their personal feelings and asking for advice (Hirsch et al. 2011).

Leaders thus help create conditions that influence youth's emotional learning. In the study of a high school theater program, Larson and Brown (2007) found that the adult leaders cultivated high standards that contributed to youth experiencing certain types of emotional episodes, such as anxiety about performing before an audience and stress in preparation for the show. Yet the leaders also cultivated a program culture in which emotions were acknowledged and discussed. They modeled and provided youth with strategies for handling emotions. Here we delve more deeply into how effective leaders help youth learn more directly from the youth's experiences of emotional episodes.

15.3   A Study of Emotional Development in Four Youth Programs

In this chapter we examine youth's processes of emotional learning in four after-school programs and how leaders support that learning. We draw on theory and empirical findings to build empirically grounded theory about how these processes play out.

The four programs in the current study all engage youth in projects where they are working toward goals. The programs involve a range of projects. At *Community House,*[1] youth engage in science learning and carry out technology projects, such as making their own web pages. At *The Station*, youth organize community events, such as music concerts. At the *Celina Boys and Girls Club*, youth plan and lead community service events. At *Unified Youth*, teens create public service announcements to disseminate ideas and information on important topics to other youth and to community members. The adult leaders in all four programs were experienced youth professionals.

We conducted structured individual interviews with adolescents and leaders in these four programs. Youth, ages 12–18, responded to questions about their experiences of

---

[1] All names of programs, youth, and leaders are pseudonyms.

anger, frustration, and other emotions in the program (e.g., "During the last month, was there a time you felt worried or nervous about your work in the program?"). For each emotional experience, they were asked what *caused* it, how it had *influenced* them, how they *handled* it, and what they had *learned*, if anything, from the experience. In separate interviews, the adult program leaders were asked to describe how they work with youth to support learning, including emotional learning. Data were analyzed using grounded theory and related techniques for qualitative data.

In the next section we examine youth's processes of emotional learning within these programs. In the following section, we analyze how leaders supported these processes.

15.4 Youth as Agents of Their Emotional Development

The youth in these four programs had many opportunities to experience and learn about emotions. Their work created conditions for emotions to occur. Youth at The Station, for example, really cared about music and wanted to put on the best shows possible. Across programs, youth were taking on complex open-ended tasks and trying to solve problems they had never encountered before (Salusky et al. 2012).

It is not surprising then, that the youth encountered a range of strong emotions while pursuing their goals. They experienced anxiety about how to proceed, frustration when peers were not helping out, and anger when someone interfered with their plans. These emotions can disrupt work, for example, by distracting concentration or provoking group conflict (Grawitch and Munz 2005). As in the study of the theater program (Larson and Brown 2007), youth also reported experiencing powerful positive emotions, including excitement about their work and satisfaction when completing a project successfully. But we are going to focus primarily on youth's learning about negative emotions, since these emotions tend to be more difficult to manage in ways that foster work and learning (Baumeister et al. 2001).

15.4.1 Learning to Regulate Emotions

Most discussions of emotional development emphasize the importance of acquiring abilities to control negative emotions (Izard et al. 2008). Youth programs provide opportunities for adolescents to develop strategies for regulating emotions in the context of meaningful projects. Let us provide an example. Debra Napolez, a teen at Unified Youth, was preparing a presentation for a big audience of people from a community organization, and she experienced episodes of anxiety. This was a large and novel task for her, and she was worried that people in the audience "weren't going to listen, that they weren't going to get anything out of it."

Adolescents are at an age when they have the potential to understand abstract psychological phenomena, like the pernicious dynamics of worry. Feelings of anxiety and worry can fuel ruminative brooding on negative thoughts and feelings

(Nolen-Hoeksema et al. 2008). But Debra gained experience dealing with these dynamics. As she worked on the presentation, she reported learning to "just stay focused on the topic. I don't go off thinking 'what if, what if that, what if this.'" When asked how she learned not to focus on what might go wrong, she explained, "I guess by doing it so many times that I just figured that that wasn't the right thing. That's what made me worried, thinking that." She had figured out a way to avoid the self-perpetuating cycle of worry. As a result of this strategy, she was able to keep on task and contribute to a successful presentation. Other youth reported similar process of observing and learning strategies for regulating anxiety. For example, Adeline Tamsin at The Station described learning to get started on a task rather than "sit around freaking out about it."

Anger is another emotion that can run out of control. It can be even more problematic than anxiety, because anger can lead to verbal or physical aggression. Youth in these programs described experiences learning to regulate anger and the related emotion of frustration that arose in their work.

Madelyn Brooks described feeling angry because other youth were not helping with a project: "The other members weren't focusing so we can get it done. I was just totally out of patience … I was about to yell some things." But rather than yelling, she stopped to reflect:

> I had to keep in mind where I was, who I was around, and who my peers were. So then I'm like, "Okay, what if we do this?" So I bring up ideas and try to get everybody back on task. It worked, because eventually we got back on task and got to work.

Madelyn and other teens in our research describe learning to brainstorm potential alternatives for dealing with negative emotions. Rather than letting her anger get the best of her, Madelyn thought about what might help get her teammates back on board, tried it, and noticed that it worked.

Alexis Roscoe at the Celina Boys and Girls Club described a different lesson about regulating anger. She became angry at herself when she had ideas for improving her project at the last minute – when it was too late to make changes. She wanted to act on her anger by yelling and giving up. But Alexis described handling it in a way that would not interfere with her work. She recalled, "I learned that you gotta kinda tone it down, keep it modest, keep it within, and just kinda let it mellow itself out until you can find somebody to talk to about the situation." She was learning new ways of managing her feelings.

The teens in our research described numerous similar situations in which they experienced anxiety and anger. They noticed the urge to yell or respond reflexively to these emotions – what emotion researchers describe as "felt action tendencies" (Fridja 1986). Yet, many youth were able to resist the felt urge and to try different strategies for managing the dynamics of anger and anxiety. They were able to recognize and accept negative emotions, breaking the self-perpetuating cycles by addressing the cause, and considering alternative ways to handle them.

We have found that teens in programs learn to regulate emotions through repeated experiences of trial, error, and reflection. They are active in deliberately experimenting with different strategies.

15.4.2   Learning to Use Emotions

Much discussion of emotional learning stops here. This is especially true when discussing the emotions of adolescents. Current adolescent scholars portray emotions as troublesome internal forces that "hijack" young people's thought processes; the message is that youth need to learn to control emotions (Dahl 2004; Steinberg 2007). But, as noted earlier, emotions have adaptive functions. Some youth spoke not only of learning to regulate negative emotions, but also of *learning to use these emotions in constructive ways*. Most salient in youth's accounts was learning to use the motivational and attentional functions of emotions.

15.4.2.1   Motivational Function

Within the current study, youth reported noticing how emotions influenced their motivation. For example, a youth explained how she was motivated by the worry she experienced in her work at the Celina Boys and Girls Club:

> Well I don't like being worried. If I can figure something out and I am worried about it, I just like plan harder. It's just something that goes on in my head. Something just clicks, "Try harder, don't give up."

Her observation fits with the concept that a key function of emotions is to motivate thoughts and behaviors related to one's goals (Izard 2009).

Another youth on a sports team in the same program described how negative emotions motivated him to learn:

> I was mad because I knew we could get to the playoffs, or the championship, if we do better. And I was scared because I didn't think we would get better. [So] I started practicing. I would practice more by myself so I could get better and release frustration. It made me practice harder.

He and other youth recognized that even if an emotion felt unpleasant, it could motivate them into positive action.

Youth also described learning about motivational aspects of positive emotions. One of the youth said she learned that if you want to have the feeling of being really satisfied you, need to keep up with your work and accomplish your goals. Similarly, in the previous study of a theater program, youth learned to use excitement to sustain their motivation in rehearsals (Larson and Brown 2007).

15.4.2.2   Attentional Function

Emotion theorists have also described the role of emotions in arousing and focusing attention. Cannon (1932) stressed their role in directing attention to basic survival needs, while more recent theorists recognize that emotions can also focus attention to higher-order goals (Gross and Thompson 2007). Teens in the four programs described learning to use these attentional functions from their work on their projects.

Alexis described learning about how the aroused state of anger can have positive functions:

> Sometimes when you're heated, at your hottest moment or your most mad moments, you come up with some stuff you wouldn't have thought of if you were just calm and mellow. Because when you get mad you see things that you didn't see: certain different things come to your mind, and you look at things differently.

She decided instead of giving up to focus on what she could do differently next time. In line with this way of thinking, Alexis's advice to others was: "Don't get angry, as angry as you normally would. Don't let it affect your work after that point. Take that being mad and turn it into something great." This ability to reflect on one's emotions and respond in constructive ways can be considered a useful and sophisticated emotional skill (Izard et al. 2008).

Other youth describe similar learning about worry. A teen who had a writing deadline for the program newsletter said that feeling worried made him "more focused." Some of the youth observed that these beneficial aspects of emotions were experienced when they felt the emotion but not too strongly. One noted that worry "shows that I actually care about doing things right, but I don't think it has to go to the extent that I feel it." This observation is consistent with research showing that a moderate level of emotional arousal fosters adaptive responding (Bradley 2000).

These adolescents were learning to *harness* the attentional and motivational properties of emotions. The youth's descriptions reflect understanding of and utilization of a core principle in affective science: that emotions have functional value and, if managed effectively, can inform and motivate progress towards goals (Baumeister et al. 2007; Schwarz and Clore 2007).

15.4.3 Conclusions: Youth's Learning Process

These youth's accounts suggest teens are not simply pawns of emotions, but can learn to stand back and consider alternative responses. They can learn to manage anger and worry in ways that allow them to focus attention on the task at hand, and work effectively with others. Even when they feel like yelling at teammates out of anger or giving up out of fear of failing, they can consider alternative possibilities and choose an approach that keeps them working towards their goals.

Of course not all youth in our research realized this potential of learning to reflect on emotions. For some, their main strategy was suppression trying not to think about what they were feeling. Some expressed difficulty managing their emotions in positive ways. For example, one youth said, "When I'm angry or frustrated, I tend to procrastinate."

Yet many were actively developing these skills. Because they were devoted to their projects, they were invested in managing their emotions in ways that would help them achieve their goals. Youth, such as Madelyn, realized that attacking others out of anger would interfere with the goals they were seeking to accomplish. They were learning to stop, analyze, and choose a constructive response. Some learned to *use* the functional properties of emotions. Through processing multiple experiences of emotion, teens are able to apply their new metacognitive potentials to develop sophisticated skills for managing emotions.

15.5   The Role of Program Leaders in Supporting Youth's Emotional Development

How can program leaders help youth with the conscious developmental processes just described? Emotional learning requires understanding abstract and complex yet powerful "felt tendencies." If youth learn through their own experience, what role can leaders play? In the analysis of our data we found that program leaders play a key role by *coaching* youth in situations in which emotions arise.

The concept of "emotion coaching" was identified in research on how parents help young children learn about emotions (Gottman et al. 1996, 1997). Emotion coaching is defined as providing supportive guidance for understanding and handling emotions. A distinguishing feature of emotion coaching is viewing negative emotions as opportunities for connection and learning, rather than as problems to be avoided. Research has shown that children and adolescents whose parents provide emotion coaching become better able to regulate anger and experience greater psychological adjustment (e.g., Katz and Hunter 2007; Stocker et al. 2007).

The research on emotion coaching to date has focused on parents. In the current study, we identified three types of emotion coaching leaders provided to youth: fostering awareness and reflection, suggesting strategies, and encouraging problem solving.

15.5.1   Fostering Awareness and Reflection

The ability to label and differentiate emotions is fundamental to developing emotion competence (Izard et al. 2008; Brackett et al. 2011). We found, first, that leaders coached youth to identify emotions and the situations that triggered them. Leaders monitored youth's emotions and called attention to them before problems erupted. Vanessa Walker, a leader at the Celina Boys and Girls Club, described how she notices when youth look upset and asks if something is troubling them. "I ask them 'Well, what happened? You're usually this way in this situation, and [today] you was down low. Talk to me. What's going on? Because I've seen that you just wasn't in it today.'" She said youth often responded by explaining what has been troubling them, such as a problem with friends or family. By asking youth to talk about how they are feeling and what situations caused them to feel that way, leaders helped youth learn to apply their ability for self-reflection to understanding emotional episodes.

Youth confirmed that leaders played this role of encouraging them to talk about whatever was bothering them. For example, a teen described how she learned from the leaders to ask others for help when she was feeling worried about her work on a community service event. "I learned not to keep it to myself and to talk about how I am feeling." She explained that the leaders "are the ones that influence me to not keep everything to myself all the time."

Rather than minimizing youth's troubles or simply telling them to cheer up, the leaders encouraged them to talk about negative emotions and interpret what caused them. These conversations helped youth learn to verbally label emotions and reflect on what may have triggered the emotions. This process is key because emotions are in many ways abstract phenomena, involving diverse visceral cues and behavioral urges, which can be difficult to recognize. Identifying the contributing causes of emotions—ranging from physical factors (such as lack of sleep) to social interactions, environmental conditions, and recalled experiences—is also a complex skill, for which coaching can be helpful.

15.5.2 Suggesting Strategies

The second approach leaders used was coaching youth to consider and apply adaptive strategies for managing emotions. Coaching on strategies was most common for anger and frustration. For example, a teen described how a competing debate team was being disrespectful and made her and her teammates angry. She explained that she learned ways to handle her anger by listening to the leaders coach another youth. "It was when another student got mad; so they just told [the student] to leave, calm down, walk around the building, come back with a better attitude and overlook what the other person says, just don't listen to them." By recommending strategies for handling anger, leaders help youth learn to consciously reflect on emotion and consider alternative responses.

A program leader at the Community House explained how she attends to youth's level of frustration and then provides various alternative strategies:

> Any time they are feeling frustrated I try to keep tabs on that and keep track of what level of frustration they are at. I mean, if they are hugely frustrated, I will tell them to go take a break or start doing something else for a little while. Or I'll sit with them and try to work through it, or pair them up with a mentor, someone who is more experienced who can help them work through it.

This leader emphasized that learning to deal with frustration is "a huge skill." Thus, she suggests a set of strategies to help youth work through their feelings of frustration.

A teen in the theater program, studied by Larson and Brown (2007), described learning from one of the leaders to deal with his frustration by "channeling it through my singing and acting." Rather than allowing frustration to get in the way of progress, the leader coached the youth to harness the motivational aspect of frustration into constructive activity. This type of coaching can contribute to youth's ability to use emotions as motivation for working towards their goals.

15.5.3 Encouraging Problem Solving

The third way that leaders coached youth was by providing encouragement to problem solve and persist in emotionally challenging situations. Leaders prompted youth to work through frustration and anxiety rather than giving up.

Ana Guzmán, a teen at Community House, described being challenged by the program leader to deal with her fear of writing:

> When [the leader] told us that we're gonna do a magazine – I hate writing, I hate it, I hate it, I hate it – and I'm like, "Oh I don't think I'm gonna be able to do the program. Because you know I've just never been good at writing and I don't think I'll make a good enough article for this." And she's like, "No, you could try, you could try."… She told me, "You just need to get away from your fear. Maybe you're not afraid of writing, but you're just stuck on the fact, 'Oh no, I suck at writing, I suck at writing,' so that's why you're scared of doing the project." That's what kind of got me excited. And then once I started working on it and looking into the topic and interviewing people, that's when I got more excited and I want to finish and everything.

Ana actually became *excited* about dealing with the fear. The leader helped transform her appraisal of the situation from a threat to a challenge. The distinction between threat and challenge appraisals has been studied in research on emotion and motivation for learning – the same situation can trigger different emotional and physiological responses depending on how it is viewed by the individual (Blascovich 2008). Challenge appraisals are associated with mastery and growth while threat appraisals are associated with fear of failure and avoidance (McGregor and Elliot 2002).

Leaders also encouraged youth to work through emotionally challenging interpersonal situations. A leader described an example of a teen, Jake, who had been elected president of the program, but wanted to give up when his friends were being disrespectful in a meeting. Jake was fearful of losing his friendships if he asserted his role. Based on encouragement from the program leader, he figured out a way to persuade his teammates to focus on getting work accomplished during the meetings. This type of coaching through difficult situations can help so that the next time youth experience frustration or fear, they may be more likely to see these emotions as a sign to problem solve rather than a sign to give up.

15.5.4   Conclusion: Leaders' Role in Youth's Learning Process

Emotions have complex, surreal effects that even emotion researchers struggle to understand; for example, they distort perception, thought, and behavior (Ochsner and Gross 2007). For this reason it may be hard for adults to directly teach young people about emotions and how to manage them. But program leaders appear to be effective in helping youth learn through their emotional experiences. Supportive leaders play the role of "guide on the side": rather than telling youth what to do, they coach. They notice and ask youth what they are feeling and why. They help youth problem-solve and develop options for how to handle emotional situations. Leaders also encourage youth to take emotional risks, for example, trying out new and thus uncertain directions in their projects, which fosters learning goals (Kaplan and Maehr 2007). These processes involve helping adolescents use their developing cognitive abilities to understand and learn from emotional episodes. As a whole, these different forms of coaching help youth understand the types of situations that trigger different emotions, interpret the complex signals and surreal effects of emotions, and develop strategies for managing them.

15.6   Conclusion

The adult "real world" that young people eventually enter requires managing complex situations. High-quality programs provide a supportive context for adolescents to develop skill sets for dealing with this complexity – including cultural competencies for working with people from diverse backgrounds (Cooper 2011) and strategic thinking skills for making plans and anticipating contingencies (Larson 2011a).

Managing emotions is one of these complex skill sets. Emotions, such as anger, frustration, worry, and excitement, arise as youth work towards their goals. These emotions bring with them their own complexities. For example, anger can disrupt work and trigger aggressive behavior. Yet these emotions can also be functional: they provide information and can help focus on attention on important problems.

Effective youth programs provide supportive environments for young people to actively engage in learning to manage these complex dynamics. Programs provide a context in which the nuanced causes and effects of emotions can be observed and discussed. We have found that youth learn about emotions through repeated experiences. They observe recurrent patterns in how their emotions change over time. They experiment with strategies, such as managing worry by concentrating on the task at hand. Repeated observation and experimentation help them learn to use the effects of emotions in constructive ways, for example, to channel frustration from setbacks into motivation to work harder.

Although youth are active agents of these learning processes, our findings suggest that effective program leaders play important roles in supporting youth's learning from emotional experiences. Leaders help youth use their developing capacity for reflection to notice how emotions influence their thoughts and behavior. They encourage youth to consider alternative strategies, to problem solve difficult situations, and to view emotions in relation to the future horizon of their work. In short, experienced leaders help support youth's agency, but they also coach youth in navigating the complexity of emotional situations.

The current study builds on previous research indicating that organized programs are valuable contexts for youth to develop social-emotional skills (Durlak et al. 2010). Yet many questions remain. How might youth's learning processes differ for other emotions, such as boredom, jealousy, and excitement? Are there certain types of emotional dynamics (e.g., those involving egocentric bias) that are difficult for young people to learn solely from direct experience? How might learning through a structured curriculum complement learning about managing emotions through coached experience? What types of professional skills and training enable leaders to effectively coach youth through emotionally challenging situations?

Understanding adolescents' development of skills for navigating a complex world is a complex task. We think it is crucial to examine how these skills develop within nuanced real-world contexts. For our topic of emotional development, we believe it important to understand how emotions are embedded in dynamic episodes. It is also essential to recognize that emotions have deep roots in early life experiences and that they are shaped by interactions with family member, peers, teachers, and other aspects of youth's lives. Future research needs to examine how these different levels of complexity influence what youth can learn in a youth development program and how they can learn it. A central point we have sought to make is that researchers – as well as program leaders and youth policy makers – should not underestimate the capacities of young people as active learners. All need to appreciate the abilities of adolescents to observe and learn from experiences in complex environments – and the important role that skilled youth professionals can play in facilitating their learning.

Acknowledgments We would like to thank the William T. Grant Foundation for its generous support of this research and the youth and adult leaders who shared their experiences with us. Additional funding was provided by the USDA National Institute of Food and Agriculture, Hatch project number 600108-793000-793323 (awarded to M. Raffaelli) and Hatch project number 600112-793000-793319 (awarded to R. Larson).

References

Baumeister, R. F., Bratslavsky, E., Finkenauer, C., & Vohs, K. D. (2001). Bad is stronger than good. *Review of General Psychology, 5*, 323–370.

Baumeister, R. F., Vohs, K. D., DeWall, C. N., & Zhang, L. (2007). How emotion shapes behavior: Feedback, anticipation, and reflection, rather than direct causation. *Personality and Social Psychology Review, 11*, 167–203.

Blascovich, J. (2008). Challenge, threat, and health. In J. Y. Shah & W. L. Gardner (Eds.), *Handbook of motivation science* (pp. 481–493). New York: Guilford.

Brackett, M. A., Rivers, S. E., & Salovey, P. (2011). Emotional intelligence: Implications for personal, social, academic, and workplace success. *Social and Personality Psychology Compass, 5*, 88–103.

Bradley, S. (2000). *Affect regulation and the development of psychopathology*. New York: Guilford.

Calkins, S. D., & Leerkes, E. M. (2010). Early attachment processes and the development of emotional self-regulation. In K. D. Vohs & R. F. Baumeister (Eds.), *Handbook of self-regulation: Research, theory and applications* (2nd ed., pp. 355–373). New York: Guilford.

Cannon, W. (1932). *The wisdom of the body*. New York: Peter Smith.

Cooper, C. R. (2011). *Bridging multiple worlds: Cultures, identities, and pathways to college*. New York: Oxford University.

Dahl, R. (2004). Adolescent brain development: A period of vulnerabilities and opportunities. *Annals of the New York Academy of Sciences, 1021*, 1–22.

Dawes, N. P., & Larson, R. W. (2011). How youth get engaged: Grounded-theory research on motivational development in organized youth programs. *Developmental Psychology, 47*, 259–269.

Durlak, J. A., Weissberg, R. P., & Pachan, M. (2010). A meta-analysis of after-school programs that seek to promote personal and social skills in children and adolescents. *American Journal of Community Psychology, 45*, 294–309.

Eccles, J. S., & Gootman, J. A. (Eds.). (2002). *Community programs to promote youth development*. Washington, DC: National Academy Press.

Fridja, N. H. (1986). *The emotions*. Cambridge: Cambridge University.

Gottman, J. M., Katz, L., & Hooven, C. (1996). Parental meta-emotion philosophy and the emotional life of families: Theoretical models and preliminary data. *Journal of Family Psychology, 10*, 243–268.

Gottman, J. M., Katz, L. F., & Hooven, C. (1997). *Meta-emotion: How families communicate emotionally*. Mahwah: Lawrence Erlbaum Associates.

Grawitch, M., & Munz, D. (2005). Individual and group affect in problem-solving workgroups. In C. E. J. Härtel, W. J. Zerbe, & N. M. Ashkanasy (Eds.), *Emotions in organizational behavior* (pp. 119–142). Mahwah: Erlbaum.

Gross, J., & Thompson, R. A. (2007). Emotion regulation: Conceptual foundations. In J. Gross (Ed.), *Handbook of emotion regulation* (pp. 3–24). New York: Guilford.

Harris, P. L., Olthof, T., & Meerum Terwogt, M. (1981). Children's knowledge of emotion. *Journal of Child Psychology and Psychiatry, 22*, 247–261.

Heath, S. B. (1998). Working through language. In S. M. Hoyle & C. T. Adger (Eds.), *Kids talk: Strategic language use in later childhood* (pp. 217–240). New York: Oxford University.

Hirsch, B. J., Deutsch, N., & DuBois, D. (2011). *After-school centers and youth development: Case studies of success and failure*. New York: Cambridge University.

Izard, C. (2009). Emotion theory and research: Highlights, unanswered questions, and emerging issues. *Annual Review of Psychology, 60*, 1–25.

Izard, C., Stark, K., Trentacosta, C., & Schultz, D. (2008). Beyond emotion regulation: Emotion utilization and adaptive functioning. *Child Development Perspectives, 2*, 156–163.

Kaplan, A., & Maehr, M. (2007). The contributions and prospects of goal orientation theory. *Educational Psychology Review, 19*, 141–184.

Katz, L. F., & Hunter, E. C. (2007). Maternal meta-emotion philosophy and adolescent depressive symptomatology. *Social Development, 16*, 343–360.

Kirshner, B., O'Donoghue, J., & McLaughlin, M. W. (Eds.). (2003). *Youth participation: Improving institutions and communities* (New directions for youth development, Vol. 96). San Francisco: Jossey-Bass.

Kuhn, D. (2009). Adolescent thinking. In R. M. Lerner & L. Steinberg (Eds.), *Handbook of adolescent psychology* (3rd ed., Vol. 1, pp. 152–186). Hoboken: Wiley.

Larson, R. W. (2000). Towards a psychology of positive youth development. *American Psychologist, 55*, 170–183.

Larson, R. W. (2011a). Positive development in a disorderly world. *Journal of Research on Adolescence, 21*, 317–334.

Larson, R. W. (2011b). Adolescents' conscious processes of developing regulation: Learning to appraise challenges. In R. M. Lerner, J. V. Lerner, E. P. Bowers, S. Lewin-Bizan, S. Gestsdottir, & J. B. Urban (Eds.), *Thriving in childhood and adolescence: The role of self-regulation processes* (New directions for child and adolescent development, Vol. 133, pp. 87–97). San Francisco: Jossey-Bass.

Larson, R. W., & Brown, J. R. (2007). Emotional development in adolescence: What can be learned from a high school theater program. *Child Development, 78*, 1083–1099.

Larson, R. W., Hansen, D., & Moneta, G. (2006). Differing profiles of developmental experiences across types of organized youth activities. *Developmental Psychology, 42*, 849–863.

Lerner, R. (2002). *Concepts and theories of human development*. Mahwah: Erlbaum.

Lerner, J. V., Phelps, E., Forman, Y., & Bowers, E. (2009). Positive youth development. In R. M. Lerner & L. Steinberg (Eds.), *Handbook of adolescent psychology* (3rd ed., Vol. 1, pp. 524–558). Hoboken: Wiley.

Mahoney, J. L., Vandell, D. L., Simpkins, S. D., & Zarrett, N. R. (2009). Adolescent out-of-school activities. In R. M. Lerner & L. Steinberg (Eds.), *Handbook of adolescent psychology: Contextual influences on adolescent development* (3rd ed., Vol. 2, pp. 228–267). Hoboken: Wiley.

McGregor, H. A., & Elliot, A. J. (2002). Achievement goals as predictors of achievement- relevant processes prior to task engagement. *Journal of Educational Psychology, 94*, 381–395.

Nolen-Hoeksema, S., Wisco, B. E., & Lyubomirsky, S. (2008). Rethinking rumination. *Perspectives on Psychological Science, 3*, 400–424.

Ochsner, K. N., & Gross, J. J. (2007). The neural architecture of emotion regulation. In J. J. Gross (Ed.), *Handbook of emotional regulation* (pp. 87–109). New York: Guilford.

Salusky, I., Larson, R. W., Wu, J., Griffith, A., Raffaelli, M., Sugimura, N., et al. (2012). *How youth develop responsibility: What can be learned from youth programs*. Manuscript submitted for publication.

Schwarz, N., & Clore, G. L. (2007). Feelings and phenomenal experiences. In A. W. Kruglanski & E. T. Higgins (Eds.), *Social psychology: Handbook of basic principles* (pp. 385–407). New York: Guilford.

Steinberg, L. (2007). Risk taking in adolescence: New perspectives from brain and behavioral science. *Current Directions in Psychological Science, 16*, 55–59.

Stocker, C. M., Richmond, M. K., Rhoades, G. K., & Kiang, L. (2007). Family emotional processes and adolescents' adjustment. *Social Development, 16*, 310–325.

Vandell, D. L., Reisner, E. R., Pierce, K. M., Brown, B. B., Lee, D., Bolt, D., et al. (2006). *The study of promising afterschool programs: Examination of longer term outcomes after two years of program experiences*. Madison: Wisconsin Center for Education Research.

Walker, K. C. (2011). The multiple roles that youth development program leaders adopt with youth. *Youth and Society, 43*, 635–655.

Chapter 16
Legal Foundations of Adolescents' Rights and Positive Youth Development

Roger J.R. Levesque

16.1 Introduction: Adolescents in Law

Adolescents increasingly emerge as a unique demographic group, as they have been deemed as having their own needs and abilities as well as constituting a particularly important time period in the life course. The legal system, however, has yet to recognize the period. Instead, the legal system essentially recognizes two periods in the life course: childhood (generally under 18) and adulthood (generally over 18). In the United States, this lack of recognition is evident in the legal system's foundation, which is Constitutional law and the Supreme Court's interpretation of it through its jurisprudence. The Court has yet to provide a determinative approach to the adolescent period, but it certainly has sought to address the intricacies of the challenges that adolescents' needs pose for their development, their personal relationships, their families, and broader societal institutions. That jurisprudence generally seeks to determine when (and how) to treat adolescents as competent adults for some purposes and as incompetent minors for others. Although laws may be found to both embrace and reject the notion that adolescents are neither children nor adults, the Court has begun to accept the concept of adolescence as a unique developmental phase requiring a separate theoretical approach. That legal development, however, clearly remains in its infancy and its outcome is far from certain. As a result, those interested in understanding the law's approach to the adolescent period inevitably face the daunting task of delving into conceptually complex sets of laws guided by some foundational principles but pervasively driven by contextual dictates.

The general failure to accept and develop what could be deemed as an overriding "adolescent jurisprudence" requires that we examine a dispersed body of

R.J.R. Levesque (✉)
Department of Criminal Justice, Indiana University, 302 Sycamore Hall,
47405 Bloomington, IN, USA
e-mail: rlevesqu@indiana.edu

C. Proctor and P.A. Linley (eds.), *Research, Applications, and Interventions for Children*   263
and Adolescents: A Positive Psychology Perspective, DOI 10.1007/978-94-007-6398-2_16,
© Springer Science+Business Media Dordrecht 2013

literature and landmark cases to identify and delineate potentially overriding assumptions, principles, and mandates. This chapter seeks to do so. This chapter examines the growing recognition of adolescents' rights relative to those of other parties, particularly of parents and others acting as adults on behalf of the state. It focuses on what that recognition actually means. The analysis reveals that, in the United States, the notion of adolescents' rights involves a movement away from a paternalistic concern with protection of the child to the notion that adolescents actually have individual rights, rights that they themselves can control. That development is of utmost significance for the simple reason that who controls a right retains considerable power, as they can exercise it and it could be used to trump the interests of others (e.g., parents). As evident in any area of jurisprudence, the development of rights relating to adolescents remains considerably complex, far from linear, and far from comprehensive.

The emerging recognition that adolescents actually can control their own rights is a truly radical development and departure from traditionally accepted ways of recognizing youth's rights, even in international contexts (see Levesque 1994). Given that this development reflects a decisive break from the past, it comes with both benefits and limitations. Progress and its limits find reflection in important generalizations that emerge from Supreme Court jurisprudence. First, when balanced against the family, particularly parents, the legal system has been and continues to be reluctant both to interfere in the family domain and to recognize that adolescents even have rights, but significant exceptions have emerged. Second, adolescents' rights tend to be most recognized and respected when balanced against the interests of the state, when the interests of parents are lessened. Third, regardless of those recognitions, when adolescents are within systems of care (families, schools, juvenile justice systems, health care, etc.), those who care have immense discretion in how to treat adolescents. Fourth, adolescents increasingly gain rights in the sense that they are protected by having their particular abilities determine, partly, their capacity to act or be treated in a certain manner in situations that might involve extreme circumstances, such as when they would receive adult punishments, when they would request intrusive health services, when subjected to maltreatment by parents, and when schools would invade their privacy very intrusively or would treat them very harshly. As no doubt obvious, these generalizations are just that, generalizations and tentative ones at that given how, as we will see, contexts matter considerably when considering the rights of adolescents.

Despite being tentative generalizations, the themes identified above provide the parameters for addressing youth's place in close relationships as well as broader society, and how youth could be treated. They provide the foundational lessons for thinking through the law's receptivity to policies that would ensure greater consideration of the principles of positive youth development that continue to emerge from developmental science. This chapter, then, not only provides readers with the necessary foundation for understanding the parameters of adolescents' rights but also delineates the practical lessons that may be learned from current jurisprudence, and their significance for those interested in making full use of developmental science findings relating to positive youth development.

16.2 Families as the Foundation of Adolescents' Rights

Without doubt, the family has long been recognized as the institution that serves as the foundation for adolescents' development, and that development includes controlling youth, even to the extent of controlling their rights. The Supreme Court has noted, for example, that it is through the family that society inculcates and passes down many of its most cherished values, moral and cultural. Among the Court's most highly-cited and followed passages is the one where it notes that "It is cardinal with us that the custody, care and nurture of the child reside first in the parents, whose primary function and freedom include preparation for obligations the state can neither supply nor hinder" (Prince v. Massachusetts 1944, p. 166). Indeed, the Court even has gone so far as to refer to parents' interests at stake in child rearing as "sacred" (Prince v. Massachusetts 1944, p. 165). These proclamations essentially distill down to the point that the legal system allows parents to structure their relationships with their children as they so choose. Although mandatory schooling laws, child labor restrictions, and the outside boundaries of abuse and neglect do limit the broad parameters of parental rights, for the most part, the state steers clear of interfering with the parental relationship. Although there may be limitations, the Court supports the view that parents are presumed to act in their children's best interest (see, generally, Parham v. J. R. 1979) and that the most effective way to ensure the integrity of family life and positive youth development is to support parents' far reaching right to raise their children as they deem fit. And such presumptions have important consequences. The most obvious consequence that we focus on is that the very notion of adolescents' rights rests on the legal system's deep attachment to honoring the potential for people to enrich and define themselves through their families by using a default rule that assumes the parental and familial relationship should be left alone. This type of honoring raises general issues that we must address to understand the rights of adolescents in families, with those having to do with what may happen when the state wishes to direct adolescents' upbringing and what may happen when adolescents make claims against parents.

16.2.1 Parental Rights Against the State

Arguably the most important case that serves as the modern touchstone for the Court's approach to delimiting the contours of parental rights (and, by doing so, also largely determining the rights of adolescents) is *Wisconsin v. Yoder* (1972). In that case, the Court made clear that the importance of the familial relationship, to the individuals involved as well as to society, stems from the emotional attachments that derive from the intimacy of daily associations, and from the role familial relationships played in promoting a way of life to be respected by the legal system. And that respect included the rights of parents to direct their children's upbringing. Specifically, in *Yoder*, the Court respected parents' rights to withdraw their teenage children from public school before the age of 14 on the grounds that the rights of parents include the right to raise children within the tenets of the Amish religion. The Court explicitly found that parents' fundamental right to freedom of religion outweighed the state's interest in educating its children through a state mandated curriculum, and the Court even did so knowing that approving the removal would result in stifling some youth's individual educational, social, and personal development. The Court reasoned that it was impossible to afford the parents' religious freedom without concomitantly affording them parental freedom because the freedom to believe and act in accordance with their religious beliefs included a basic relational right, the right to raise one's children in accordance with those beliefs. Importantly, the case gained significance not only in the area of education (which now permits parents to remove children from school at any age) but also other areas as well, especially those that would involve potential conflicts between parents and the state in efforts to determine what would be in children's best interests.

Importantly, *Yoder* had followed a long line of important cases, known as the parental rights cases, which had culminated in *Yoder* itself. The Court previously had reasoned that liberty included the right of parents to control the education and upbringing of their children, and the government should not unreasonably intrude on this liberty. That liberty was protected under the Fourth Amendment's Due Process Clause, which provides that no state shall "deprive any person of life, liberty, or property, without due process of law". In doing so, the Court not only had recognized the right but also had stated its high importance. Such recognition is of significance in modern constitutional law in that when rights are deemed to be of high importance, such as their being fundamental rights, they receive considerable protection from interference (see Levesque 2008). That protection means much for not only the rights of the parents but also the types of rights that youth might have within as well as outside of their families.

The Court originally had noted the importance of parental rights, in *dictum*, in *Meyer v. Nebraska* (1923). The issue before the Court in *Meyer* involved the right to learn a foreign language in school. The Court used that case as an opportunity to note that its jurisprudence historically had reflected Western civilization concepts of the family as a unit with broad parental authority over minor children and that it was the right of parents to choose their children's education and upbringing. After identifying the right within the realm of liberty, the Court set a high standard for infringing on these rights by stating that any statutes restricting the education of children should not be arbitrary and need to have a reasonable relationship to an end "within the competency of the state to effect" (Meyer v. Nebraska 1923, p. 400). Based on that standard, the Court found that the state could not bar the students from learning all foreign languages in schools when parents were not against the education unless the legislature could identify a harm that would come from such learning. Most importantly, the Court stated that the "legislature has attempted materially to interfere … with the power of parents to control the education of their own" (Meyer v. Nebraska 1923, pp. 400–401). The Court found unpersuasive the state's rationales for limiting the rights of parents. That type of language, and the Court's findings, set the tone that legislatures and courts should not unreasonably interfere with the parental decisions in a child's education, very broadly defined to include the child's general upbringing.

The Court most notably would repeat its *Myer* reasoning in *Pierce v. Society of Sisters* (1925), a case in which the Court rejected laws requiring children to attend public schools. In *Pierce*, the Court took the opportunity to state more firmly the notion that parents have the responsibility to guide their own household and that such responsibilities were basic in the structure of our society. Parents have this responsibility because they have the duty to understand how to "prepare [their children] for additional obligations" (Pierce v. Society of Sisters 1925, p. 535). The Court stated that the legislature could not "unreasonably interfere[] with the liberty of parents and guardians to direct the upbringing and education of children under their control" (Pierce v. Society of Sisters 1925, pp. 534–535). This liberty only can be "abridged by legislation which has … [a] reasonable relation to some purpose within the competency of the state" (Pierce v. Society of Sisters 1925, p. 535). Such a restriction on legislation protects the liberty of parents from arbitrary intrusions and serves as the rationale for giving parents the right to direct their children's upbringing. As a result, the case set forth that a parent's duties and rights are parallel with one another. Also importantly, the case affirms the notion that states only can interrupt this right when the protection of children's interests falls within a state's competency. The state was not deemed generally competent or well-suited enough to raise children on its own, so it created a protected zone of family privacy supported by the parental rights doctrine that permits a state to infringe on these rights only for a compelling reason and only insofar as that infringement is necessary to protect the state's interest.

16.2.2 Adolescents' Rights Against Parents

In approaching the rights of adolescents within families, the Court generally has not sought to disentangle the parents' interests from those of their children. Even cases where there could be direct conflict between parents and their children, such as when parents are seeking to institutionalize their children, the Court has sided with the parents. That was the general rule announced in *Parham v. J. R.* (1979), which involved the institutionalization of minors for mental health care. Theoretically, everyone has the right to not be involuntarily institutionalized, and they can be committed involuntarily only if states follow strict due process protections. In *Parham*, however, the Court noted that the child's "interest is inextricably linked with the parents' interest in and obligation for the welfare and the health of the child" (Parham v. J. R., p. 600). The Court acknowledged that "some parents may at times act against the interest of their children … but [that] is hardly a reason to discard wholesale those pages of human experience that teach that parents generally do act in the child's best interests" (Parham v. J. R., pp. 602–603). Given the parents' attachment to the child, the Court approved of considerably reduced protections from commitment to institutions. As the *Parham* case made clear, parents have a considerably broad right to shape their children's development, including the emotional development adolescents.

In a few rare instances, the Court has seen it fit to somewhat backtrack from the position that parent and child are one for legal purposes (and that parents control the rights of their minor children). Most notably, the Court did so in *Troxel v. Granville* (2000). In that case, the Court found that grandparents may have a right to visit their grandchildren against the wishes of a parent, if it is in the child's best interest. But the Court was very clear in noting that efforts to interfere in the family required the state to operate from a (rebuttable) presumption that parents do act in the best interest of their children. Although finding that parents may have their right to control their children infringed by considerations of children's own rights, what this case supported was the general rule that parents are presumed to be fit to raise their children; once unfitness has been established (and sometimes merely alleged), a court may interfere and impose its own views of what would be in the child's best interest (just as the Court had ruled in *Parham*). What the *Troxel* case again confirmed, then, is that parents have enormous discretion in controlling their children's upbringing and that they retain that right even in instances where it otherwise may be in their children's best interests to form relationships with and be influenced by others.

The *Troxel* approach reflects the Court's effort to balance the rights of parents with those of others outside of the family, but it also reflects the Court's effort to balance the rights of parents against other societal interests, most notably the harm that would come to society if children were harmed. As in criminal law, for example, the harms that victims suffer actually are harms against the state (it is the "state" vs. a defendant, not a defendant against the victim; see Levesque 2006). In a real sense, it is the harm that society would suffer if children were not raised properly that gives the state the ability to infringe on the rights of parents. In the language used above, protecting citizens from harms falls within the state's area of competency, and that competency gives it the interest to intervene in families and it is that interest that is balanced against the rights of parents and family privacy. Given the high interest given to parental rights and their control over their family, the state needs to ensure that it infringes in a way that protects the assumption that parents are raising their children appropriately, an approach that has important consequences for when and how a state can intervene in family life (see Levesque 2008, 2010).

The health and safety of children have long served as supporting the state's interest to pierce the private family realm and influence how parents raise their children. The leading Supreme Court case that both confirmed and continues to support this proposition is *Prince v. Massachusetts* (1944). In *Prince*, the Court upheld the enforcement of child labor laws against a 9-year-old girl and her guardian aunt who were convicted of "selling" Jehovah Witnesses' publications on the public streets. The guardian challenged the conviction on First Amendment freedom of religion grounds, buttressed with a claim of parental right as secured by the due process clause as articulated in *Meyer*. The Court acknowledged and accepted the aunt's claim of parental right; however, the right was trumped here by the state's broad *parens patriae* power to limit a parent's authority, even in matters of religion, in order to protect the child's welfare. Even if it would have been argued that no specific harm would come to the child in this instance, the state was deemed to have acted within its legitimate powers in the manner it had devised broad child protection policies affecting all children. Perhaps with some hyperbole given *Prince*'s fact pattern, the Court added: "Parents may be free to become martyrs themselves. But it does not follow they are free, in identical circumstances, to make martyrs of their children before they have reached the age of full and legal discretion when they can make that choice for themselves" (Prince v. Massachusetts 1944, p. 170). Despite this broad language supporting the state's power to intervene, the Court clearly stated that the government cannot intervene whenever it so desires just because there are concerns about family life; the Court deemed such an interventionist state as "repugnant to American tradition" (Prince v. Massachusetts 1944, p. 603). The Court reasoned that the relationship between the parent and the child is a relationship having its origins entirely apart from the power of the state and the Court has held steadfast to that distinction (see Levesque 2008). As a result, the Court requires a connection between the government's interference into the family and the need to protect the child from danger or unhealthy decisions.

Prince established that parental authority is not absolute and that parental authority can be restricted if doing so serves the interests of a child's welfare. That general rule has led to the development of a three-prong legal standard to determine whether a child should be removed from his or her parents when there are allegations of child maltreatment (Levesque 2002a, 2008). First, the state generally must provide proof of imminent danger to the physical health or safety of the child. Second, the state must determine whether the child's remaining with the parents is contrary to their welfare. Lastly, the state generally must make reasonable efforts to prevent the removal of the child from their parents. This balancing is of significance in that it is, in a real sense, a balancing of the parents' fundamental right to raise their children as they see fit against the state's responsibility to protect its minor citizens from harm when they lack the capacity to protect themselves. The minor's interests may be at stake but, legally, the balancing of interests occurs between the parent and the state. A state may infringe on parental rights only for compelling reasons and only insofar as that infringement is necessary to protect the state's interests.

Prince may have helped to develop the law that would govern disputes between the rights of parents and the state's ability to intervene on behalf of the child, but it left open the state's role in protecting the parent's claimed right to control their child against a claimed constitutional right of the child. Among the most difficult and challenging cases that have involved the pitting of parental rights directly against those of their children have been cases dealing with minors' rights to abortions and other very invasive medical procedures. The leading case in this area, *Bellotti v. Baird* (1979) laid the foundation for this area of law as well as the foundation for other cases that would attempt to balance the rights of parents against those of their children in situations involving potential conflicts between the constitutional rights of parents and the constitutional rights of their children.

Bellotti involved the Court's review of a Massachusetts statute requiring parental consent for abortions on unmarried minor women with a provision allowing the minor to petition a judge if one or both of her parents refused consent. Allowing that the constitutional rights of children are not co-extensive with those of adults, and recognizing a constitutional parental right against undue, adverse interference by the state in parental authority to direct the rearing of their children, the Court reasoned that the rights of parents needed to weigh heavily in these situations. It reviewed key parental rights cases in this area as it recognized the duty of parents to prepare the child for "'additional obligations'… including the inculcation of moral standards, religious beliefs, and elements of good citizenship" (Bellotti v. Baird 1979, pp. 637–638). It further reasoned that "[l]egal restrictions on minors, especially those supportive of the parental role, may be important to the child's chances for the full growth and maturity that make eventual participation in a free society meaningful and rewarding" (Bellotti v. Baird 1979, pp. 639–640). Nonetheless, the Court concluded that:

> [t]he unique nature and consequences of the abortion decision make it inappropriate 'to give a third party an absolute, and possibly arbitrary, veto over the decision of the physician and his patient to terminate the patient's pregnancy, regardless of the reason for withholding consent.'… We therefore conclude that if the State decides to require a pregnant minor to obtain one or both parents' consent to an abortion, it also must provide an alternative procedure whereby authorization for the abortion can be obtained. (Bellotti v. Baird 1979, pp. 642–643)

The Court, then, required a state to provide an alternative route for minors to petition a court if they wanted to have their rights recognized. That petitioning included their ability to demonstrate that they were mature enough (i.e., enough adult-like) to make what would amount to an adult decision. Importantly, the Court also found the Massachusetts judicial by-pass procedure unconstitutional, since the judge may still refuse to authorize the abortion when s/he concludes that an abortion would not serve the best interests of the minor even after finding that the woman is mature and well-informed enough to make, and has made, a reasonable decision. The Court required that the judge, upon finding the adolescent mature enough to make the decision, leave the decision in her hands. In a real sense, the Court recognized that some adolescents can be mature enough to make adult decisions, meaning decisions without needing their parents' consent.

The result of the *Bellotti* rule, and those following it (see Levesque 2000), is that minors who can be deemed mature can exercise rights without their parents' consent or even their notification. This rule may seem to be quite broad and permit adolescents' considerable control over their own rights. However, the rule only applies in situations in which adolescents can claim that they have a constitutional right that inherently conflicts against the rights of their parents. Indeed, *Bellotti* is known for clearly articulating why minors pervasively do not have rights against their parents and, equally importantly, why their rights are not co-terminus with those of adults. In reaching that conclusion, the Court identified three important reasons why children's constitutional rights are not equal to adults' rights: "the peculiar vulnerability of children; their inability to make critical decisions in an informed, mature manner; and the importance of the parental role in child rearing"

(Bellotti v. Baird 1979, p. 603). Although clearly limiting, the rule also had the benefit of highlighting what a minor would need to demonstrate in order to be able to control their own rights: that the right at stake was a fundamentally important (constitutional) one; that exercising that right would not place them in a peculiarly vulnerable situation; that they are able to make critical decisions in an informed, mature manner; and that the recognition of their rights would not necessarily interfere with their parents' roles (e.g., they could be deemed to no longer need their parents' support or getting their parents' support would be problematic for the child). *Bellotti* makes clear, then, that the Supreme Court retains a high regard for the rights of the parents in directing the family unit, but the Court also seeks to respect the independent rights of children who can be deemed more adult than child-like.

16.3 The Rights of Adolescents Outside of Families

Although the foundation of adolescents' rights certainly rests in the family, and adults within the family presumptively control the rights of adolescents, it remains to be determined how adolescents' rights would figure in institutions outside of the family. In those contexts, we do find general rules that parallel adolescents' rights within families. Namely, adults pervasively tend to control the rights of adolescents, barring instances that would place adolescents in harms way. Also as with families, just as adolescents' rights against parental rights are not fully developed, their rights are not fully developed when they conflict directly with those of adults outside of families. These general trends and recent developments are notable in contexts highly relevant to the everyday lives of adolescents – public schools, juvenile justice systems, and health care systems. The rights of adolescents in other institutions, particularly those deemed private as a matter of law (private schools, religious institutions, private clubs, recreational activities), are pervasively not developed, and that lack of development tends to be attributed to the presumption that adolescents have minimal rights (barring abuse) in such institutions, that those institutions essentially can act as families and that they can do so for the simple reason that they would not be in them without their parent's permission. It is that presumption that grants institutions broad freedoms because (1) it is assumed that parents approve of what the institutions are doing and (2) parents are the ones whose rights generally are involved in these instances (not those of adolescents because parents control the rights of adolescents). These general rules were elucidated over the past half-century. Prior to that, there had not been much thought given to the rights of adolescents. Although important, the developments have been far from even, and understanding that uneven development provides a good foundation for understanding the nature of adolescents rights, including possible developments relating to them.

16.3.1 Adolescents' Rights in Public Educational Systems

Parents may retain the right to control their children's educations, but once they
have their children attend public schools, parental rights become considerably
diminished in that regard. As a result, an important issue arises in terms of the
respect that should be given students' own rights when they are in schools, even
including whether they even have the type of rights that should be respected. The
Supreme Court has addressed a variety of issues relating to the broad questions of
whether adolescents have rights within schools and, if so, to what extent adolescents
do control them and to what extent they do need to be respected. Leading cases in
this area are important to examine not only because they are so illustrative but also
because schools are a primary contexts in which adolescents find themselves, and it
also happens to be a context particularly ripe for interventions conducive to positive
youth development (Levesque 2002b).

A long line of cases have provided important statements regarding the rights of
youth in schools. The general rule that emerges from these cases is that schools
essentially act as parents, which means that they have considerable discretion but
that discretion finds limits especially at extreme cases (e.g., schools may not be
abusive). But, even those extreme cases are known for the incredible extent to which
they provide school officials with discretion to develop the minds and personalities
of youth. Despite that recognition and when considering public schools, the issue
arises as to the extent to which students do have rights when those right arguably
would involve constitutionally protected rights (such as free speech) and those
rights would be exercised in the context of a state controlled system (involving state
action, which automatically initiates the need to protect constitutional rights, unlike
private situations like families). Supreme Court precedent, including the most recent
on this matter, reveals how school officials retain the general right to make curricular and administrative decisions, and those matters end up considerably significant
given that much of schooling falls under those two types of decisions.

The earliest cases specifically had recognized students' right to protection from
governmental intrusion in students' right to engage in speech and right to protection
from government-compelled speech. In *West Virginia State Board of Education v.
Barnette* (1943), for example, the Court used unusually powerful language to find
"that no official, high or petty, can prescribe what shall be orthodox in politics,
nationalism, religion, or other matters of opinion or force citizens to confess by
word or act their faith therein" (West Virginia State Board of Education v. Barnette
1943, p. 642). The Court found a school's requirement that all students salute the
U.S. flag an unconstitutional exercise of governmental authority. In the following
case that was thought to be a bellwether of future cases that would give students
more rights, the Court delineated even more strongly its commitment to students'
rights. In *Tinker v. Des Moines Independent Community School District* (1969),
which involved a school's prohibition against students' wearing black arm bands to
protest the Vietnam War, the Court struck down the ban as it found that students
may not be confined to the expression of "officially approved" sentiments (Tinker v.

Des Moines Independent Community School District 1969, p. 511). According to this approach, schools should encourage students to participate in the learning process, rather than impose values. Although *Tinker* became the Court's leading case of the late 1960s, as it harkened back to the notion that democracy demanded respect for "hazardous" freedoms and that students had a right to those freedoms, the Court eventually retreated from this image of democracy and would place the power to guide and direct democracy squarely on the schools – on local school officials and teachers. The Court did so by ceding the authority to regulate curricula and the school environment to the schools.

In curricular matters, for example, the Supreme Court has announced that school boards essentially retain complete discretion in deciding the values it wishes to transmit. The leading case in which the Court asserted this blanket claim, *Board of Education, Island Trees v. Pico* (1982), actually was one in which the Court had ruled against school officials. In that case, a school board had removed a slew of books from its library and justified the removal on the basis that they were "anti-American, anti-Christian, anti-Semitic, and just plain filthy" (Board of Education, Island Trees v. Pico 1982, p. 857). The Court found that school boards could not remove books based on partisan politics. Although clearly limiting the powers of school boards, the Court did so in a way that left the power of schools quite expansive. Most notably, schools still had discretion to remove books based on educationally relevant criteria. Indeed, the Court granted schools with the broad authority to determine which books it could place in the library in the first instance. The Court construed the school board's rights as "vitally important 'in the preparation of individuals for participation as citizens' and…for 'inculcating fundamental values necessary to the maintenance of a democratic political system'" (Board of Education, Island Trees v. Pico 1982, p. 864). In curricular matters, the Court concluded that school boards "might well defend their claim of absolute discretion" to transmit community values (Board of Education, Island Trees v. Pico 1982, p. 869).

The cases that followed firmly shifted the control of school governance in the direction of school officials. In *Bethel School District No. 403 v. Fraser* (1986), a 17-year-old senior delivered a sexually charged speech nominating a fellow student for elective office. The Court affirmed that students' constitutional rights in public school settings are more narrowly defined than those of adults in other settings. The limitation allowed school officials to curb forms of speech deemed threatening to others, disruptive, and contrary to "shared values" (Bethel School District No. 403 v. Fraser 1986, p. 683). Importantly, the Court reiterated its focus on community standards and the inculcative function of schools. Public education must inculcate "fundamental values necessary to the maintenance of a democratic political system" (Bethel School District No. 403 v. Fraser 1986, p. 681). Included in these values is tolerance of diverse and unpopular political and religious views that must be balanced against the interests of society in teaching the bounds of "socially appropriate behavior" (Bethel School District No. 403 v. Fraser 1986, p. 681). The power of school authorities, acting as the inculcators of proper community values, was supported and developed further in *Hazelwood School District v. Kuhlmeier* (1988). In *Hazelwood*, students alleged that their free speech rights had been violated when the principal deleted two objectionable articles from a school newspaper. One article had addressed issues of teen pregnancy and the other had described the impact of parental divorce on students. The *Hazelwood* Court upheld the authority of school officials to control the content of school-sponsored speech based on "legitimate pedagogical concerns" (Hazelwood School District v. Kuhlmeier 1988, p. 273). The Hazelwood majority emphasized the role of schools as the primary vehicles for transmitting cultural values and their discretion in refusing to sponsor student speech that might be perceived as advocating conduct otherwise inconsistent with "the shared values of a civilized social order" (Hazelwood School District v. Kuhlmeier 1988, p. 272).

It took the Court nearly two decades before it would revisit students' rights, and the Court used the opportunity to confirm that students do not enjoy much free speech in public schools. That case, *Morse v. Frederick* (2007), involved school officials' permitting students to leave school grounds to watch the Olympic Torch Relay pass through their city. Once camera crews arrived from area news channels, Joseph Frederick and his friends unfurled a 14-ft banner which read "BONG HiTS 4 JESUS". When Frederick rebuffed the principal's request to take the banner down, he was subsequently suspended from school for 10 days. The Court declined to apply *Tinker's* "substantial disruption" standard and instead held that "[t]he 'special circumstances of the school environment' and the governmental interest in stopping student drug abuse … allow[s] schools to restrict student expression that they reasonably regard as promoting illegal drug use" (Morse v. Frederick 2007, p. 408). Despite a vigorous dissent, the case stood for yet another example of the limits placed on the expressive rights of students. The cases further installed school authorities as the inculcators of proper community values; schools were to determine community standards and the inculcative function of schools in the manner they wished to teach the bounds of socially appropriate behavior.

The Court also has granted local school officials with immense discretion in the manner they discipline students, and in doing so the Court has affirmed that it more narrowly defines students' constitutional rights in public school settings than it does those of adults in other settings. Two examples are illustrative. The first example emerged when the Supreme Court directly addressed the constitutionality of schools' use of corporal punishment in *Ingraham v. Wright* (1977). In *Ingraham*, two assistant principals and a principal disciplined students with brass knuckles and a large wooden paddle. For apparently minor infractions, if infractions at all, several students had been subjected to repeated beatings on their legs, arms, backs and necks; the punishments were so severe that some students were sent to the hospital for painful bruises diagnosed as hematoma, swollen arms requiring pain medication, lumps on their heads requiring surgery, and for coughing up blood. Some of these students brought suit in federal court arguing that the paddling was "cruel and unusual punishment" and that students should have a right to be heard before suffering physical punishments. After losing at their initial trial and at the Court of Appeals, the students appealed to the Supreme Court, where they also lost. The Court held that the cruel and unusual punishment clause of the Eighth Amendment applied only to criminal punishments and thus provided no protection against the imposition of corporal penalties by school authorities. The Court further held that the procedural due process guaranteed by the Fourteenth Amendment did not require schools to provide notice and a hearing before the application of physical discipline. Rather than being found in the basic principles of the Constitution, the protections were to be found at the local level – in the openness of the school, the professionalism of those who impose punishment, and the civil and criminal remedies available to those who get too severely beaten. As a result of *Ingraham*, states can and many of them do impose corporal punishment in their schools, a remarkable position given that even imprisoned criminals cannot be subjected to corporal punishment (Levesque 2006).

The second example of schools' immense power to control students and of the Court's leaving matters to local decision makers involves policies that permit schools to infringe on students' privacy to determine whether they are using drugs. Two Supreme Court cases are directly on point, and both confirm the move toward granting school officials increased authority and offer considerable discretion to school officials in their effort to control student behavior. The first case, *Vernonia School District 47 J v. Acton* (1995), involved a challenge by a seventh grader who was ineligible to play football because he and his parents refused to submit him to mandatory random drug testing – a policy that had been endorsed unanimously by parents in a public meeting called to address drug usage in the school. The Court found that the drug-testing program did not violate the Constitution even though the program involved suspicionless random drug testing for students who participate in school athletics. The Court ruled individualized suspicion unnecessary. The Court emphasized that school officials exercised their duties as state actors, an authority that was "custodial and tutelary, permitting a degree of supervision and control that could not be exercised over free adults" (Vernonia School District 47 J v. Acton 1995, p. 655). The Court even took the decision beyond its immediate context to conclude that "when the government acts as guardian and tutor the relevant question is whether the search is one that a reasonable guardian and tutor might undertake" (Vernonia School District 47 J v. Acton 1995, p. 655). Rather than move toward protecting the privacy of students, the Court took the opportunity to expand school officials' discretion in the next case, in *Board of Education of Independent School District No. 92 of Pottawatomie County v. Earls* (2002). In that case, the Court expanded *Vernonia* to include students who participate in any type of competitive extracurricular activity and essentially removed the need to show that there was a particular need to test students. The suit in *Earls* was brought by two students, one who was a member of the show choir, the marching band, the Academic Team, and the National Honor Society and another who sought to participate in the Academic Team. They alleged that the policy violated the Fourth Amendment, which requires reasonable searches and seizures, most likely supported by warrants and probable cause. They also argued that the school district had failed to identify a special need for testing students who participate in extracurricular activities, and that the policy neither addressed a proven problem nor promised to bring any benefit to students or the school. The Court found that it was not unreasonable to force all students to submit to random drug testing as a condition of participating in school activities, that the schools' interest in ridding their campuses of drugs outweighs students' right to privacy, even when the school had not shown that the school was marked by a drug problem or that the targeted students were suspected of drug use. These cases reveal that the Court does struggle to find the proper balance between the rights of individual students and the needs of school officials; but the Court continues to broaden the authority of public schools to control the development of youth, including the school environment.

Even when the Court has found that students have protected liberty interests, it still leaves immense discretion to schools. Two examples again are illustrative. *Goss v. Lopez* (1975) involved the suspension of 75 Ohio high school students, including Lopez, for 10 days because of they allegedly had destroyed school property and had disrupted their learning environment. At that time, Ohio state law provided schools with the right to suspend problem students without a hearing. A number of students, through their parents, sued the board of education, claiming that their right to due process had been violated when they were suspended without a hearing. Eventually, the Supreme Court held that when students are suspended from school, even for short periods of time, they are entitled to basic due process protections: notice and opportunity to be heard. The Court found the need for these protections because the students had, under state law, the right to a public education; the Court also continued and found that students had an interest in protecting their reputations, although it did not clearly note the source of that interest. To avoid injustice and damages to their reputation based on allegations of misconduct, the Court held that the students may present their side of the situation prior to suspension. This opportunity included: oral or written notice of the charges, an explanation (if students deny the charges) of the evidence against them, and an opportunity for students to present their side of the story. Although the recognition that students' educations do implicate the Constitution is nothing that should be dismissed, the protections granted students actually were surprisingly minimal. The Court again evinced a need to protect local decision makers as it found that students' rights could be protected by an informal hearing that presumes most disciplinary decisions correct and that grants final authority to school officials. The Court did not, for example, give students a right to an attorney, a right to cross-examine witnesses, a right to call witnesses, or a right to a hearing before an impartial person. In instances like these, the Court finds nothing improper with having local school officials serve as the arbiters of students' rights.

The other case that exemplifies the broad power granted to school officials, even when the Court finds that students have recognized rights, is *Davis v. Monroe County Board of Education* (1999), involved Title IX legislation. In *Davis*, a 5th-grade girl was harassed by a fellow 5th-grade male student. Although the student and her mother complained to several different teachers who witnessed the harassing behavior, as well as to the school principal, no action was taken, and the harassment continued until criminal charges were brought successfully against the offender and litigation was brought to stop the behavior. Lower courts had granted the school summary judgment, a ruling that finds that the party alleging a claim has no legitimate cause of action. In determining whether there existed a private right of action against school districts for student-on-student harassment, the Court noted that congress had based its authority to enforce Title IX on the spending clause. This clause, however, only permits a funding recipient, such as a school district, to be held liable if the recipient has notice of potential liability. Notice of liability, according to the Court, exists and allows for a private right of action for monetary damages when school districts act with deliberate indifference to acts of student-on-student sexual harassment of which the school has actual knowledge. In *Davis*, the Court held that the school's refusal to respond to the complaints could potentially constitute deliberate indifference. Given the challenges in determining legitimate harassment claims, the Court further required that the harassment be so severe, pervasive, and objectively offensive that it denies educational opportunities and benefits at that school. This three-pronged standard, however, is very difficult to meet and creates an environment in which schools have very little incentive to create proactive sexual harassment prevention policies (Levesque 2000). As a result of the reduced obligations placed on local decision makers, students are likely to continue to face a significant amount of sexual harassment in school. Thus, although there may be benefits to supporting school official's discretion, there certainly appears to be instances in which doing so remains problematic.

Despite the high level of deference and discretion left to school officials, the Court has not given school officials free reign. Some of the cases reviewed above reveal potential limits well. But, two other leading cases, both involving searches of students, reveal important twists on some of the key limits placed on schools, with the upshot of these limitations revealing, again, school's immense discretion in how they treat youth. In *New Jersey v. T. L. O.* (1985), the Supreme Court set forth the standard for determining whether a search of a student by a school official violates the Fourth Amendment. The case involved a female student whose purse was searched after school officials found her smoking in a school restroom. When school officials searched the purse for cigarettes, they uncovered marijuana and other evidence suggesting that she had been dealing marijuana. Considering the constitutionality of the search, the Court held that public school officials are governed by the Fourth Amendment because they act as representatives of the state, not merely as surrogates of the parents. Although this was a major recognition that students have enforceable rights in the school context, the Court declined to hold school officials to the long-established probable cause standard regulating searches and instead balanced the student's privacy interests against the government's need to enforce order. As a result, the Court held school officials to a reduced standard as it ruled that the search of the purse was reasonable because it was "justified at its inception" and the method was "reasonably related to the objectives of the search and not excessively intrusive in light of the age and sex of the student and nature of the infraction" (New Jersey v. T. L. O. 1985, pp. 341–342, 347). Thus, the Court held that schoolchildren do maintain a legitimate expectation of privacy that must be weighed against the government's need for the search. But, the Court recognized that the school context provided an exception, a special need, to the general protections from state conducted searches and seizures.

In the most recent case in this area, the Court affirmed the limits of school officials' ability to control its students. That case, *Safford Unified School District No.*

1 v. Redding (2009), involved the strip search of a 13-year-old girl for prescription drugs. The search, which uncovered no contraband, ended when the student, in the nurse's office, was asked by the nurse and an administrative assistant (both female) to strip down to her bra and underwear and then pull out her underwear and pull her bra to the side and shake it, partially revealing her breasts and pelvic area. In holding the strip search to be unlawful, the Court applied the standard it had set in *T. L. O.* and determined that, although the indignity of the search did not make it unlawful, the intrusiveness of the search outweighed the degree of suspicion about drug possession. It held the search unreasonable in its scope. Most importantly, however, the Court in *Safford* recognized the student's subjective expectations of privacy and refused to quibble over the precise details of the strip search. The Court held that any search that moves beyond the outer clothing and belongings is categorically distinct and requires special justification. Adolescents are uniquely vulnerable to embarrassment from an intrusive strip search, the Court continued, and thus should be protected by a subjective expectation of privacy prohibiting uncomfortable and frightening searches, even when the breasts and pelvic area are not fully exposed. The Court's recognition of the need for limits, and the need to respect subjective expectations of privacy, certainly are important; but, focusing on making this a categorical exception draws away from the case's potential reach. Making one categorical exception leaves other instances outside of the announced protection. Still, it is clear that students retain rights to privacy in school and that those rights generally are reduced as school officials have considerable discretion in searching students, and using the fruit of those searches against students (see Levesque 2002b).

16.3.2   Adolescents' Rights in Juvenile and Criminal Justice Systems

While the rights of youth within schools have developed in a manner that provides school officials with considerable discretion, the juvenile justice system explicitly has been viewed as taking a different turn. Indeed, the leading Supreme Court cases in this area evince a move away from providing juvenile justice personnel discretion that had served as the very foundation of the system. The context also has led to the creation of some of the most comprehensive efforts to address youth's own legal rights. A close look at those rights, however, reveals a system still fraught with discretion, with the major exception of rules relating to how and whether juveniles enter the system. A similar look at how the criminal justice system treats youth reveals a similar trend, with increasing concern about the protections youth have before they would enter the system but also, unlike the juvenile system, clear cases that involve the types of punishments youth can receive. In a real sense, this area of law reveals immense discretion, with the exception relating to extreme punishments that may not be imposed readily (if at all) on adolescents explicitly because of their status as adolescents.

Efforts to recognize the rights of youth began with the creation of a juvenile justice system that would treat youth differently from adults. The creation of juvenile courts and systems focusing on youth's needs was the product of the nineteenth century "child-saving movement". That movement, in part, sought to rehabilitate youth in the name of benefitting both them as well as society. The shift made full use of the concept of *parens patriae* that permitted the state to provide supervision and control over delinquent youth. Charged as essentially acting as parents (since parents whose children were delinquent were viewed as having failed, hence permitting the state to intervene at least temporarily), the system explicitly sought to ensure the child's best interests as it focused on protection and treatment of the child and not on punishment. The focus on treatment and protection is what provided the rationale for the immense discretion had by juvenile justice system personnel, as their duties were deemed as most appropriately executed if they had the requisite freedom to act as parents would, with little limitations on their rights.

Given the philosophical foundation that served to build the juvenile justice system, the legal developments that emerged from this area were, and in many ways continue to be, remarkably impressive. Most notably, in *Kent v. United States* (1966), the Supreme Court first stressed the importance of procedural protections for juveniles. In *Kent*, the Court held that a juvenile court could not transfer a juvenile to an adult criminal court without following certain procedures, including holding a hearing and providing effective assistance of counsel and a statement of reasons. The Court emphasized that, although the statute in question gave the juvenile court "a substantial degree of discretion" it did not confer "a license for arbitrary procedure" (Kent v. United States 1966, p. 553). This case was of significance for recognizing not only that adolescents had rights but also that they had the right to be tried in juvenile rather than adult court, that they had the right to the system that embraced discretion and served to rehabilitate youth.

Having decided that juveniles have a right to procedures before being removed from juvenile court jurisdiction, the Court then addressed the important group of rights that would be implicated in giving juvenile court jurisdiction over the youth in the first instance. It was that case, *In re Gault* (1967), that is seen as the watershed case that revolutionized the rights of adolescents. That case involved considering the detention of a 15-year-old boy who was deemed juvenile delinquent and sent to a state industrial school. His serious offense was a prank phone call, of an "adolescent nature", to a neighbor. For that misbehavior, Gault was sent to be institutionalized until age 21 (given that he was 15, that was considerably much longer than the penalty he would have received had he been an adult, which would have been 2 months maximum). The Court took the opportunity to highlight the importance of procedural protections for youth, and reversed the juvenile court's decision. The Court held that certain due process rights apply equally to both juveniles and adults, such as the right to counsel, adequate notice of the charges (comparable to the notice given in criminal or civil proceedings), the privilege against self-incrimination, and the right to confrontation and sworn testimony by witnesses available for cross-examination. The Court sought to introduce procedural regularity, fairness, and orderliness into the juvenile system, emphasizing that "unbridled discretion [was] a poor substitute for principle and procedure" (In re Gault 1967, p. 18). Given the panoply of rights that were recognized, it is unsurprising to find that *Gault* is viewed as having revolutionized the rights of youth by recognizing that they have basic, due process rights similar to those of adults.

Despite the above developments, the early promises of procedural rights for youth articulated in *Kent* and *Gault* still remain considerably unfulfilled. Juveniles can be held to adult accountability standards but denied similar constitutional rights. For example, in *Schall v. Martin* (1984), the Court approved of the state's considerable discretion to determine when to detain juveniles before hearings and trials, when compared to the detention of adults, on the rationale that juvenile detention can be deemed rehabilitative, for their own good (an argument that would not work for adults, see Levesque 2006). In addition, in *McKeiver v. Pennsylvania* (1971), the Supreme Court held that juveniles have no constitutional right to a trial by jury in the juvenile court's adjudicative stage, a lack of protection meant to help secure the discretion of juvenile courts. Equally importantly, the *Kent* protections do not apply to transfers to adult court that do not require hearings, such as automatic transfers or those leaving the discretion to prosecutors. And, *Gault* itself did not provide the right to appeal, a rather significant limitation given that it does leave juvenile courts with immense discretion and reveals how the juvenile court remains a judicial anomaly – imagine an adult court system that did not grant adults the right to appeal a trial judge's decision to a higher court. Given the potential reach of due process rights, the cases understood as revolutionizing and confirming the due process protections of juveniles certainly remain strikingly limited.

In terms of juvenile's rights, arguably the most important limitation that emerges from the above cases is that they focused on the process rather than the treatment that juveniles would receive once they were in the juvenile or criminal justice system. Focusing on the actual treatment of juveniles – what they receive once adjudicated delinquent or deemed as having offended, reveals that the system retains immense discretion. As with the school context, the Court protects adolescents from extreme treatments. In this context, the Court has removed minors from being considered eligible for specific types of extreme penalties. Two cases are illustrative, as they highlight the Court's limitations on what the state can do in extreme cases and, at the same time, gives states considerable leeway in that they permit a broad array of dispositions in the states' efforts to address juvenile justice. Indeed, the cases involved the treatment of juveniles who had been waived to adult court; so they still leave much unsaid about the treatment that juveniles may have in juvenile court systems.

The two illustrative cases involved the permissibility of adult-like punishments. The first illustrative case of the limits placed on the state's treatment of juveniles involves juveniles in adult courts. That case, *Roper v. Simmons* (2005), announced that it is unconstitutional for juveniles to receive the death penalty, a case that overturned an earlier decision, 16 years earlier, that had upheld subjecting juveniles to the death penalty (see Stanford v. Kentucky 1989). Importantly, the Court relied on studies demonstrating that adolescents performed worse than adults in their decision making competence and indicated that, relative to adults, adolescents were less able to consider alternative decisions. The Court eventually noted that adolescents are often perceived as immature and irresponsible, susceptible to peer pressure, and have not yet attained the attributes of a fully developed character. Emphasizing adolescents' vulnerability and comparable lack of control over their immediate surroundings, the Court concluded that the differences between juvenile and adult offenders are too marked and well understood and that they counseled against risking irreversible adult punishments. The second case, *Graham v. Florida* (2010), involved the imposition of life sentences without parole for non-homicide crimes committed by juveniles. The Court found such punishments as constituting cruel and unusual punishment and therefore unconstitutional. The Court followed similar reasons it had in *Roper*, which was that juveniles are not fully developed, do not have a moral sense to the same extent as adults, and that those differences required the legal system to provide them with the possibility that they could change (hence, not permitting life sentences without parole for non-homicide cases). What the Court essentially did was recognize adolescents' lessened culpability, including ability, and the appropriateness of treating adolescents as children, not like adults. This view likely has important implications for the general rights of juveniles in other contexts, but at least for here it still leaves open other types of punishments in the adult system and it does not disturb the types of dispositions that juveniles may receive in the juvenile justice system, a system that remains fraught with immense discretion (and criticisms for being, for example, inappropriately harsh on particular groups, such as girls and minority youth).

Focusing on what happens to adolescents once they are in the court system and their punishments should not detract from the systems that lead minors to them, such as the police and other investigating systems. As may be expected, the legal system in this context often is of two minds when it deals with minors. Generally, however, adolescents are treated as adults, in the sense that they have the full protection of adults. For example, when considering the right to move about public streets unencumbered by state intrusion, the Court protects that right absent probable cause to believe criminal activity is afoot. The Court has assumed, often without discussion, that children have the same Fourth Amendment rights as adults (see California v. Hodari D 1991; Florida v. J. L. 2000). What this means, of course, is that they do not have added protections from searches due to, for example, their reduced level of maturity and how they might interact with authority figures and may more readily waive those rights. In the Court's most recent case in this area, *J. D. B. v. North Carolina* (2011), the Court did allow for considering a youth's minority status in interrogations, but it is clear that it is not mandated. As a result, this area of law serves as an example of how granting adolescents' full rights (meaning equality with adults) may well not be in their own best interests.

16.3.3 Adolescents' Rights in Health and Medical Care Systems

The legal system typically views adolescents as not capable of making medical decisions on their own volition (Levesque 2000). The reason for this is that parents are deemed as having the right to control their children's medical decision making on the assumption, for example, that they will act on their child's best interests and that adolescents do not have the maturity (ability) to make important, life changing decisions. On grounds quite similar to those supporting juveniles' exclusion from extreme forms of punishment when they are in adult systems of punishment (that they are not necessarily mature, subject to peer influence, incapable of making important decisions), the legal system acts paternalistically as it seeks to protect adolescents from potential harm.

What is quite unusual about the general rule regarding minor's access to medical care is that it is fraught with numerous important exceptions. Those exceptions may well swallow the general rule. For example, a common exception includes emancipation, which results in viewing the minor as an adult given that their status assumes that they are able to make decisions without parental consent. Exceptions also include emergencies, which permit health providers to provide treatment on the assumption that they would do what a parent would do in emergency situations and, equally importantly in law, to protect providers from liability. Exceptions also emerge due to the nature of the service that would be provided, with the most invasive and life-changing typically requiring parental consent. That exception may involve a recognition of an adolescents' decision-making capacity but it is equally likely involves situations that would involve threats to public health, such as the protection from diseases or the burdens that come from sexual activity. For example, adolescents generally can obtain non-invasive contraception (e.g., condoms) and medical treatment for sexually transmitted diseases without parental consent. This exception rests on the rationale that it promotes access to treatment and prevents the spread of disease by eliminating the deterrent of having to inform parents of sexual activity. If the medical procedure is to be more invasive, adolescents also may be able to control their access to it by an exception known as the mature minor doctrine, which figures prominently in understanding adolescents' rights (as noted above in the case of Bellotti v. Baird 1979). Undoubtedly, the general rule prohibiting access to care leaves one to wonder why it still exists and why there is such a profound attachment to it.

The numerous exceptions are important, especially the mature minor doctrine that permit minors to give consent to medical procedures if they can show that they are mature enough to make the decision on their own. But the exceptions remain limited. All of the exceptions, for example, tend to take into account the age and situation of the minor to determine ability to control their own rights. For example, the mature minor rule especially is used for minors who are 16 or older, understand the medical procedures in question, the minor has engaged in adult-like behavior, and the procedure is not serious – all of which reduce the need for parental involvement. Even in contexts where adolescents are deemed to have fundamental rights at stake, such as the rights to access abortions, it is difficult to view their rights as fully adult-like given that they may require a court proceeding to demonstrate their maturity and ability to make important decisions on their own. Adults simply are assumed to be mature, and mature adolescents can be far from free to exercise their rights if they only can do so by being declared able by a court. Again, imagine a system where adults have to obtain a judge's permission to exercise a right (such as access to a physician); such a situation would not be deemed as granting adults considerable freedom. Arguably even more limiting, the reality is that adolescents may have access to care but not actually gain it due to, for example, costs; and if they do gain access, the utility of access varies depending on the nature of the needed services. These limitations highlight well the very practical limits that can face theoretical developments.

What the above developments translate into is the principle that adolescents can be treated very differently, either as adults or as children, in health care arenas. In the health care contexts, adolescents typically are excluded from decision-making but they may well be able to decide on their own volition whether to make use of a service depending on a variety of factors, including the procedure's intrusiveness and irreversibility. Despite important developments in adolescents' legal rights, then the vast majority of adolescents are treated as children for the purposes of health care.

16.4 Conclusions: Lessons Learned for Promoting Positive Youth Development

The law's approach to adolescents and their rights rests on four fundamental points. First, the legal system relies on the presumption that parents possess what adolescents lack in maturity, experience, and capacity for judgment required for making life's difficult decisions. Second, the legal system also relies on the long held recognition that natural bonds of affection lead parents to act in their adolescents' best interests. Third, when parents fail, the state intervenes to act as parents should, which grants the state considerable discretion in controlling the rights of adolescents. Lastly, despite the above three foundational points, the legal system exhibits an increasing interest in recognizing that adolescents can have the capacity to make thoughtful and informed decisions for themselves and can be empowered to make legally binding decisions on their own; it also exhibits a tendency to offer adolescents the power to control their own rights even when they may not need to prove that they have adult-like capacities, such as when society benefits from having adolescents hold the power to make certain decisions. As we have seen throughout this chapter, these are important generalizations but they are fraught with complexities and exceptions, all of which make difficult efforts to draw simple and clear implications.

Although legal developments relating to adolescents' rights likely will never result in simple rules, important lessons emerge from the above fundamental points. The conclusions highlight the need to take parents and families seriously as we consider shaping environments that would be conducive to positive youth development. Clearly, parents must be involved not only because of what they do within their families but also because of the control that parents can exert when their children are outside of families. Although they must be involved, however, the legal system does set important limits on what they can do. Similarly, the legal rules show how legal systems increasingly provide public institutions, such as schools, with considerable autonomy, but that autonomy comes with important strings attached to it. Schools must seek to develop students' educated capacities, and the Court properly has seen fit to require schools to promote rather than stifle civic attitudes that prepare students for living in democratic, pluralistic, and civil communities. Similarly, the need to control institutions like those dealing with maltreated children, those in need of health care, or those deemed delinquents reveals the assumption that the state is acting on youth's best interests and preparing adolescents for becoming independent, productive, responsible, and law-abiding citizens. Those assumptions provide considerable room for enlisting the assistance of developmental sciences through, for example, making full use of the discretion bestowed on state officials when they interact with and treat youth. And the assumptions are particularly significant in that they coincide with the key principles and goals identified as critical for fostering positive youth development. Fostering positive youth development, then, means recognizing that the legal system affords parents, families, and institutions like schools opportunities to shape adolescents' lives, and the legal system seeks to ensure that they do so responsibly and actually in ways consistent with the ideals of positive youth development.

Lessons also emerge in terms of the need to reconsider conceptions of rights. There is now a real sense that the legal system simply cannot give youth full adult rights, as doing so can have dreadful consequences and actually be against adolescents' best interests. In turn, this recognition means that recognizing and ensuring adolescents' rights means moving beyond simple and well accepted conceptions of rights to consider, for example, that adolescents may need specialized support systems for them to even realize that they do have rights, let alone exercise those rights freely. This recognition raises the key point that sometimes reaching a similar end can require that adolescents be treated differently from adults. It also raises the thorny and controversial issue that in order to achieve similar ends for some adolescents, some of them may need to be treated differently from their peers.

Lessons also include the need for engaging in different research. Given how the legal system approaches adolescent capacity, for example, researchers need to reconsider how best to approach it as well, as they need to recognize that adolescents' capacities in law can rely as much on the interests of others as on the adolescents themselves. In other words, adolescents' relative capacities are not determined through science alone; they require considering laws and policies; they require developmentalists to take the law seriously. The need for developmentalists to reconsider their lines of research appears to gain significance given the Court's apparent willingness to consider findings from developmental sciences. Even if a close look at cases where the Court does consider such findings reveals that the science may not have been that persuasive, the Court's consideration emerges as momentous and provides important opportunities for researchers to develop research that the Court would find authoritative enough to influence its jurisprudence.

Arguably the most important lesson to emerge when considering adolescents' rights is that focusing on one arena for their development is fraught with peril. Even when the Court recognizes rights and can charge ahead with reform, for example, the reform may be short-lived or actually counterproductive. Focusing on parents to secure adolescents' rights brings with it is own limitations. Similarly, even though arguably the most radical change in conceptions of adolescents' rights has been the recognition that adolescents have rights against their parents as well as against potential state actions, that change has not always led to intended outcomes. History reveals that many reforms originally deemed liberating and ground-breaking sometimes end up being much less so in the long run. This reality leads us to the conclusion that the most important developments in adolescents' rights will emerge and sustain themselves if they can infiltrate multiple constituencies that have interests in adolescents' effective development. In the end, the current understanding of adolescents' rights highlights the important roles that all must play in fostering rights in a myriad of contexts, and the need to figure out exactly what adolescents' rights are before we can start taking them seriously.

References

Bellotti v. Baird, 443 U.S. 622 (1979).
Bethel School District No. 403 v. Fraser, 478 U.S. 675 (1986).
Board of Education of Independent School District No. 92 of Pottawatomie County v. Earls. 536 U.S. 822 (2002).
Board of Education, Island Trees v. Pico, 457 U.S. 853 (1982).
California v. Hodari D, 499 U.S. 621 (1991).
Davis v. Monroe County Board of Education. 526 U.S. 629 (1999).
Florida v. J. L, 529 U.S. 266 (2000).
Goss v. Lopez, 419 U.S. 565 (1975).
Graham v. Florida, 130 S.Ct. 2011 (2010).
Hazelwood School District v. Kuhlmeier. 484 U.S. 260 (1988).
Ingraham v. Wright, 430 U.S. 651 (1977).
In re Gault, 387 U.S. 1 (1967).
J. D. B. v. North Carolina, Supreme Court No. 09–11121 (2011).
Kent v. United States, 383 U.S. 541 (1966).
Levesque, R. J. R. (1994). The internationalization of children's human rights: Too radical for American adolescents? *Connecticut Journal of International Law, 9*, 237–293.
Levesque, R. J. R. (2000). *Adolescents, sex, and the law: Preparing adolescents for responsible citizenship*. Washington, DC: American Psychological Association.
Levesque, R. J. R. (2002a). *Child maltreatment law: Foundations in science, policy and practice*. Durham: Carolina Academic Press.
Levesque, R. J. R. (2002b). *Dangerous adolescents, model adolescents: Shaping the role and promise of education*. New York: Plenum/Kluwer.
Levesque, R. J. R. (2006). *The psychology and law of criminal justice processes*. New York: Nova Science.
Levesque, R. J. R. (2008). *Rethinking child maltreatment law: Returning to first principles*. New York: Springer.
Levesque, R. J. R. (2010). The law's response to child maltreatment. In M. P. Koss, J. White, & A. Kazdin (Eds.), *Handbook of violence against women and children* (Navigating solutions, Vol. 2, pp. 47–69). Washington, DC: American Psychological Association.
McKeiver v. Pennsylvania, 403 U.S. 528 (1971).

Meyer v. Nebraska, 262 U.S. 390 (1923).
Morse v. Frederick, 551 U.S. 393 (2007).
New Jersey v. T. L. O., 469 U.S. 325 (1985).
Parham v. J. R., 442 U.S. 584 (1979).
Pierce v. Society of Sisters, 268 U.S. 510 (1925).
Prince v. Massachusetts, 321 U.S. 158 (1944).
Roper v. Simmons, 543 U.S. 551 (2005).
Safford Unified School District No. 1 v. Redding, 129 S. Ct. 2633 (2009).
Schall v. Martin, 467 U.S. 253 (1984).
Stanford v. Kentucky, 492 U.S. 361 (1989).
Tinker v. Des Moines Independent Community School District, 393 U.S. 503 (1969).
Troxel v. Granville, 530 U.S. 57 (2000).
Vernonia School District 47 J v. Acton, 515 U.S. 646 (1995).
West Virginia State Board of Education v. Barnette, 319 U.S. 624 (1943).
Wisconsin v. Yoder, 406 U.S. 205 (1972).

Printed in Great Britain
by Amazon

36746644R00170